WESTERN HERBS
ACCORDING TO
TRADITIONAL
CHINESE
MEDICINE

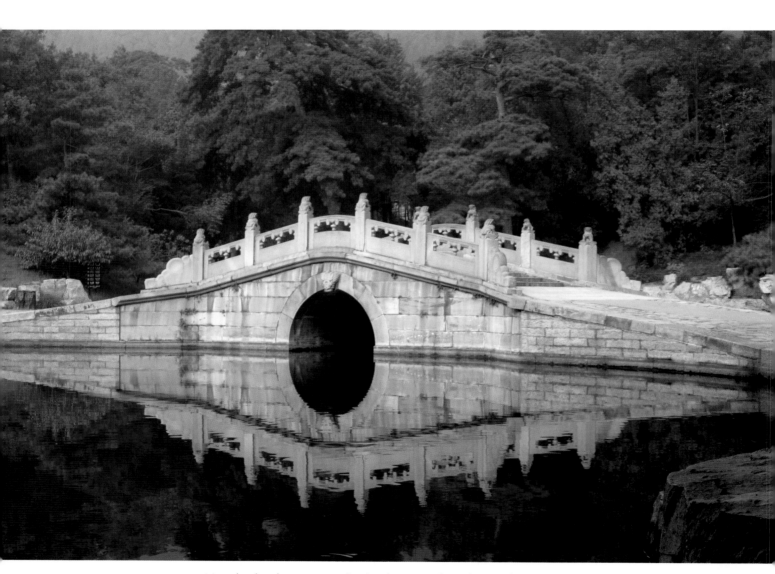

May this book serve as a bridge between the cultures of East and West.

WESTERN HERBS

── ACCORDING TO ──

TRADITIONAL CHINESE MEDICINE

A PRACTITIONER'S GUIDE

Thomas Avery Garran, MTOM, L.Ac.

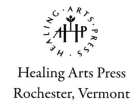

Healing Arts Press
Rochester, Vermont

Healing Arts Press
One Park Street
Rochester, Vermont 05767
www.HealingArtsPress.com

Healing Arts Press is a division of Inner Traditions International

The photographs of damiana *(Turnera diffusa)* on pages 183 and 184 were taken by Mimi Kamp and used by permission of the photographer.

The glossary definitions of Chinese medical terms are derived from *A Practical Dictionary of Chinese Medicine* by Nigel Wiseman and Feng Ye and used by permission of Paradigm Publications, Brookline, MA.

Note to the reader: *This book is intended as an informational guide. The remedies, approaches, and techniques described herein are meant to supplement, and not to be a substitute for, professional medical care or treatment. They should not be used to treat a serious ailment without prior consultation with a qualified health care professional.*

Library of Congress Cataloging-in-Publication Data
Garran, Thomas Avery.
  Western herbs according to traditional Chinese medicine : a practitioner's guide / Thomas Avery Garran.
      p. ; cm.
  Includes bibliographical references and index.
  ISBN-13: 978-1-59477-191-0 (hardcover)
  ISBN-10: 1-59477-191-X (hardcover)
  1. Herbs—Therapeutic use. 2. Medicine, Chinese. 3. Materia medica, Vegetable. I. Title.
  [DNLM: 1. Phytotherapy—methods. 2. Materia Medica. 3. Medicine, Chinese Traditional—methods. 4. Plants,
Medicinal. WB 925 G238w 2008]
  RM666.H33G39 2008
  615'.321—dc22
                                                                                    2007030808

Printed and bound in India by Replika Press Pvt. Ltd.

10 9 8 7 6 5 4 3 2 1

Text design and layout by Jon Desautels
This book was typeset in Garamond Premier Pro with Futura used as a display typeface.

To contact the author of this book, please visit his website at **www.sourcepointherbs.org.** Alternatively, you may mail a first-class letter to the author c/o Inner Traditions • Bear & Company, One Park Street, Rochester, VT 05767, and we will forward the communication.

CONTENTS

PART TWO
THE MATERIA MEDICA

APPENDICES

FOREWORD

By Michael Tierra, L.Ac., OMD

A key principle of herbal practice holds that it is more important to know who has a disease than to merely know the named disease. Thus, traditional herbalists typically prescribe based on an energetic assessment (diagnosis) of the patient that becomes the basis for subsequent treatment and guides the selection of specific medicinals.

Another essential prinicple by which I have always practiced is to know the plants in one's own vicinity. A few books have been written purporting to assign energetic classifications—flavor and *qi*—to herbs from around the world. While it is remarkable how much similarity exists among worldwide traditional medical systems—from traditional Chinese medicine and ayurveda to Egyptian, ancient Greco-Roman, and even Central American herbalism—it is important that the energetics assigned to an herb take into account the context of the medical system in which it is used. For instance, an herb such as berberis (barberry) is considered hot in ayurvedic medicine but cold in traditional Chinese medicine (TCM); honey is viewed as lubricating in TCM but drying in ayurveda. Thus, an energetic system without its systematic cultural context will lack the therapeutic precision and accuracy it is intended to have.

With this book, Thomas Garran makes an important contribution to both TCM and our understanding of the energetics of Western herbs. Thomas's extensive commitment to the study and practice of TCM—as well as his intimate familiarity with indigenous plants throughout North America—makes him uniquely qualified to write such a book. The system of herbal energetics Thomas uses is based on the diagnostic assessment methodology employed in the practice of TCM, which forms the basis of what I described as "planetary herbology" in my book by the same name. Thomas has studied and worked closely with me for many years, steeping himself in medicines from the earth by gathering, making medicines from, and using plants found as natives, weeds, and garden cultivars in the West.

With the thousands of herbs known and used by practitioners of Chinese medicine, one may wonder what is the value of learning and incorporating Western (non-Chinese) herbs, let alone the indigenous herbs of a distant continent, into Chinese medicine. Consider the fact that Chinese immigrants were the first non-native people to recognize the value of North American ginseng *(Panax quinquefolius),* which resulted in extensive trade between the two continents from the seventeenth century to the present—and this is just one of many integrations of non-Chinese plants into Chinese medicine by the Chinese themselves. Today North American ginseng is one of the three hundred or so herbs studied and used by TCM practitioners around the world. Further, chamomile, one of the best-known Western herbs, is valued for its calmative and digestive properties and deemed "a bandaid for the stomach" by Western herbalists, yet has virtually no use in TCM practice.

The following are some of the many other good reasons for TCM herbal practitioners to incorporate and use Western herbs, especially herbs native to their own region of practice:

1. Some North American native or other Western plants may be more effective for certain conditions than their Chinese counterparts.

2. Herbalists should learn how to prescribe and use herbs that are already familiar to the local population, rather than exclusively use exotic plants from a distant continent.

3. In the event that a specific herb from a distant source becomes unavailable, it is prudent to know the uses of local plants. As a byproduct, this will also foster respect for our local resources and can encourage the sustainable use of both local and distant plant populations.

4. Bodies may tend to respond better to locally available herbs. Though this is not always true, finding health resources (and, I might add, food) closer to where we reside is a good practice to cultivate overall.

There are many more good reasons to use local plants, including what for many of us are purely aesthetic reasons. The point is, in my opinion, that it is vitally important for herbalists to know and use the plants of their own regions, and it is to encourage such ends that this book is intended. With great affection and some pride, I heartily recommend Thomas Garran's book to all serious herbalists seeking to understand how to use North American and other non-Chinese herbs in clinical practice.

Michael Tierra, L.Ac., OMD
Founding member of the
American Herbalists Guild (AHG)
Author of *The Way of Herbs,*
Planetary Herbology, and
East-West Herb Course

FOREWORD

By Z'ev Rosenberg, L.Ac.

Back in the 1990s, Thomas Garran blew into town, fresh from his studies with Michael Tierra in Western and Chinese herbal medicine, to gain his Master's Degree in Oriental Medicine at the school at which I teach, Pacific College of Oriental Medicine. He quickly became a legend in San Diego, taking groups of students out to the desert and mountains for herb walks. He would train them in gathering and storing herbs, as well as preparing them as medicines. He had the flash and bravado of a pirate (Johnny Depp, anyone?), but had the knowledge to back up the chutzpah.

The many centuries and textual traditions of Chinese herbal medicine developed in the numerous indigenous cultures of the Chinese subcontinent, from the Tibetan highlands to the warm, humid coastal plains of the south and east. The herbs were found in the wild, cultivated in home gardens, tasted, added to cooking, and used as medicines by common folk and physicians alike. In the "new lands" of the Americas, Chinese medicine has taken root as a powerful complement and alternative to biomedicine and its pharmaceutical drugs. However, we are still largely dependent on herbs imported from mainland China, and have not found an effective way to access the vast storehouse of medicines growing both in the wild and in cultivated gardens across this massive continent. Therefore, anyone who wishes to study the venerated Chinese herbal tradition is largely cut off from seeing the plants growing in their native habitat. Practitioner and student alike are unable to experience growing, foraging, and preparing fresh, local herbs as medicine, and this removes an entire level of experience that cannot be substituted by memorizing the uses of desiccated herbs in glass jars. Also, we cannot take for granted that the supply of herbal medicines from China will not be disrupted by trade sanctions, pollution, and loss of habitat to urbanization as well.

Happily, many Chinese herbs are already growing in the Americas, from forsythia fruit and honeysuckle flower to clematis vine, from schizandra fruit to kudzu vine. Here in San Diego, I was able to catalog eighty-six Chinese herbs growing among the flora at the zoo! Many more Chinese herbs will be cultivated here over time as demand increases. Already, such companies as High Falls Gardens are making available fresh, live, organic Chinese medicinals, and I hope this trend will continue.

While other books have attempted to tackle the subject of Western herbs using Chinese criteria, Thomas's book is the most fully realized. Having a mastery of both Western and Chinese herbal traditions, Thomas has succeeded in cross-referencing Western herbs to Chinese sources wherever possible, and his terminology and descriptions are clear and concise without needless obfuscation. He has inspired and reawakened my own interest in wildcrafting herbs in Taos, New Mexico and in our Californian mountains and canyons. I hope this book will attract a broad readership and great success. It is a necessary beginning for a journey we must all undertake for the future of Chinese medicine in the West.

Z'EV ROSENBERG, L.AC.
CHAIR OF DEPARTMENT OF HERBAL MEDICINE
PACIFIC COLLEGE OF ORIENTAL MEDICINE,
SAN DIEGO, CALIFORNIA

PREFACE

Using Western herbs within the paradigm of traditional Chinese medicine is a controversial undertaking, but one that I believe is important. The path I've followed, first as a student and later as a practitioner and teacher, has led me to a unique understanding of herbs, one that convinced me there is great value in attempting to integrate the insights and knowledge from two great herbal traditions. The primary motivating force behind this work is actually a desire to redefine the understanding of the plants I have presented here. I have used the insights and knowledge on the healing properties of these plants gained from the Western herbal tradition to guide me to their use, and the wisdom from the Chinese medical paradigm as a framework in which to redefine the Western herbal understanding. Thus the expression of the work herein is, in part, an integration or fusion of East and West. I prefer, however, to see it more as an alternate way of looking at much of the same herbal healing information. Please note that some of the clinical data comes from my own or colleagues' personal experience. Our data may differ somewhat from the currently available literature.

During my early years studying plant medicines I took many herbs and even gave some to friends. I remember one instance of trying to give two friends horehound tea. They had been traveling and had bad coughs. The tea was bitter and they did not want to drink it, but I assured them (trustingly) that this tea would help. Magically, it did!

When I decided to take herbal medicine more seriously, I encountered these same herbs again, and many more. My main teachers were Michael Tierra, L.Ac., OMD, and Christopher Hobbs, L.Ac. With his great love for the native plants of the western United States and the rest of the Western materia medica, Christopher Hobbs inspired me to learn field botany and study Western herbs, especially native plants. I can't thank him enough for instilling in me a love for plants from the medical botanist's point of view. This is a way to be intimately connected to the plants and understand them in ways that can only be appreciated while they are alive and growing in the wild.

At the same time, I was learning about Chinese medical theory for the first time. Although I had studied martial arts and was aware of some basic Asian spiritual ideas, the new language of Chinese medicine was intriguing. My teacher in this was Michael Tierra, who inspired in me a fascination with clinical herbalism. Fortunately for me, he too has deep roots in Western herbalism and the Western materia medica.

I spent the next three years trying to understand what these two fine men were teaching, while com-pleting their herb program at the American School of Herbalism. For the next two years, I worked with Michael at the East West Clinic, learning to practice Chinese medicine according to Michael's eclectic style, which includes the use of Western herbs. After more than two years of practicing on my own, I went on to earn my Master's degree in Oriental Medicine, in the meantime teaching, developing, and practicing the material set forth this book.

It is my hope that with this book I will do justice to the teachings I received from Michael and Christopher, as well as many others along the way. By developing these ideas and bringing to you the first presentation of Western herbs in the familiar language and format of our Chinese medicine materia medicas, I acknowledge all of you who have supported and schooled me along the way. May each who reads this find a gem that allows him or her to help relieve human suffering.

To contact me, access herbal resources, or view an extensive collection of medicinal plant photographs, please visit my website:

www.sourcepointherbs.org

THOMAS AVERY GARRAN

ACKNOWLEDGMENTS

Many people have supported the hard work that went into this book, in many different ways. All of them have been teachers to me, but I would like to recognize a few with whom I have studied intensively. Michael Tierra, Christopher Hobbs, Z'ev Rosenberg, and Bob Damone: You have been the most influential of those I call teacher. Barbara Nigel, for first introducing me to and teaching me the value of martial arts and Chinese wisdom, I thank you.

I am blessed to have some special people in my life that I can call both colleague and friend. Many of you helped in various stages of this work with reading and suggestions. Ben Zappin, David Winston, Bill Schoenbart, and Paul Bergner, to you I am indebted. Garth Reynolds and Tommy Lee, thank you for the work you did with much of the translation found here—you made life a little easier. Although many have helped me along the way, any and all mistakes found in this text are entirely of my own making and I take full responsibility for them.

Thank you to Richo and Mache Cech of Horizon Herbs for allowing me to come and take many of the photographs found in the book.

To my patients, I extend a special thank you. It has been an honor to have walked on your path while we worked together. Thanks also to all the students I have had through the years, for listening when I was rambling and asking questions for which I had no answer. Mahalo to La'akea, for all of your help during the final stages of writing this book.

To the good folks at Inner Traditions • Bear & Company, a very special thanks. From Jon Graham, who first saw the value of the work and got me through the preliminary stages; to Jeanie Levitan, who managed the whole thing; to Laura Schlivek, whose eye for detail brought into focus all my blood, sweat, and tears; to Evelyn Leigh, who did some of the most painful work in the project and asked some of the finest questions; to Peri Champine, who was patient with my art issues and despite all that created a fine product; to Jon Desautels who designed the interior; and to all the rest of the unsung heroes in the good green state, a heartfelt thank you. Without you, this book would still be a group of files on my hard drive.

And finally, outside the plant world and the publishing world, thanks to the many who have helped in various supportive ways over the years: the mother of my beautiful children, Julie Maloney; my little brother, Steve Garran; my father and mother, Tam and Sheila Garran; and most of all, the most special gifts anyone could ask for, my two girls Aralia and Mara. To all of you, thank you.

INTRODUCTION

*In [prescribing] medicinals, what is vital is not variety
but the choice of what is effective.*

LIU YI-REN,

THE HEART TRANSMISSION OF MEDICINE

Classifying Western herbs into the Chinese medical system is no easy task, and I offer this book as a stepping-stone toward a more complete understanding of how Western herbs can be classified according to the Chinese medical paradigm. Chinese medicine's way of looking at plants is very different from ours and is, as it would be with any culture in the world, largely based on the Chinese cultural worldview, which is simply different from the Western paradigm.

The basic concepts of *qì* and *yīn-yáng* are the building blocks used to construct an entire system of medicine. These building blocks contain the fundamental ideas that govern how Chinese herbalists understand medicinal plants. I have attempted to cultivate the understanding within myself so that I could do a work such as this justice. Thanks for joining me on this path.

I was motivated to take on the challenge of creating such a work because I felt a need for it in my own practice. I started writing things down to help organize the material for myself, and it wasn't long before I realized that a book was forming. Of course, I also had significant influence from my teachers, one of whom is Michael Tierra, author of *Planetary Herbology* and the first to attempt this type of work. Thus, what I am trying to do in writing this book is not new; Chinese medicine has absorbed many herbs from around the world into its own system. Plants are created equally in the eyes of nature. It is this understanding that

1

allowed Taoist monks and master herbalists to assess and classify each plant according to the principles of Chinese medical theories.

I wrote this book primarily as a reference for practitioners of Chinese medicine. Those who want to incorporate Western herbs into their practice will find it helpful. The book can also serve as a reference for Chinese medicine practitioners whose patients are taking Western herbs. A word about the term "Western herb" as used in this book: This is a broad term that I will discuss in more detail later, but in general, a Western herb is any medicinal plant used in the Western herbal tradition that is not of Asian origin.

The herbs described in this text are those I employ regularly in clinical practice. Most of them are in common use and easily procured. However, I have also included some less frequently used botanicals that are native to the western United States; these reflect the region in which I practice and are an important contribution to this text. Research, while important, cannot make up for a lack of practical experience. Therefore, all of the material set forth in this book has a basis in my own clinical experience. In some cases, the impetus for an idea came from another practitioner or teacher, but you will find nothing within the pages of this book that I have not observed in my own clinical practice.

Throughout history, Chinese medicine has seen many transformations, most of them reflective of the times. These transformations have molded traditional Chinese medicine into one of the most comprehensive systems of medicine in the world. The Western world began ingesting bits of Chinese medicine over the last several decades; it has only just begun to digest them. This movement to the West has transformed the practice of Chinese medicine anew. The transformation has grand potential, but we must be wary. Like those who came before us, we must stay true to the origins of Chinese medicine. The nature of this evolving system requires an astute understanding of the classics and how they relate to current medicine. For the first time in history, many people are looking at Chinese medicine from "outside the box," from different cultural experiences and reference points. As the West adopts Chinese medicine, it is essential that we shepherd the transformation of the medicine.

I see my work as a continuation and evolution of the ideas set forth in *Planetary Herbology,* by Michael Tierra, and, to some extent, in *The Energetics of Western Herbs,* by Peter Holmes, and in *Botanical Medicine,* by Dan Kenner and Yves Requena. *Planetary Herbology* gave us a glimpse into the basic Chinese classification of many Western herbs. I believe Michael Tierra opened the door to what is possibly the greatest transformation in the contemporary Chinese medicine materia medica, at least in the West. *The Energetics of Western Herbs,* although in many ways a scholarly work, is often confusing, as Holmes valiantly attempts to resurrect the energetic system of ancient Greece and combine it with principles of Chinese medicine.* Rather than giving the reader an insight into the Chinese energetics of Western herbs, however, the reality is that Holmes has created an entirely new system. *Botanical Medicine* attempts to classify Western herbs using a Five Phase model, and, although an excellent book, does not give the Chinese herbal practitioner much to work with. Finally, the most recent addition to the mix is Jeremy Ross's tome, *Combining Western Herbs in Chinese Medicine*—a book that in the end leaves the Chinese medicine practitioner wondering how to fit the medicinals presented into his or her own practice.

None of these texts is true to any one system, and I believe that is one of the differences that set my work apart. In this book, I have done my best to stay within the confines of the Chinese medicine paradigm to explain both the herbs and the human body. You will find only rare mentions of Western biomedicine. Furthermore, I have tried to adhere to the terminology set forth by Nigel Wiseman and Feng Ye in their book, *A Practical Dictionary of Chinese Medicine.* The impor-

---

*Please refer to the first volume of Peter Holmes's *The Energetics of Western Herbs* for an excellent account of the old system of energetics used by Western herbalists and how it compares with the Chinese system.

tance of this terminology cannot be overstated. I hope those not familiar with Wiseman and Feng's work will take an opportunity to peruse a vocabulary that, in my opinion, could serve as an incredibly helpful standard to which we can all look in order to clarify the meaning of Chinese terms that have been translated into English. Wiseman and Feng's choices of English words sometimes may seem terse or obscure. However, the words were chosen to best approximate the actual Chinese term, an incredibly difficult task.

This topic is highly contentious, and a brief discussion is warranted to clarify the reasoning behind my decision to use Wiseman and Feng's terminology. Knowledge transfer from one culture to another is a difficult process. A clear understanding of the terms used in the culture from which the material is coming is critical to facilitating that process. To enhance the transfer of knowledge, *A Practical Dictionary of Chinese Medicine* attempts to define a standard set of terms. This is not meant to imply that *all* Chinese doctors use *all* terms in exactly the same way. However, when we have a standard, we have a place to start. If one needs to deviate from the standard when transferring knowledge, one can simply note that they are doing so and define the difference, and the reader will be able to easily understand the material. In writing this book, I have applied Wiseman and Feng's standard terminology so that there should be no question about what I am discussing. All of the terms relating to Chinese medicine used in this book can be found in *A Practical Dictionary of Chinese Medicine*.

Many Western practitioners have previous training in the healing arts before beginning their study of Chinese medicine. Some have a background in modern biomedical training, while others come from a traditional style of healing, many of which include herbs. Those who come from Western herbal training, no matter what style, find that using herbs from China represents a move, in part, away from their roots as traditional healers. Many Western herbalists are taught to use plants from their own bioregions and even their own gardens. For Western practitioners of Chinese herbal medicine,

the herbs come from very far away, and frequently we don't feel a connection to the plants as living entities. Although this last issue may not be particularly germane to the practice of Chinese herbal medicine, it is often important to the trained Western herbalist.

As an herbalist who comes from a traditional Western background and now primarily practices Chinese medicine, I believe incorporating Western herbs will be essential for the progression of Chinese medicine, principally in the West (North America and Europe). For the North American or European practitioner of Chinese medicine, understanding how Western medicinals work within the Chinese medical paradigm is important for several reasons. First, it is essential to have a reference point when assessing a patient who may be taking Western medicinals. Second, the expansion of the materia medica to include plants that are not only of native origin, but also generally available as clean, high-quality material, often either wildcrafted or organically grown, cannot be overlooked. Understanding plants from other parts of the world may also help practitioners better serve patients. More is not necessarily better, but variety does give us the opportunity to choose the best possible medicinal. In *The Heart Transmission of Medicine*, Liu Yi-ren states,

> The subtlety in prescribing medicinals is like that of commanding an army. What is decisive is not the amounts of armies but putting them to their best use. In (prescribing) medicinals, what is vital is not variety but the choice of what is effective.[1]

He goes on to describe one hundred and forty-six medicinals by making one statement about each, asserting a unique quality for each medicinal. His fine text, which has been translated into English by Blue Poppy Press, not only adds variety to our materia medica, but also, more importantly, adds plants that have very specific uses, which allows us as practitioners to apply Liu Yi-ren's statement to the fullest.

Patients often come to the clinic asking about herbal products, frequently Western herbal products, that they have either purchased or seen advertised. It is imperative to understand these medicinals from the Chinese paradigm. How do you assess a patient who is taking Western herbs? If he or she were taking Jade Windscreen Formula *(yù píng fēng sǎn)* or just plain *huáng qí (Astragalus membranaceus)*, you would understand how these herbs might affect his or her health and could factor this information into your diagnosis and treatment. Further, you would feel comfortable advising the patient about the possible benefits or risks of taking these or any Chinese herb or formula. One function of this book is to assist you with these important questions in your clinical practice.

For those of us who live in the West (North America or Europe), there are many other good reasons to make use of Western plants. Probably the most important of these is conservation of resources. Most Western herbs employed in the United States are either native to North America or are European herbs that have now naturalized or are cultivated here. The same is true in Europe, where some North American native herbs are cultivated. This is not meant to imply that herbs from China or anywhere else are inferior. However, I believe the majority of organically grown Western herbs are superior in quality to most Chinese herbs. There is a rich materia medica in your back yard. It may not always be easy to procure herbs from distant lands, and they are certainly not getting any cheaper. Further, it takes an enormous amount of resources to ship herbs around the world.

As practitioners, we look constantly for answers to clinical questions. The essence of the art of clinical herbalism is understanding which medicinals to use in a given situation, and in what combination. This book offers more tools for the practitioner's toolbox. The plants I have chosen to include were not selected randomly. Rather, they are a group of herbs from the Western materia medica that I believe will add specific meaning to the already large materia medica of Chinese medicine. It is my hope that my work will provide a welcome springboard for deepening the tradition of Chinese herbal medicine.

HOW TO USE THIS BOOK

This book is divided into two parts. The first explains the methodology I have used to incorporate Western herbs into Chinese medicine, as well as a brief introduction to some essential medicine-making techniques.

My methodology for incorporating herbs from outside the Chinese materia medica is something of an evolving process. I have done my best to logically lay out the method I used, and offer it as a model for those who may want to embark upon such a project themselves. While my methods have been helpful in guiding me, I do not necessarily expect everyone to follow them as dogma. For those who wish to use my work as a model (or not), I am always open to discussion and willing to consider ways to improve on the process.

I offer the medicine-making section of this book as a brief and general overview to familiarize the reader with the types of products mentioned in the text. The medicine-making discussion is not meant to be exhaustive, nor is it meant to serve as a manual to train students in the techniques involved in producing medicines from plants. It is intended mainly as brief but helpful information for those in the Chinese medicine field in the West, who are generally not well trained in this aspect of herbal medicine.

The second part of the book is the materia medica, organized according to major categories used in the Chinese materia medica. I have listed the plants in order of my frequency of use. This ordering is somewhat arbitrary and not static, so don't read too deeply into it. My choices are based primarily on my personal preferences and are not meant to imply that any one plant is necessarily more important than any other. Some of you may find that you prefer some plants to others, and thus the order would be different for you.

The herb entries included in each category are organized as follows:

Plant name: Each herb entry is headed with the common (English) name for the herb. After that, I've listed several different names for the plant, including scientific (Latin) binomial and family name, pharmaceutical

Latin, and other common names (Chinese as well as English, if possible). For those not familiar with pharmaceutical Latin names, here is a brief explanation. A pharmaceutical Latin name is based on the scientific plant name (Latin binomial) used in botany, with some changes to the spelling of the ending according to rules of the Latin language. In addition, a word is added to denote the plant part used for medicinal purposes. These words include *radix* (root), *rhizoma* (rhizome), *flos* (flower), *folium* (leaf), *semen* (seed), and *planta* (whole plant). As an illustration, the pharmaceutical Latin name for valerian *(Valeriana officinalis)* rhizome and root is Valerianae Officinali rhizoma et radix.

Flavor and *Qi*: This section describes the flavor and *qi* I've assigned to the herb. These designations are intended for use as guides to help you understand how to apply the plant in a clinical situation. Again, my designations should not be considered absolute. When looking over different materia medicas of Chinese medicine, one will find plenty of variation. I expect that while some readers will agree with my choices, others will disagree with me occasionally, and others will find little agreement. In the end, this is not of critical importance and will not be consequential to the main body of work presented. Whether a plant is warm or slightly warm may be a matter of potential dispute, but in the end, is more a theoretical than practical question. Please see the section on flavor and *qi* under The Construction and Use of a Materia Medica for more information on these properties.

Channels Entered: Under this heading you will find the primary channels as I have assigned them according to Chinese medicine. Again, there are some who might dispute these assignments, but this is a matter of debate even in standard materia medicas. Furthermore, the assignment of channels to medicinals is in itself debatable and of limited use. I offer these assignments as a starting point for those who apply this understanding as part of their practice.

Actions: This section focuses on the biomedical, physiologic, and traditional Western herbal actions of the plant, providing a Western (generally scientific) understanding of how the herb works. I have drawn most of this information from the latest data available, and this is one of the only places in the text that you will find biomedical descriptions of the plants' properties.

Functions and Indications: Here I set forth the functions of the herb from a more or less strict Chinese medical perspective. I have purposely omitted any reference to biomedical actions in this part of the monograph. The indications included here are traditional indications, with few exceptions. These exceptions occur when I have found the medicinal useful for other conditions after analyzing it from the Chinese medical perspective, or when I have adopted specific uses from teachers or colleagues. Thus, some of the uses found in this book are "new" (in other words, not found in the traditional books). A note on terminology: Patients often come to the clinic with an allopathic diagnosis, but I frequently use the terms "concretions and conglomerations" to refer to nonpalpable masses such as fibroids, ovarian cysts, and the like. This diverges somewhat from the traditional use of this term. However, I believe there is no other way that makes clinical sense to describe these conditions in terms of Chinese medicine.

Cautions: Any relevant cautions are presented here, from either a Chinese or biomedical perspective.

Dosage and Preparation: Here I have provided dosages for the most common methods of preparation for each herb. Because tinctures are very popular in the West and commonly used in Western clinical herbology, all of the herb entries give tincture dosages. I have also included a description of what good-quality dried plant material should look, smell, and taste like when it arrives in your clinic. This may vary greatly depending on the company you buy from and how they prepare the herbs. In this section, I have also included *páo zhì* for some of the herbs. With this strict use of the word *páo zhì*, I am referring to preparations such as honey mix-fried licorice, steamed rehmannia, and so forth.

Major Combinations: This part of each herb entry

provides suggested ways to combine the herb with other Western herbs, Chinese herbs, or Chinese formulas in order to treat specific conditions. This section is very important for two reasons. First, it shows us how practitioners before us have combined the herbs; many of the Western herb combinations are found in the traditional literature. Second, it offers ways to combine Western herbs with Chinese herbs and formulas. These are combinations I have found to be effective in clinical practice.

Commentary: In this section you will find a wide array of information, from historical use by Native Americans, early American physicians, ancient herbalists, and European practitioners to specific comments about the plant in question. Botanical notes, specific biomedical indications, listings in official pharmacopoeias, and sustainability issues are also covered here.

Translation of Source Material: This section, found in some but not all of the monographs, is a translation of available material on either the same or related species used in Chinese medicine. All of this material came from the *Grand Dictionary of Chinese Medicinals,* 13th edition *(Zhōng Yào Dà Cí Diăn)*. The purpose of including this information is to give you some idea of what Chinese authors have said about the medicinals

and allow you to compare it to what I have written. All of this translation was done after I wrote the book, as I did not have access to the material prior to writing the book. Thus, the translated material has not had any significant effect on the material I have presented. Sometimes it confirms what I have written; sometimes it does not.

Beyond the Main Body of the Text

Appendix 1 includes brief descriptions of herbs that grow in the West and are either analogous to commonly used Chinese herbs or, in some cases, the same species. Although many of these plants are unavailable on the market because they are not used in Western herbology, this is a valuable reference for anybody wishing to expand their appreciation and use of the plants growing in their region.

Appendices 2 and 3 provide a cross-reference, in table format, for the Latin, common (English), and, when possible, Chinese names of the medicinals discussed in this book.

Appendix 4 contains a glossary of terms important to understanding the material in the text. All of the terms pertaining to Chinese medicine are from *A Practical Dictionary of Chinese Medicine* by Nigel Wiseman and Feng Ye.

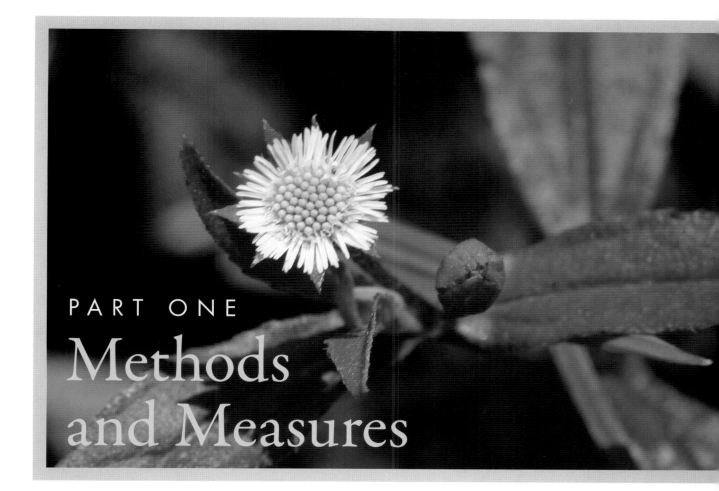

PART ONE
Methods
and Measures

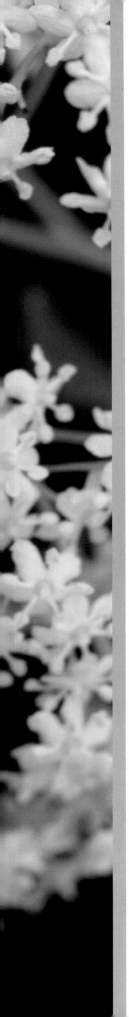

UNDERSTANDING WESTERN HERBS FROM THE CHINESE MEDICAL PERSPECTIVE

One of the advantages of the Chinese medicine materia medica over the Western materia medica is that it represents the culmination of thousands of years of clinical data. In the West, much of our herbal knowledge includes large gaps of time during which information was not passed on, or when entire lines of understanding were broken. Consider the Native American tradition and how little is known about how these people used plants, or think of the four-humors system of Western–Arabic medicine. Over time, with a continued and unbroken chain of doctors who used many of the same herbs, the Chinese were able to build and record an extensive and specific materia medica based on an ever-evolving system of medicine. Although Chinese medicine has changed through the years, the basic theories have remained more or less the same through the millennia. That being said, it is important to remember that there is also a large body of literature concerning the use of herbs in the West, and with the current resurgence in herb popularity, there will undoubtedly be much more.

Many materia medicas written in the West, especially the popular ones, are largely regurgitations of work done in the past. Moreover, the theories of Western biomedicine are in a constant state of flux; what is true today may well be false tomorrow. I am sure that replication of materia medicas also occurred in Chinese medicine, but instead of getting more general, as some of the (popular) Western materia medicas have, the Chinese materia medicas have become more specific. In the West, works such as Scudder's *Specific Medication* show just how specific Western herbal medicine can be. However, many of the popular Western materia medicas are written according to generalities. For example, if you look up "cough" in most Western materia medicas, you will find listed many herbs that are good for cough, but little differentiation among the different herbs or the different types of coughs for which they may be appropriate. There are some good, professionally oriented materia medicas (and a few popular ones) that avoid this pattern. However, looking in a Chinese materia medica, one will find more or less the same number of herbs listed for cough as in the Western herbal, but find that they are differentiated into categories according to the type of cough to be treated, an obvious asset for the practitioner.

Another difference between Chinese and Western materia medicas is that there is much more emphasis in Chinese medicine on the use of formulas and combinations (polypharmacy); the old formulas from Western herbalism are rarely used. This may have to do with the fragmented history of herbal medicine in the West.* In Chinese medicine, where some of the same formulas written two thousand years ago are still used and discussed today, the idea of formulation and herb combinations is critical to practice.

The term "Western herb" as used in this book has broad meaning. The majority of these herbs are native to Europe, the Middle East, and North America. Others that are commonly used hail from Africa, South America, and the South Pacific. Many plants from Asia also have been incorporated into various systems of Western herbology. There has been trade of herbs and spices between Asia and Europe since the beginning of the Common Era. Herbs such as ginger, car-

---

*Read *Green Pharmacy* by Barbara Griggs for an excellent account of the history of herbal medicine in the West.

damom, and cinnamon were among the earliest traded into some parts of Europe. As early as 65 CE, there was enough cinnamon in Rome for a year-long funeral rite for Poppaea, Nero's wife.

Likewise, various herbs used in Chinese medicine come from other parts of the world. As early as the seventh century, herbs such as frankincense, myrrh, dragon's blood, and aucklandia came from the Middle East.[1] In 667 CE, Christian missionaries from Daqin brought opium from Europe.[2] Between the fifth and thirteenth centuries there was much trade between China and other Asian countries, the first of which were India and Vietnam. From Vietnam came coix, aquilaria, clove, amomum fruit, fennel fruit, black pepper, long pepper, alpinia, alpinia fruit, zedoraria, erythrina bark, cinnamon bark, turmeric, momordica seed, evodia fruit, sappan wood, and areca fruit. Finally, from the Americas came American ginseng, corn silk, echinacea, and now perhaps a few more. Some herbs used in Chinese medicine grow here in the West as native plants, nonnative weeds, or cultivars. These include glehnia, eclipta, cyperus, honeysuckle flowers, and round-leaf vitex.

In a lecture I attended once, the teacher stated that Chinese herbs must be stronger because we generally use the top three hundred to four hundred herbs from a materia medica of around five thousand substances, and that the Western materia medica represented "the best fifty herbs from a choice of one hundred to two hundred." I am quite sure this person merely misspoke. Those familiar with the Chinese materia medica know that the list of five thousand substances to which the speaker referred consists of 15 to 20 percent animal and mineral products. Further, the first book I reached for on Western herbs, *Potter's New Cyclopaedia of Botanical Drugs and Preparations,* by R.C. Wren, F.L.S., discusses nearly five hundred and fifty botanical medicines. Thousands of botanical medicines not mentioned in this book are used by practitioners throughout the Americas, Europe, and Australia. In fact, tens of thousands of plants are used throughout the world as medicine. Certainly, some of those are stronger, or even better or more applicable to specific conditions than others in use. However, there is no correlation between potency and the country or region in which the herbs grow. Ultimately, the herbs we choose to treat a specific pattern or condition should not be based on their country of origin as much as on their ability to treat the patient and relieve suffering.

The importance of clear terminology to describe medicinal plants and their actions has been an issue in Western herbal medicine through the years. This is evidenced in the monograph on echinacea from *King's American Dispensatory,* originally published in 1899. Professor King states,

> The day is rapidly approaching when these qualifying terms [Author's note: e.g., antiseptic and alterative] will have no place in medicine, for they but inadequately convey to our minds the therapeutic possibilities of our drugs. Especially is this so with regard to such terms as alterative, stimulant, tonic, etc. If any single statement were to be made concerning the virtues of echinacea, it would read something like this: "A corrector of the depravation of the body fluids," and even this does not sufficiently cover the ground.

There is a striking resemblance here to the way ideas about medicinals are expressed in Chinese medicine. This is particularly interesting because *King's American Dispensatory* is without question the most comprehensive materia medica written in American history.* This monumental piece of literature stands as the epitaph of Eclectic medicine (an important plant-based system of medicine that flourished in the United States from the mid-nineteenth into the early twentieth century), even though it was revised for the last time in 1898—forty years before the last Eclectic medical school closed its doors. Perhaps the Eclectics

were moving toward a more energetic understanding of botanical medicine. Unfortunately, because of various factors that contributed to the decline of botanical medicine in North America, we'll never know for sure.[†]

THE CONSTRUCTION AND USE OF A MATERIA MEDICA

Creating a materia medica of Western herbs using the language of Chinese medicine is no small undertaking, and I certainly do not consider this work absolute. However, I feel strongly that the material herein is an important step toward uniting the roots of Western herbalism with Chinese medicine. The old English proverb says it simply: "Both together do best of all."

I have studied many materia medicas. The information gleaned from this study, combined with the experience of my teachers, my own experience, and the experience of fellow practitioners is the basis for my viewpoint on individual herbs in the Western materia medica. Because I am a trained Chinese herbalist, the idea of combinations *(duì yào)* is important to me; thus I try to incorporate this concept with Western herbs in as much detail as possible. Many of these combinations come from historical references. Because some of the combinations are new, I admit that I have less data on them than I would have liked to have. However, I have tried everything described in this book and found that it worked to my satisfaction, or I would not have included it.

When I initiated this work, I first outlined what I had learned from teachers and from my clinical experience. I looked through patient files to see how I had used specific herbs for specific Chinese diagnoses, and determined whether or not the patient had responded in the way I expected. This was a difficult process, as I use polypharmacy and it was not always easy to see how a single herb or combination of herbs affected a person. However, with careful study, patterns began to arise, and what at first was obscure began to come clear.

---

*Professor John King, a giant in Eclectic medicine, was the original author of this book. Two other leaders of the Eclectic movement—Harvey Wicks Felter, M.D., and John Uri Lloyd, Phr.M., Ph.D.—completed the third and final revision of the eighteenth edition.

---

†To learn more about these factors, including the infamous Flexner Report of 1910, I strongly suggest reading *Green Pharmacy* by Barbara Griggs.

The next step was to research how these plants have been used in their native systems of medicine. I have drawn heavily on the work of the American physicians of the nineteenth and early twentieth centuries in the Physio-medical and Eclectic schools of medicine. Much of my understanding of the Western herbal tradition is based on the body of clinically based information they amassed. I find many of the much older European texts to be a bit obscure and cumbersome. This does not mean that I have not referenced some of the great classical herbalists, such as Culpeper, Gerard, Parkinson, Dioscorides, Galen, and even Hippocrates, but only that their contributions do not make up the bulk of the material presented herein. This stands in marked contrast to the tradition of Chinese medicine, in which the classics are heavily weighted.

When considering the five flavors and *qi* of herbs, I considered not only the actual taste as it occurs in the mouth, but also the physiological response each herb produces in the body. I am trained in the culinary arts, and the idea that the flavor of an herb can suggest something about how it acts physiologically has always intrigued me. In my early days as an herb student I spent hours on end tasting herbs, trying to understand how the Chinese came up with the flavors they ascribed to each herb. At first, I was often befuddled, because my mouth could not taste the flavors listed in the texts. I then learned that taste means more than mere flavor in the mouth, and that it has more to do with effects on physiological function than anything else. In other words, in order for a plant to be ascribed a particular taste, it had to perform the action representative of that flavor. With this understanding, I was able to train my palate and my body to taste the five flavors (plus bland) of Chinese medicine. These actions are clearly laid out in the theories of Chinese medicine: Acrid flavors disperse and move; sweet flavors supplement, harmonize, and sometimes moisten; bitter flavors drain and dry; sour flavors astringe and stop or prevent leakage; salty flavors purge and soften; and bland flavors leach dampness and promote urination.

Michael Tierra, Peter Holmes, and Dan Kenner had already done much work in ascribing the five flavors to Western herbs, and I have translated some Chinese sources describing the flavors, *qi,* actions, and indications of some of the herbs found in this text. However, I took it upon myself to decide how I would ascribe flavors and *qi* to the herbs, based on my own clinical experience and many hours of meditation, before referencing any other work. This allowed me to consider each herb clearly without outside influence; I could then sit down and compare my ideas with the other available material to decide how to present each medicinal in this book. It is important to note that flavors and *qi* within the Chinese materia medica often differ, at least somewhat, from book to book.

Next, by looking at symptom groups (i.e., how symptoms can be grouped to show a pattern, as defined by Chinese medicine) I was able to get ideas about how the actions of the medicinals relate to the Chinese concepts of how the body works. Coupled with the five flavors and *qi,* these ideas gave me the basis for the majority of the work I've presented in this book. This involved a tedious process of reviewing many texts and looking for similarities as well as discrepancies, and then comparing and contrasting these with my own experiences and the experiences of my teachers and colleagues. However, it was also an extremely interesting process of learning and discovery. For example, I found that some Chinese books described applications for Western herbs that were nearly the same as Western applications, though they used different words to explain the clinical picture and diagnosis.

Some herbs were easier to figure out than others. Lobelia, for instance, was a struggle, because it has such a wide range of uses—some seemingly contradictory. In contrast, herbs like usnea were relatively easy. Throughout the process, I applied my ideas in clinical practice and occasionally made changes and modifications to the text according to what I observed. I also asked certain colleagues—those with training and experience with both Chinese medicine and Western herbs—to read through drafts and critique my work, and consequently made some additions and changes based on their input.

In conclusion, although it was challenging, I believe my process was far easier than the one Chinese herbalists underwent to classify Chinese herbs. I say this because I had a base of literature from which to work and teachers to guide me. In the early days of Chinese medicine, practitioners had much less to work with and probably even needed to experiment with their patients in order to get a clear understanding of how specific medicinals worked.

EASTERN VS. WESTERN WAYS OF WORKING WITH HERBS

There are a number of differences in the primary methods by which herbs are employed in Chinese and Western systems of herbal medicine. Most of these relate to either preparation or formulation styles. Gaining a better understanding of how these methods differ gives us insight into the healing systems the plants have been used in for millennia. I believe this insight helps us create the paradigm shift necessary to understand the use of medicinal plants that currently fall outside the traditional Chinese materia medica through the eyes of Chinese medicine.

Formulation is the main mode in which Chinese herbalists use botanicals, a concept that is often overlooked in Western herbology, at least as evidenced by many of the popular products available in health food stores and markets. When Chinese herbalists see a patient, they generally think of formulas that might be helpful for that particular patient, whereas the Western herbalist is more likely to think in terms of individual herbs that may prove beneficial to the case. Both ways of seeing have inherent benefits, but being able to see with an eye from each perspective is perhaps most useful of all. On the one hand, there are formulas that may address the pattern(s) at hand, while on the other, there may be specific herbs that can be used to modify the representative formula to best suit the individual case. The Chinese herbalist formulates in this way as a matter of course, but many Western herbalists strive for simple, to-the-point prescriptions. This keeps formulas small and makes it easier to pinpoint potential prob-

lems and thus determine how to make changes to a particular formula. Further, the bulk of Western formulas are acutely focused on the treatment principle to treat a specific disease rather than a constellation of symptoms that make up the patterns of Chinese medicine. For example, the formula may address only an acute manifestation of a disease, with little consideration for other symptoms that make up underlying patterns and may be contributing to the acute illness.

Western herbal preparation methods are also somewhat different from those employed in Chinese medicine. The most significant difference is the large amount of tinctures dispensed in the West, compared with a relatively insignificant number of tinctures dispensed in China. In Chinese medicine the vast majority of preparations are water extracts and, recently, an ever-increasing number of powdered extracts (especially in Taiwan). The bulk of the water extracts are simple decoctions. This means the herbs are simmered in a pot of water for the appointed amount of time, strained, and drunk. (Some notable exceptions are uncaria [gōu téng], mint [bò hé], agastache [huò xiāng], and a few other aromatics, which are added for the last five minutes of decoction or sometimes incorporated as powders into a finished decoction.) In spite of this fact, there is a very long tradition of medicated wines in Chinese medicine, dating back to at least the Shang Dynasty (1766–1122 BCE).[3] Furthermore, Chinese herbalists widely prescribe powdered or solid extracts, which are basically nonexistent in Western herbal practice (with the exception of modern phytomedicines that make up a relatively small part of many clinicians' repertoire).

Powdered or concentrated extracts are relatively new to Chinese medicine, having been introduced from Japan in the late 1950s. These are pharmaceutical-grade water extracts. Although some traditional tinctures are made in Chinese medicine, as far as I know, few are used in modern Chinese medicine. In contrast, the variety of extraction methods used in the West, from cold-water infusions to percolation extracts, is symbolic of our worldview. These extraction processes are scientific, based on particular "active" chemical constituents and how best to extract them. It is this information that defines how each medicinal is prepared.

According to Chinese medicine, "a *little* alcohol warms the center and supplements the *qi* while at the same time it raises clear *yáng* and quickens the blood" and ". . . alcohol opens the blood vessels, wards off cold *qi*, arouses the spleen and warms the center, and moves (i.e., makes more capable) the power of medicinals."[4] Although the small quantity of alcohol prescribed as part of a tincture is infrequently an issue, alcohol cannot be overlooked as an energetic force and must be carefully considered for each patient. Alcohol has an energetic force of being "upbearing and dispersing, heating and also dampening."[5] This must be taken into account before we send our patients out of the office with any preparation that contains alcohol.

It is important to note that I have not found tinctures very effective in supplementation therapy, particularly when supplementing *yīn* or blood. Because many *yīn* supplementing herbs tend to be heavily weighted with polysaccharides and other sugars that are water soluble, not alcohol soluble, the use of alcohol in a preparation impairs the ability of the solvent (water) to do its job effectively. Further, because of the warm, dispersing energy of the alcohol, it can evaporate or disturb *yīn*. Conversely, because of this warming and dispersing energy, alcohol is well suited for clinical applications such as treating cold-damp, most wind diseases, and, when used carefully, *yáng* or even *qi* vacuity. However, tinctures may be safely and effectively applied in other clinical pictures, as detailed in the materia medica section of this book.

Another major difference between Eastern and Western herb preparation methods is that Western herbalism has largely lost what is known as *páo zhi* in Chinese medicine. This term has a much broader meaning in Chinese than is often understood in the West. I use it here in the narrower way it is commonly understood in the West—that is, to indicate specific ways of preparing medicinals that change their functions and indications (e.g., honey mix-fried licorice).

Páo zhi, which translates as "processing of medicinals," relates to any method used to prepare medicinals for clinical use. Although the phrase refers to any process important in preparation, including washing and cutting, when we think of *páo zhi* we generally think of processes like honey mix-frying, steaming, or ginger-processing. These are methods used to prepare medicinals prior to their final processing for ingestion by the patient. These methods of treating herbs were once common in Western herbal medicine, and there is evidence of such use in Native American medicine as well as other systems. For example, in his *Complete Herbal and English Physician*, Nicholas Culpeper had this to say about caraway: ". . . some of the seed bruised and fried, laid hot in a bag or double cloth to the lower parts of the belly, easeth the pains of the wind colic." Some of the other older herbals of Europe, such as Parkinson's and Salmon's, discuss similar preparations.

I have a great deal of interest in the subject of traditional Chinese *páo zhi*, likely due to my background in the culinary arts, and have tried to adopt some of it into my practice. Most of the techniques are quite simple and add an interesting dimension to the flavor and *qi*—and thus the functions and indications—of the final preparation. A beloved chef once told me, "Each dish needs a special touch of love, because that energy can be felt by the patron who eats the dish." I believe that some of these special preparations can be influenced in an energetic way through the hands of the person who prepares them. Throughout the book, you will find descriptions of Western medicinals with which I have experimented using some of these techniques. I have included only the ones I use on a regular basis and believe to be useful in clinical practice. Undoubtedly, there are many more ways to prepare these and other plants, and I hope to reveal more of them in the future.

WESTERN HERBAL PREPARATIONS

This section is a brief introduction to some of the different ways Western herbs are prepared. It is meant to help familiarize practitioners, particularly Chinese herbalists, with the variety of preparations available to them when using Western medicinals. I hope it also inpires some to learn to make a few of these preparations in order to offer patients hand-crafted products, tailored to their specific needs. However, even if you decide you don't want to make them yourself, this section will serve as an overview of how the medicines are prepared and will allow you to make good decisions when purchasing them from the many fine companies who specialize in such products.

Western herbs are prescribed in many forms, the most common of which are alcohol-based tinctures. The popularity of tinctures is generally due to ease and patient compliance—the same reason many Chinese medicine practitioners use powdered and liquid extracts. I have found that including Western herbs in traditional teas in combination with Chinese herbs is not only effective, but also an excellent way to integrate them into the practice of Chinese traditional herbology. Furthermore, I often go one step beyond that and prepare my own tinctures of Chinese herbs to use in formulas with my favorite Western herbs. I find this an excellent and powerful tool in the clinic. Unfortunately, to my knowledge, there is not a good source for powdered extracts of Western herbs (unless you are prepared to purchase large volumes), and the process of preparing them is far too time consuming for most private practitioners. For those who are interested, however, the next chapter describes a number of basic medicine-making techniques that may be applied with either Western or Chinese herbs.

Tinctures are extracts made using alcohol and water as solvents to extract and hold the "active constituents" in a liquid solution. This is an excellent way of extracting and taking herbs. Water is the best-known solvent, and alcohol is a close second. Other solvents used include glycerin, which is similar to alcohol as solvents, and vinegar. Vinegar is not a very good solvent for most herbs, although it does work rather well for a few. Several large companies and a slew of smaller regional companies provide most of the tinctures on the U.S. market.

The appropriate percentage of alcohol in tinctures varies greatly, because the constituent base of medicinal plants varies dramatically. All alcohol-based tinctures contain a minimum of 18 to 20 percent alcohol to eliminate the possibility of spoilage, unless either glycerin or vinegar is also added. For instance, nettle leaf consists of mostly water-soluble constituents, and therefore requires only a minimal amount of alcohol for extraction and preservation, perhaps only 25 to 30 percent. Other herbs, such as milk thistle seed, require the strongest alcohol available, usually 95 percent, since its major constituents are soluble only in alcohol. This is also true for resinous herbs. Resins are alcohol soluble rather than water soluble, so herbs that contain these substances require a higher percentage of alcohol to make a proper extraction.

Tinctures may be made with either fresh or dried herbs. Most companies use dry herbs for many of their extracts because it is easier to work with dry plant matter than fresh. Fresh material must be processed immediately to ensure that the herbs will not spoil and that the extraction is of the highest quality. Some herbs simply process better when fresh; others process better dry. There are many opinions about which method is best, and the debate will probably continue as long as tinctures exist, but I believe that in most cases, fresh is best. Unfortunately, fresh material is not always available, or the dry material available is actually better than the available fresh material (a decision made at the discretion of the company producing the extract). Further, whether fresh or dry is best may vary according to the therapeutic application. For example, an extract of fresh ginger is more dispersing to the exterior, while an extract made from dried ginger is more appropriate for warming the interior.

Many commercially available tinctures provide a ratio of herb to liquid extract on their labels. This information is useful, but not well understood by many consumers or even many practitioners. A ratio of 1:5 or 1:3 represents the amount of herb to solvent in the product. In other words, for a 1:5 extract (the standard tincture ratio), "1" represents the amount of herb and "5" represents the amount of solvent or menstruum (a technical term describing the solvent or liquid that will dissolve the medicinal properties of the herb). This means for every 1 gram of herb, 5 milliliters of extract are produced. This may seem foolish. Why would anyone "water down" the herbs? Why not make tinctures in a ratio of 1:1, or even 5:1, for that matter? The reason tincture is generally made at a ratio of 1:5 is that it takes that much solvent to completely extract the constituents from the plant. Liquid extracts in a ratio of 1:1 or 5:1 are concentrated in the lab. These extracts are more potent and usually reserved for professional use, as they are very concentrated and the difference between a therapeutic and a potentially dangerous dosage is much smaller than it is with a standard tincture.

A few companies produce a number of other types of liquid extracts. A fluidextract is one in which the herb is represented in the extract at a 1:1 ratio. This means that every milliliter of extract represents 1 gram of herb. This type of extract should have a much stronger flavor than a tincture made from the same herb and should require a lower dosage to achieve the same therapeutic effect. These extracts, although more potent, are not generally found in the consumer-based retail market because of their strength and the potential that exists for a layperson to use them improperly. These extracts are also more labor intensive and therefore more expensive.

A pill or powder is generally the least desirable way to take herbs, partly because of the poor quality often available to the consumer. This is not to say that all pills are poor quality. However, many of the most commonly available herbal pills are made by grinding the herbs into a powder, then pressing them into a form using a binder, a process that leaves a lot to be desired. The potency of powdered herbs diminishes dramatically over a short time. There is also some question about the body's ability to absorb herbs in powdered form (rather than extracted; see below), as they require the digestive tract itself to extract the medicinal components. Since so many of our patients have digestive difficulties, this could present a real problem for some. Further, the amount of physical matter the patient actually ingests is generally quite small, leading to dosage issues because it can be difficult to ingest enough pills to get an appropriate dose of the medicine. This is not to meant to imply that pills and powders made this way are useless, only that there are better ways to take herbal medicine that are more effective and less wasteful.

Pills made from extracts are much more desirable. Many pills available on the market, including those little round black Chinese tea pills, are made this way. Solid extracts are made by first making a liquid extract and then evaporating the solvent, leaving behind only the principal part of the medicinal extracted by the liquid solvent. These extracts generally hold up better to the elements than powdered herbs, and their potency is also dramatically better. Extracts are more easily absorbed in the digestive tract. Some companies combine powdered herbs with extracted herbs in pills, which is a good way to keep the cost of the product reasonable, since pills made from extracted herbs are bound to be more expensive.

A large number of other herbal preparations are also available on the Western market, from salves and creams to cosmetics made with herbal extractions. There are a few general rules to heed when considering the vast number of products appearing on Western shelves. If the product contains herbal extracts along with a bunch of substances that appear to be single chemicals, buyer beware. Many products incorporate a few herbs so the manufacturer can claim the product is "natural" or "herbal." If the herbal extract is made with a plant from the rain forest, buy with the caveat that hundreds of acres of rain forest are being destroyed on a daily basis. Is the product you are buying contributing to this deforestation? If the product is made with a "special patented extraction process," beware. This is generally a marketing scheme; there are only so many ways to extract an herb. If the company claims you will have overnight therapeutic success or that the product cures the incurable, stay away. "Obviously!" you may say, but these schemes work on unsuspecting people every day (even professionals) with all kinds of products.

HERB QUALITY

Herb quality is a vitally important issue. In the Chinese herb market, it is often difficult to procure what most Western herbalists would call excellent quality herbs, even though there are a few excellent Chinese herb companies. This is due, in part, to the differences in quality preferences among practitioners, but also to shipping and handling of plants. Chinese herbs are grown halfway around the world and then shipped here by boat, which may greatly impact their quality. Western herbalists are trained to reject poor quality herb material, whereas until relatively recently, Chinese herbalists haven't had much choice. Fortunately, this situation is changing, but there is very little instruction in Chinese medicine schools concerning herb quality. There is also some question about what "good quality" means when it comes to Chinese herbs. Chinese medicine practitioners native to China often favor some herbs over others; unfortunately, this may have more to due with the company (family) with which the herbs originated than with the quality of the herbs themselves. Fortunately, the difficulty is being overcome through importation of high quality material from China and, on a small scale, via cultivation efforts here in the West.

Herbs are medicine and should be treated as such; therefore quality is of utmost importance. Whether they are intended for internal or external application, quality plays an important role in determing the difference between products that work well and products that don't. Bulk herbs sold in the health food stores and to practitioners in America today too often are not of the highest quality. There are several reasons for this. Most important is the manner in which the herbs are processed for sale. When an herb is gathered—either from the wild or the field—it should be dried as quickly as possible without overheating. Herbal material should be dried in as whole a form as possible, then cut into a size for easy storage. To ensure quality of roots and rhizomes, they must be sliced before drying so they dry rapidly. In the commercial Western herb market, most plants are processed using a method called "cut and sift." This means that the dried herbs are run through a hammer mill and cut to a size that will pass through a small sifter. This makes the herbs easier to package, but is problematic because a large amount of plant surface area is exposed to air. The exposure to air allows for greater oxidation, and the quality of an herb processed in this way will decline much faster than that of herbs left in larger pieces. This is a very important issue in the American market, one all practitioners should be aware of and concerned about.

The quality and therapeutic value of an herb greatly depends on when it was harvested, so it is important to try to determine whether the plant was harvested at the correct time or past its prime. It is difficult to answer such a question when the herb has been cut and sifted into small pieces. An herb that has been broken into larger pieces (leaving the leaf as whole as possible, for example) will retain its medicinal value longer. Thus, powdered herbs represent the least desirable way to purchase herbs. Powdered herb is very difficult to assess for quality and can be adulterated easily. For example, an expensive herb like goldenseal, which is oversold and quickly becoming endangered in the wild, might be cut with an inexpensive herb like turmeric. Companies will grind herbs for you as a service, but make sure they are grinding it for your order and not simply pulling off the shelf a product that may have been sitting around—already ground—for months.

Although uncommon, sometimes there are questions concerning the proper identification of plants sold in bulk. I personally have been in herb shops that were selling mislabeled plants, but fortunately, this is not a major problem.

There are a few main ways in which to check the quality of bulk herbs. Aside from the size of the cut, which should be as large as possible, take a look at the herb itself. Is it green? The aboveground portion of a plant such as peppermint should be green with a strong peppermint scent, not brown and musty. If the material in question is a root or rhizome, it should be free of dirt and not discolored. Flowers should retain their brilliant colors and come as whole as possible. The amount of moisture is also important. Herbs should not be overdried and crumbly, nor should they be moist, lending themselves to the development of mold.

Smell is also a clue, as the smell of a given herb could be its most distinctive characteristic. My teachers always encouraged us to smell the plants, because olfactory memory is excellent. Not all herbs have a strong smell, but the ones that do should retain a good portion of that original smell. Herbs that do not have an inherently strong odor often smell somewhat "earthy," but should never smell moldy, stale, or musty.

Finally, the most crucial test is taste. All herbs have flavor, and many have particularly distinctive flavors. When herbal material gets old, it changes in a way that speaks to your tongue.

CULTIVATED VS. WILDCRAFTED HERBS

Wildcrafted plants are those that are harvested from the wild. This type of plant material may also sometimes be called "wild-harvested," "wild," "custom-wildcrafted," or any variety of other names suggesting that the herbs were not cultivated. They grow in their natural habitat without supplemental water or fertilizer. Because the wildcrafter (the person who picks the herbs) often needs to travel to harvest the herbs, they are sometimes picked when they are not at their peak. However, this is not always the case and one should not assume it to be true; most often the medicinals are picked at the appropriate time. Cultivated herbs are those that are grown via various agricultural techniques. Many forms of agriculture may be employed to cultivate herbs; the primary ones include organic, biodynamic, and woodsgrown, as well as more conventional methods. These plants are grown in the field, can be given special attention, and can be harvested at just the right time.

What is the difference between cultivated and wildcrafted herbs in the clinic? Are wildcrafted herbs any better or more potent that cultivated herbs? What environmental impacts are caused by our use of wildcrafted herbs? What environmental hazards are posed by the commercial cultivation of herbs? All of these questions are important, and, in today's increasingly active herb market, all of them must be answered if these plants are to remain available to us. Some of the questions are particularly critical if we are concerned with ecology and the preservation of natural resources.

Unlike China, with its long, essentially unbroken history of herbal medicine, the West (particularly the United States) is only now coming to understand the agricultural aspects of herbal medicine. Since the late 1980s, significant momentum has been building to cultivate more herbs for the rapidly growing herb market. Many farms have been able to supply herbs that have been under great strain in the wild, including echinacea and others. This effort has helped to slow the decimation of wild herb populations. Other herbs, such as goldenseal, did not enjoy the same fate. The difficulty in cultivating this herb and the length of time it needs to grow before harvest hampered the development of farming practices for this herb, leading to a rather rapid decline of this species in its native habitat. Fortunately, due to the efforts of some very dedicated herbalists and farmers, goldenseal is being preserved and is now cultivated in commercial quantities.

In writing this book, I realize that I am bringing into the spotlight a group of wild herbs that has not been in demand among a large group of practitioners. With this in mind, I felt it necessary to include a discussion of the important topic of sustainability in this book. I cannot express this strongly enough: It is imperative that we, as herbalists, be aware of the plants and their status in their natural habitat. I realize that we cannot all be completely educated on the details of each plant we use. However, we should know the issues and know where we can get more information if we need it. United Plant Savers is an excellent organization dedicated to the preservation of native species in the United States and abroad. Contact them to request a list of plants that are in danger, and use this information to guide your purchase of Western herbs.

I am often asked if cultivated herbs are less potent than wildcrafted herbs. This is a difficult question to answer. I start by explaining that a very large percentage of Chinese herbs are cultivated, and they work. However, it is important to consider the way in which the herbs have been cultivated. If they are given an overly rich diet and an abundance of water, their potency will be decreased significantly. If they are treated in the way their natural habitat would treat them, I believe that their potency can be more than adequate. In all honesty, I view wildcrafted plants as better than cultivated plants in terms of potency and clinical value. However, the impact that harvesting the wild species has on wild plant populations is, in many cases, less than favorable. It is critical that we have a long-term vision and an understanding of how to produce herbal medicines in a sustainable manner. If we pick out the wild populations, we will have destroyed a natural resource, one that is very valuable and may never be replaced.

With all of these issues in mind, I believe it is critical that we herbalists rely on cultivated herbs and stay away from wildcrafted herbs as much as possible, unless we are sure they are being harvested using sustainable practices. This will encourage further development of farming, making available a larger selection of medicinals from this source and increasing the quantity of those already available.

HERBAL
MEDICINE MAKING

Herbal medicine making is the art of plant pharmacy. The word pharmacy means to prepare, preserve, and compound medicines. This is also the fundamental definition of the Chinese term *páo zhi,* which translates literally as "processing of medicinals." Western students of herbal medicine learn basic medicine-making techniques as part of their training, unlike most Chinese herbal medical students. In this chapter, you will find some basic instructions for preparing the medicines discussed in this book. Some of these preparations are simple and you will have no trouble making them, while others (such as percolation tinctures) are more difficult and require time and practice to produce good medicines. Since the cost of many commercial products is, in my opinion, completely outrageous, learning how to make some basic herbal preparations confers a cost advantage. Further, when you make your own medicines, you can be confident that you are giving your patients excellent remedies that are individualized to their needs.

Another benefit of creating your own medicines is that you can make preparations that are not available commercially, such as poultices, suppositories, and tinctures of less frequently used native plants, as well as honey mix-fried or wine-fried versions of Western herbs. I realize that many people do not have the time to make their own preparations, especially busy practitioners. Nonetheless, I feel it is important to know the basics of how the medicines are prepared and what they contain. Be patient, and good luck.

INFUSIONS AND DECOCTIONS

Infusions and decoctions are water-based herb extracts, often commonly called "teas." They differ in one essential way: Infusions are prepared by simply pouring water over a medicinal and allowing it to sit for a prescribed length of time, whereas decoctions are "cooked" in water for a given length of time. Infusions are most appropriate to use when plants are delicate or aromatic, while decoctions are important for plants (or parts of plants) that are sturdy and must be cooked to impart their medicinal qualities into the water.

Infusions

There are two main types of infusions, hot and cold. Hot infusions are made by pouring boiling water over dry or fresh herb and steeping. This method is used for lighter plant material, such as flower and leaf that is delicate and may contain essential oils that would evaporate in a decoction. To make a hot infusion, pour boiling water over a single herb or mixture of herbs in a cup, or teapot, or tea strainer. (The ratio of herb to water varies greatly; please refer to herb monographs for specific information.) Allow the vessel to stand, covered, for 3 to 30 minutes. The length of time is primarily determined by the plant, which has a lot to do with what you are trying to extract. Flower petals require a very short infusion time, while aromatic roots, such as aucklandia, will require a much longer steeping.

Cold infusions are used less frequently, but when applied properly, can be of equal therapeutic value. Cold infusions are useful for processing herbs containing constituents that may be sensitive to heat. For example, heat destroys the cyanogenic glycosides in wild cherry bark, so the bark is infused overnight in cold water. Apricot kernel contains the same compounds, which is why it is ground and added at the end of a decoction rather than simmered the entire time. According to Western preparation methods, this medicinal would be best prepared as a cold infusion, left to soak overnight, and then added to the prepared tea as needed. Herbs with a high starch or mucilage content are also better extracted with cold water.

A CLASSIC DIAPHORETIC INFUSION

Elder flowers	1 part
Peppermint	1 part
Yarrow	1 part
Boiling water	20 parts

Place the herb in a pot, pour boiling water over it, and allow to stand for 30 minutes. This infusion should be drunk warm by the cupful as frequently as desired. Instruct the patient to bundle up to encourage diaphoresis. This formula, a good example of a classic infusion, is useful for colds and influenza with symptoms such as sore throat and fever with little or no sweating. For chills, add 1 to 3 parts fresh ginger to the above formula.

A REFRESHING REFRIGERANT

A sun tea is an infusion made by putting herbs in a jar and placing it into the sun for several hours. This can be a fun and delicious way to enjoy the cooling properties of an herb on a hot summer day.

Fresh borage leaves	100 g
Fresh borage flowers	1 handful
Fresh lemon balm	75 g
Bitter orange	25 g
Rose hips	25 g
Tincture of cinnamon (optional)	to taste

Place all ingredients except tincture of cinnamon in 3 liters of fresh water in a glass container. Cover the container and leave it in the sun for 4 to 6 hours. Add the tincture of cinnamon at the very end, after you've strained the tea. Start slowly; the flavor can sneak up on you, and once it's in there, it's impossible to remove. Some people like to add a little honey to this recipe.

Decoctions

In Western herbalism, decoctions are generally reserved for tougher plant parts, such as roots and barks. This is not so in Chinese medicine, in which most herbs are decocted for long periods of time, with a few exceptions, notablyaucklandia and agastache. For Chinese herbalists, it is important to note that certain herbs that are often decocted, such as those mentioned above, should probably be infused or decocted for shorter periods of time. Herbs such as rose buds and albizia flowers should not be decocted at all lest their *qi* be scattered.

To make a decoction, place the herbs in a pot (ceramic, glass, or stainless steel) with water. A typical prescription is 75 to 150 g of herb to 900 to 1300 ml of water. Bring this to a boil, then reduce heat and allow to simmer for 20 to 50 minutes. Strain and discard the herb. This should leave two to four doses of about 1 cup (225 ml) each. Sometimes, herbs prescribed for decoction are boiled twice, the two decoctions are then combined, and the tea is taken over two or even three days. This technique is sometimes employed in Chinese herbal medicine when supplementing herbs are prescribed for long-term use. During acute disease, the dose of both herbs and decoction is often higher and the herbs are usually only boiled once.

TINCTURES, FLUIDEXTRACTS, AND LIQUID EXTRACTS

Tinctures, fluidextracts, and liquid extracts are all extracts that include alcohol, either as a solvent or preservative. Tinctures are the most commonly available of these preparations at health food stores and supermarkets. The professional preparations available to Chinese medicine practitioners are almost exclusively liquid extracts, *not* tinctures. Basic descriptions of each type of extract follow.

Tinctures

Tinctures are liquid extracts made by submerging raw herb in a solution of alcohol and water (in other words, a hydro-alcoholic solution). The "active" ingredients are absorbed into the menstruum (the water and alcohol) by either of two methods, maceration or percolation.

Maceration Tinctures

Maceration tinctures employ a technique of soaking or steeping herb material in a solvent. The solvents generally used are alcohol and water. When preparing tinctures, it is best to use pharmaceutical grade alcohol (95 percent). Some use vodka or other types of alcohol, but this can be problematic, and as a general rule of thumb, I don't recommend it. Remember, if you use cheap (read "poor-quality") alcohol, you will have poor-quality tinctures.

Maceration tinctures are made by grinding (dry) or chopping (fresh) herb and adding a specific solvent (menstruum). The general proportion of herb to solvent is 5 parts of menstruum for 1 part dry herb or 2 parts of menstruum for 1 part fresh herb. To make a tincture, combine herb and menstruum in a tightly closed jar, keep in a moderately warm place for two weeks, and (if dry herb was used) shake the jar on a daily basis. (Shaking is necessary only for dry plant preparations.) After this period, press out the liquid from the spent herb (or marc), filter it, decant it into a bottle for storage, and store it in a cool dry place. (Amber glass bottles are excellent for protecting tinctures from light damage.) *Always label your medicines!* The label should have some basic information such as the name of the plant, the ratio of solvent to medicinal, percentage of alcohol used, whether it is a fresh plant tincture or a dried plant tincture, and the date prepared.

As an example, here are instructions for making a dry-plant kava tincture. Grind 100 g dry kava *(Piper methysticum)* to a moderately coarse powder. Combine this powder with 500 ml of 70 percent alcohol (30 percent water) and shake thoroughly. Label the jar and put it on a shelf. Each day, give that bottle a good shake to thoroughly mix the contents. At the end of two weeks, strain off the liquid and filter it. You will have a 1:5 tincture of kava containing 70 percent alcohol. This may also be expressed as a 20 percent tincture using 70 percent ethanol and 30 percent water.

A fresh plant tincture is made in a similar manner, with a couple of exceptions. A fresh plant tincture does not need to be shaken as frequently, and fresh plant tinctures are usually ready to be strained after about ten days, a little earlier than those made with dry plant material. Although some commercial manufacturers grind the fresh herb material into a slurry before tincturing, it is necessary only to chop it into small pieces.

Percolation Tinctures

Percolation is a method of preparing tinctures that, although technically more difficult than maceration, is considered better because it totally exhausts the plant material of all available medicinal properties and tends to make a more concentrated preparation. The method requires a little more equipment, and weights and measures must be very accurate. In addition, the preparation technique can be somewhat finicky from herb to herb. However, many herbalists generally consider this method the best. Popularized in the early and mid-nineteenth century, percolation was and still is preferred by many companies for the quality of the finished product. Although the process takes some practice and special equipment, the results are worth the mistakes along the way. The quantities of herb and solvent to use, as well as other factors such as the degree of fineness of the powdered plant, will vary with the plant being extracted. While such specifics are beyond the scope of this book, there are some standard references for this information, such as *Remington's Practice of Pharmacy* (see bibliography).

Percolation is a multistep process. As an example, let's suppose we want to make a percolation using 1000 g dried herb; the amount of menstruum will vary according to the ratio of the finished product, and this will vary according to the needs of the specific plant being processed. In this case, a 1:3 finished product will require just over 3000 ml of menstruum. First, the herb must be powdered to the proper degree of fineness or coarseness, which, again, will vary from plant to plant.

Then, some of the prescribed menstruum is poured over the herb, but only enough to completely moisten (not soak) the herb. This mixture must then sit and macerate for 6 hours in a tightly covered container. At the end of this time, the mixture is transferred into a percolator—essentially, a cone-shaped funnel with a valve at the bottom to regulate the flow. This equipment is available at many chemical supply houses and from some herb supply websites. A coffee filter is placed at the bottom to keep the powdered herb from draining from the bottom spout. This transfer is likely the most critical step in the entire process. The herb must be packed into the percolator, loosely enough that the menstruum to be added can flow slowly and evenly through the percolator, but tightly enough that the menstruum does not run through too quickly. This takes practice, and the process will differ with different plants. If one is to become expert at this method, he or she must be willing to experiment and make mistakes.

Once the herb is packed into the percolator, a piece of coffee filter is placed on the top of it. More of the menstruum is then poured over the herb, until it begins to drip from the bottom of the funnel. The valve is then closed and the mixture allowed to macerate again for 24 hours. At the end of this period, the valve is opened, allowing a slow drip to occur. Now more menstruum is poured over the herb, until the prescribed amount is achieved. When the prescribed amount of menstruum has dripped from the cone, the product is bottled in an amber bottle, labeled, and stored in a cool, dry place for future use. Percolations can be made in the standard tincture ratio of 1:5, but often they are made in ratios of 1:2.5 to 1:4. This method can also be used to produce 1:1 fluidextracts (discussed below). These preparations are more concentrated, allowing for smaller doses, but have the same therapeutic value.

Percolation is a more complex method for making tinctures than maceration, and the process takes time and patience to master. Although percolation is the official method of preparing a tincture, as specified by the United States Pharmacopoeia and other standard references, maceration works equally or nearly as well.

If you are interested in medicine making, however, you will find this method fun and preferable in many cases. Be aware that percolation is not appropriate for plants that are very resinous.

Fluidextracts

The percolation method just described can also be used to create fluidextracts. A fluidextract is a 1:1 extract, meaning that every 1 milliliter of extract represents 1 gram of raw herb. Percolation affords a way to completely exhaust the raw plant material to make a very concentrated medicine. This method of making fluidextracts was probably most influenced by John Uri Lloyd of Lloyd Brothers Pharmacy in the latter part of the nineteenth century.

The process begins the same way as a normal percolation. The 1000 g of herb is moistened and placed in the percolator. After the herb has macerated, the valve is opened, letting a slow drip occur, and more menstruum is poured over the plant material, until the prescribed amount (875 ml) has dripped out. This amount is reserved while the process continues. The next 100 ml is collected and reserved. This process—collection and reservation of 100 ml of menstruum—is continued until the menstruum exits the percolator colorless and tasteless. The final collected portion (generally less than 100 ml) is reduced over *low* heat in a double boiler until a thick syrupy consistency is achieved, or until it is reduced to the point of being nearly gone. To this reduced volume add the last reserved portion of menstruum (100 ml) and mix thoroughly. Continue this process, reducing if necessary, so that you end up with 125 ml to add to the first reserved portion of 875 ml. Filter and bottle the final product. *Always label your medicines!*

Liquid Extracts

Liquid extracts may be made by several means, some of which require more that one process to make a single product. For example, a liquid extract may be composed of both a decoction and a maceration. The final product is one that is generally highly concentrated but has a low alcohol content. The majority of

American-made Chinese herbal products are liquid extracts. These products employ a significant amount of high-tech equipment to produce a very concentrated product. However, because of the use of alcohol and pressure during production, these extracts may not always accurately represent the original formula.

A relatively simple way to make this type of liquid extract involves a method sometimes called double extraction, which is appropriate for many different herbs. The advantage of these products is that the process allows extracts made with water and heat to be added to a tincture, thus allowing for a greater spectrum of chemical constituents to be extracted. One simple method of double extraction utilizes both a tincturing method and a decoction (water extraction) to make an extract that is appropriate for producing liquid extracts of certain medicinals without high-tech equipment.

To make a double extraction, the herb is first extracted using either the maceration or percolation method. Start the double extraction with a high alcohol concentration, adding about 10 percent vegetable glycerin to the mixture (the glycerine is added before maceration and sometimes after percolation). Glycerin is used because a water extract will be added at the end of the process, and the final product must have an alcohol content above or around 20 percent for preservation. The glycerin will also help keep solutes in a stable suspension when the alcohol and water extracts are combined; the combination of alcohol and water extracts tends to cause precipitation of solids due to the nature of the relationship between alcohol and water.

Next, the marc is decocted, making a very concentrated decoction. The two extracts—the tincture and the decoction—are then mixed together and strained. The final extract will have an alcohol content between 20 percent and 30 percent. This is especially good for the Chinese herbs, partly because they are traditionally prescribed as decoctions, but also because the alcohol helps preserve them for storage. It is important to remember that when we make these types of extracts we are using a solvent—alcohol—that extracts properties from plants that traditionally were not extracted.

Thus, the extract may not be exactly the same as the traditional water-based preparation, potentially changing the way the plant works as medicine.

POULTICES

Poultices are topical preparations intended for external application to cuts, scrapes, rashes, and other skin irritations or inflammations. They may be made with fresh or dried herbs. The most commonly used herbs are those with healing and anti-inflammatory properties, such as comfrey or plantain. However, many other herbs may also be incorporated into poultices. These include herbs with strong heat-clearing properties, like goldenseal and California figwort, or strong dispersing properties, such as prickly ash and cayenne.

Combining herbs for an external poultice formula is much like creating a formula for an internal prescription. The main difference between an external and internal formula is that most external preparations are not aimed at producing a systemic effect. Rather, the prescription is directed specifically at the local area to which the poultice is applied. Most poultices are directed at the surface and just below, while others are intended to penetrate more deeply—for instance, into deep muscle tissue, tendons and ligaments, or even bone. Poultices formulated for drawing actions or other internal effects are sometimes called plasters. The mustard plaster—a classic preparation of mustard seeds applied to the chest to loosen congested phlegm—is probably the best known example of this type of preparation.

When preparing a poultice with fresh herb, the herb should first be macerated. Traditionally, healers chewed the plant material, formed it into an appropriate shape, and applied it to the area needing treatment. This obviously is not appropriate for clinical practice, but is handy to know if you're in the woods and your young child falls and scrapes his or her knee or elbow. Alternately, chop the herb finely and then macerate it in a mortar and pestle or a similar instrument. Sometimes the addition of a little water will help to create the pastelike consistency you need. Once you've

achieved the right consistency, apply the poultice to the wound and lightly cover with a bandage. The bandage is meant merely to keep the poultice in place and should allow for proper aeration of the wound.

If you're using dry herb material, first grind or crush the herb into a powder. To this powder add small amounts of water until you obtain the proper pasty consistency. (This process will differ with different herbs and combinations of herbs, so you may have to experiment to get the consistency you want.) Instead of water, you may also add tincture to supplement the formulation.

Here's a quick poultice formula that utilizes a tincture to moisten the plant material. Grind 5 g comfrey root to a powder. To this powder add sufficient quantities of yarrow tincture to make a thick paste. This paste can now be applied as a poultice to the affected area. Remember to change the poultice frequently (at least twice a day) to ensure proper healing.

SUPPOSITORIES

A suppository, sometimes called a bolus, is an excellent method of introducing herbs to the anus, rectum, or vagina. There are many pathogenic influences for which a bolus is useful, including hemorrhoids and damp-heat with or without toxin.

This simple preparation can be made with very low-tech equipment. The bolus itself is made of cocoa butter and ground herbs or solid extracts. Liquid extracts are not appropriate for inclusion in suppositories, because the end product must be firm enough for insertion into the anus or vagina. The amount of cocoa butter will vary greatly, but in general I find about 20 to 25 percent cocoa butter in the final preparation to be sufficient.

To make a suppository or bolus, first create molds out of tin foil by wrapping foil around a sterile piece of glass or stainless steel about the size of a pen. Carefully slide the mold off, pinching it off at one end. Try to preserve the integrity of the walls of the mold, which will make the bolus easier to insert later on. (Premade molds are also available from pharmacy supply houses.)

Next, grind herbs or solid extract to a fine consistency. This consistency is important, as it will allow for the smooth insertion of the bolus. Then *gently* heat the cocoa butter until it becomes liquid. Using a double boiler will help ensure that you don't burn the cocoa butter. Slowly add the herb mixture to the cocoa butter until the mixture is about the consistency of a syrup. (When in doubt, use a little more cocoa butter than herb.) Pour the mixture into the prepared molds and allow it to cool and harden. I prefer to store suppositories in the refrigerator to reduce the chance of spoilage or melting in hot weather.

To use the suppository or bolus, simply cut off about 3 cm (approximately 1 inch), remove the tin foil and insert the cocoa butter–herb mixture. The treatment should be applied at night since there is a chance of leakage as the cocoa butter melts. Advise the patient about this possibility and suggest he or she take proper precautions. For example, a woman may want to wear a menstrual pad when using a bolus in the vagina; a rubber baby mat under the sheet or an adult diaper may also be used. Such precautions are rarely necessary, however, as only a small amount of material will leak out.

INFUSED OILS

An infused oil is an oil in which herb has been macerated in order to extract desired constituents. Thus, an infused oil is not very different from a tea or tincture, except that it uses oil as a solvent instead of water or alcohol. Infused oils can be made in two ways. You may rely either on the heat of the sun to extract the herb, or you can infuse the oil using artificial heat, such as in a Crock-Pot or double boiler. Infused oils can be made from fresh or dry plants. Fresh plants generally contain more of their essential constituents, which are likely to be present in higher concentrations. However, if you are making an infused oil from fresh plant material, it is best to let the herb dry for a day or so. This will allow for some water to evaporate from the plant, reducing the chance of spoilage.

To infuse oil with an herb, first place the herb in the jar. It is generally best to fill the jar about ¾ full, leaving enough room to completely cover the plant with oil to prevent spoilage. If you are using fresh herb, chop it up well and be sure to use sufficient pressure to stuff it into the jar. Next, add enough oil (olive and sweet almond are my preferences) to cover the herb by about 2 to 3 cm (approximately 1 inch). If you are using dried plant material, let it stand for one to two hours after covering it with oil. The dry herb will absorb the oil, and you will need to add more oil to again cover the plant material by 2 to 3 cm. Stir the mixture well with a clean spoon, being sure to work out all of the air bubbles. This is very important with either fresh or dry plant material, but especially with fresh, because any air that remains will contribute to spoilage of the oil infusion.

After you have removed all the air from either the dried or fresh plant material, and (in the the case of dry herb) it has absorbed all the oil it will hold, add enough oil to cover by 2 to 3 cm. Cover the jar with a brown paper bag and put it in the sun for about two weeks. If you have used fresh herb, open the jar daily when it is at its hottest and sponge out any moisture that has condensed on the lid of the jar. This will rid your preparation of unwanted water and further reduce the chance ·of it spoiling.

At the end of two weeks, strain the oil, decant it into an amber bottle, label it with the name of the herb, the type of oil used, and the date pressed, and store it under refrigeration. For a fresh plant infusion, strain out as much oil as possible without allowing water to get into the strained portion. Watch carefully while decanting the oil from the water to be sure to not pour any water into the decanted oil. The remainder of the herb can be squeezed and allowed to drip for an hour or two before decanting. Keep this last bit of oil separate from the rest and use it first, as it will have a tendency to contain small amounts of water that inevitably remain after the decanting process and thus will spoil more easily.

When employing artificial heat, use the same basic method, but note that the amount of time the herb will need to steep in the oil will be only 24 to 48 hours, a significantly shorter period. Be careful not to overheat the oil, as this will damage both the oil and the herb and cause it to spoil more easily. A temperature between 37 and 41 degrees C (100 to 105 degrees F) is best. Some herbs may benefit from an additional solvent to assist in the infusion process. This solvent is generally alcohol, which must be decanted off at the end, as already described. Michael Moore, one of our great contemporary herbalists, includes an excellent discussion of this preparation technique in his *Medicinal Plants of the Pacific West.*

> Grind up 1 part (by weight of herb), place it in a container with a top, moisten it thoroughly with ½ to ¾ part (by volume) of pure ethanol or 90 percent rubbing alcohol, and let it set covered for at least two hours. Place it in a blender, cover it with 7 parts (by volume) of vegetable oil (preferably olive), and blend the hell out of it. Blend it until the side of the top is warm, turn it off, and pour it through a cloth inside a strainer placed over a bowl. Squeeze out all the oil and toss the remnants.[1]

SALVES

A salve is a semisolid preparation for external application, made with beeswax, infused oils, and various other ingredients as desired, such as cocoa butter or essential oils. Lip balm is a specific type of salve, but is a good example with which everyone is familiar. Making a salve is quite easy if the infused oils are already prepared. Simply warm the oils (gently, to protect them) to a point at which they will melt the beeswax, adding about 40 g of beeswax to every 200 ml of oil. Test the hardness of the salve by taking a small spoonful out and letting it cool. If you find the mixture is not hard enough when it has cooled completely, simply add small amounts of beeswax until you achieve the proper hardness. It is better to check the hardness earlier than later, as adding more oil to the salve to soften it up is undesirable. If you don't have prepared infused oils on hand, make the oils using the artificial

heat method described earlier. After straining the oil, simply add the necessary amount of wax and pour it into jars. Allow the salve to cool, then cover and label. Salves are quite durable and can last for several years if stored in a cool, dark location.

POWDERED EXTRACTS

Sometimes called solid extracts, granulated extracts, or concentrated extracts, powdered preparations have been used in Western herbal medicine for at least one hundred and fifty years. However, these preparations are not commonly found in the Western herbalist's clinic, unless he or she is prescribing modern phytomedicines in pill form. Essentially, powdered extracts are dehydrated liquid extracts, which can be made with water, alcohol, or any other solvent. However, the use of some types of solvents, such as hexane, may be inappropriate because they may leave behind residues during the dehydration process. The extracts we get from China or Taiwan are most, if not all, dehydrated decoctions.

In a nutshell, the process for manufacturing these extracts involves brewing a decoction and then removing the water by various dehydration techniques. What is left behind is the solid portion of the decoction, or simply the components of the herb that were soluble in water. This solid portion is then combined with a specific amount of starch in order to bring it to the desired ratio, which is 5:1 in most cases. Manufacturers maintain this ratio for all medicinals so that when practitioners use the preparations in formula, they will have a consistent product with which to work. Such a preparation represents a decoction quite well, and when combined with warm water, it nearly exactly represents a decoction.

Making powdered extracts without the use of some expensive equipment is difficult and time consuming. One major problem is that any herb containing essential oils must be processed in a closed system to prevent the evaporation of these volatile components. Thus the decoction must be made in such a way that the evaporating essential oils can be captured and reintroduced to the final product; otherwise the final product will be inferior.

Very few extracts of this type are produced in the West today. Powdered extracts are made of some of the best-selling herbs, such as black cohosh and feverfew, but they can be purchased only in large quantities. This represents a large gap in the medicinal herb industry in the West, but this is slowly changing.

MIX-FRYING WITH SOLID AND LIQUID ADJUVANTS

Chinese medicine has a long history of preparing medicinals with the addition of substances such as honey (as in honey mix-fried licorice), vinegar (as in vinegar mix-fried cyperus), wine (as in wine mix-fried *dāng guī*), and wheat germ (as in wheat-germ mix-fried atractylodes), to name only a few. Many other such preparations are also used, including steamed rehmannia and steamed ginseng. However, I will not cover these latter products here, as their preparation requires some specialized knowledge and they are generally readily available. On the other hand, although some of the mix-fried products mentioned earlier are also generally available, a plethora of medicinals that might benefit from such treatment are not available from purveyors. These can be processed relatively easily and will add significant clinical effectiveness to formulas. I have taken to some of these methods, partly because of my culinary background, but also because I believe they are important in the Chinese tradition and give us the opportunity to work a little more of our *qi* into the formulas. For more information on making these preparations, I recommend the book *Pao Zhi: An Introduction to the Use of Processed Chinese Medicinals* (see bibliography). Note here that these processing methods are not unique to Chinese medicine. I found several references to similar preparations in older Western materia medicas, such as *Culpeper's Complete Herbal and English Physician*.

Honey Mix-Fried Medicinals

Add a small amount of honey to a wok and heat on medium-high heat until the honey begins to boil. Slowly add the medicinal to be processed until the herb is coated evenly with the honey. Generally, a ratio of 25 to 40 parts of honey to 100 parts of herb will work well. Mix the material in the wok until is gains a golden-brown color and is no longer sticky to the touch. (Note: This material will be extremely hot, so do not stick your finger directly into the wok or try to pick a piece of the herb out without the assistance of tongs.) Remove the material to a clean surface to dry. The honey must get quite hot in order for this to work, because you essentially are making candy with the sugars in the honey. If the honey isn't hot enough, it will be very sticky and hard to deal with in a jar. If is made correctly, it will cool to a hard, somewhat crunchy consistency. Be careful not to burn the honey; this will turn the product black and significantly lower its quality.

Mix-frying with Wine or Vinegar

Although the finished product may be different, the process for mix-frying with wine or vinegar is almost the same as that used for mix-frying with honey. The difference is that when processing with vinegar, you should use a ratio of 15:100 vinegar to herb, and with wine, 40:100 or 50:100 wine to herb. Soak the medicinal in the liquid until it is completely absorbed. You will probably have to shake the mixture to ensure an even distribution of the liquid in the medicinal. Put the plant material into the wok and heat on medium-high heat until it is dry, being careful not to burn the herb. If some of the material seems to be browning faster than the rest, which may happen if the liquid was not evenly distributed in the dry plant material, try to remove it with tongs. Then add all the material back into the hot wok at the end to ensure that all the material is completely dried. Moist product will tend to spoil once it is put into a jar.

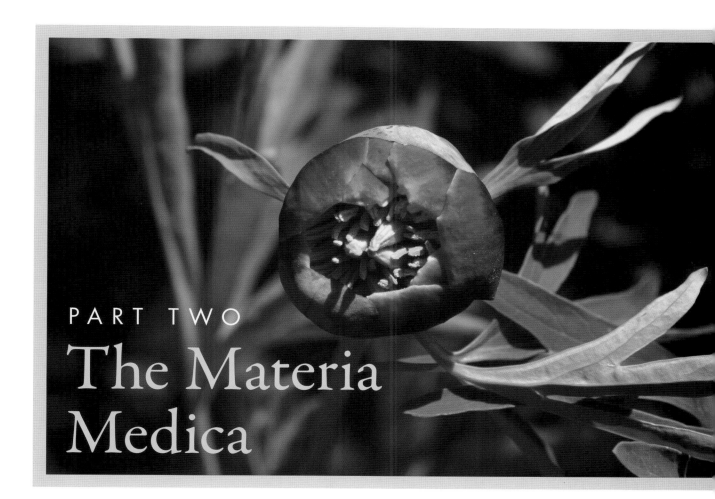

PART TWO

The Materia Medica

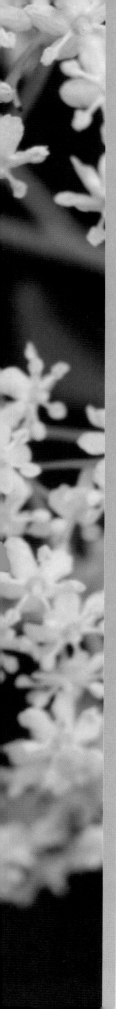

HERBS THAT RESOLVE THE EXTERIOR

Herbs that resolve the exterior are used mainly to halt the progression of an external pathogen through the surface (the skin and muscles) and relieve the symptoms that occur due to the response of the *wèi qì* to that pathogen (for example, fever and chills). There are several ways to accomplish this, including resolving the exterior with coolness and acridity, resolving the exterior with warmth and acridity, resolving the flesh, outthrusting papules, and coursing the exterior, as well as several combinations of supplementation and exterior-resolving techniques.

The primary way to resolve the exterior is through diaphoresis (causing sweating), which includes resolving with cool/acridity and warmth/acridity, as well as resolving the flesh. This method of treatment may also be a part of supplementation and exterior-resolving combination approaches. This category includes herbs with a primary function of inducing sweating; some that fit this description are yarrow, elder flowers, California spikenard, and wild ginger.

Although diaphoresis is the main method of resolving the exterior, sweating need not always be necessary to resolve the pathogen. The method of outthrusting papules *(tòu zhěn)* encourages rashes and measles to come to completion. Another method of resolving the exterior without evoking sweating is called coursing the exterior *(shū biǎo)*. In this method of treatment, causing diaphoresis is not necessary, so although the medicinals may or may not cause sweating, sweating is not requisite for the resolution of the exterior. Herbs that fit in this category are American ephedra and thyme. Another herb with this function listed in the text is echinacea.

There are three combination methods for supplementing and resolving the exterior: enriching *yīn* and resolving the exterior, boosting *qì* and resolving the exterior, and assisting *yáng* and resolving the exterior.

These therapeutic methods use both supplementing medicinals and medicinals that resolve the exterior. Some herbs may be used to treat both branches. Among herbs discussed in this text, both California spikenard and elderberry may be used in this way.

Cool Acrid Medicinals that Resolve the Exterior

The primary action of herbs in this category is to resolve exterior heat patterns. Symptoms include sore throat; heat effusion; thirst; slight aversion to cold; possibly a red tongue with dry, thin, white fur; and a floating, rapid pulse. Within this category you will find herbs that have a strong diaphoretic action, such as yarrow *(Achillea millefolium),* and others that have a weaker diaphoretic action, such as thyme *(Thymus officinalis).* Both of these herbs are excellent at clearing heat. Garden sage *(Salvia officinalis),* while not as strong at clearing heat, is excellent for complications due to damp pathogens. While it is diaphoretic when taken hot, it can stop sweating when taken cool. Like yarrow, elder flower *(Sambucus* spp.) has strong actions to induce sweating and clear heat. It can be used when wind and heat invade the lung, both during initial stages and if the pathogen gets trapped (lodged) and causes wind-heat sores.

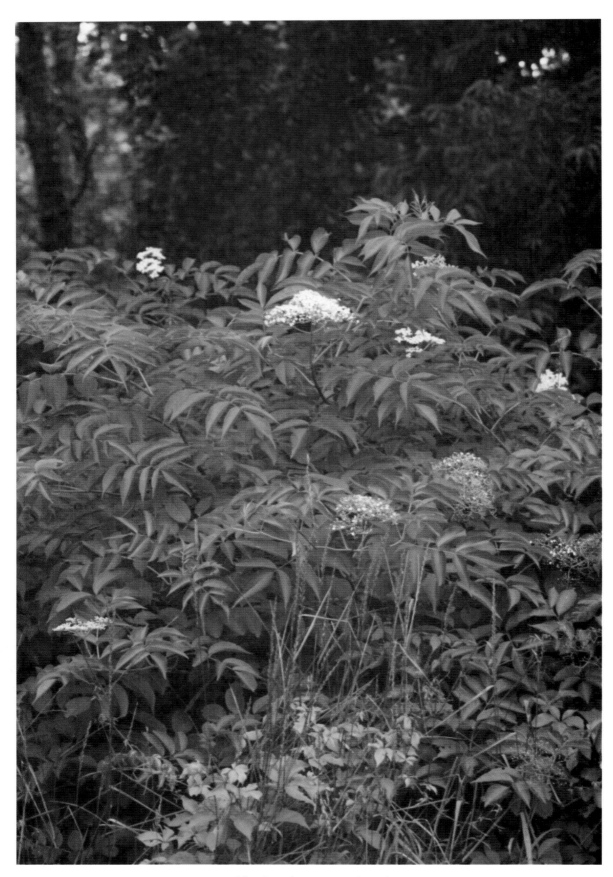

Elder *(Sambucus canadensis)*

Elder

Sambucus nigra, S. mexicana,
S. canadensis

Caprifoliaceae

Sambuci flos et fructus

Also called blue or black elderberry

Flavor and *Qi*: acrid, bitter, cool
Channels Entered: lung, bladder, liver
Actions: flowers and berries are alterative, antibacterial, anti-inflammatory, antiviral, diaphoretic

Functions and Indications

- ***Disperses wind-heat.*** Elder flower is used for the treatment of fever, cough, and a sore, red, swollen throat. These actions apply to elder flowers, and, to a lesser extent, the berries. Elder flower is a premier diaphoretic and is among my favorites for the initial stages of wind-heat. For this purpose, combine equal parts elder flower with yarrow and peppermint and make a strong infusion. Drink two cups before a hot bath and another right after, then curl up in a warm bed and sweat. You will undoubtedly feel better in the morning.

- ***Clears heat, relieves toxicity, dries dampness, and vents rashes.*** Elder flower is applied in the treatment of rashes that are edematous and red (such as erysipelas). For this purpose, the concentrated juice of the berries and/or the flowers may be used. Elder's acrid nature works to dry dampness and vent rashes; the bitter nature effectively clears heat and relieves toxicity. This medicinal can also be useful for liver heat that causes the liver *yáng* to upbear with symptoms of sore throat, red eyes, lung abscess, and sores on the upper torso and head.

CAUTIONS

Use elder with caution in weak, cold, *qi*-vacuous patients.

Dosage and Preparation

Flowers, 1–6 g in infusion or light decoction; berries, 3–30 g in decoction; either flowers or berries, 2–4 ml tincture. Tincture should be made fresh.

Gather flowers in mid-to-late summer when they are completely open. Take care when drying them so they don't turn brown. Good-quality dried flowers should be aromatic, have a light cream color, and contain few stems.

To make syrup, simmer the berries, press out the juice, and add sugar. This syrup has come into much favor in recent years since a study published in 1995 showed that the berries have antiviral activity against influenza. The syrup makes an excellent addition to a cough syrup, adding both flavor and medicinal value. Elderberries also have traditionally been made into wines and cordials.

Pollen collected from elder flowers has long been included in cosmetic preparations. Elder flower pollen is smooth and silky on the skin and adds a particularly soothing quality to skin preparations, including lotions. To collect pollen, gather flowers, lay them on screens to dry, and catch the pollen that falls through.

Major Combinations

- Combine with echinacea, sarsaparilla, sassafras, and cleavers for damp-heat rashes.

- Combine with mullein and red clover for wind-heat cough.

- Combine with Mulberry Leaf and Chrysanthemum decoction *(sāng jú yǐn)* for initial stages of wind-heat with strong heat effusion, sore throat, and cough.

- See entry for yarrow for combination to use in external attack of wind-heat.

Commentary

Hippocrates was the first to mention this plant in his writings, recommending it in the fifth century BCE as a laxative, diuretic, and gynecological remedy. Other early physicians, including Dioscorides, Pliny, and Lonicerus, also wrote about it.

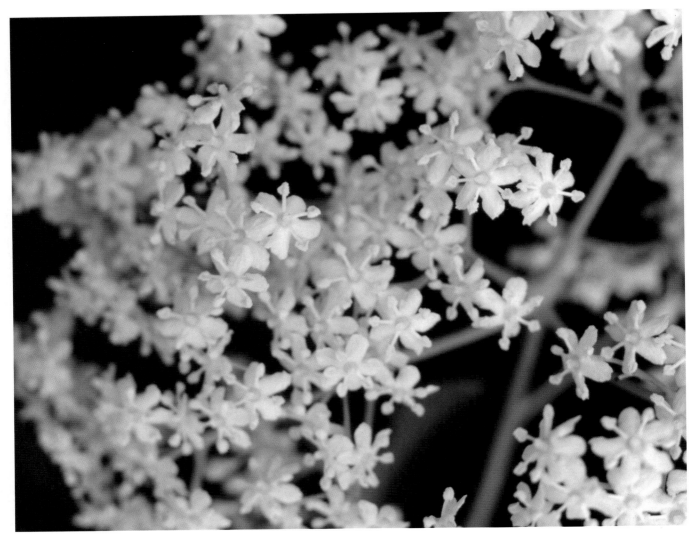

Elder flowers *(S. mexicana)*

The ancient Druids and pagans in Europe thought the elder was a mystical tree. There are said to be fairies that protect the elder, so it is important to give this plant particular respect when approaching it in the wild. Elderberries have actions similar to those of the flower, but they were traditionally used more often as a food. People have made delicious wine and pies from them for millennia. Dipped in batter and fried, the flowers also make a surprisingly good fritter.

Although significant research on elderberry has been undertaken over the last decade, I rarely use the berries, sticking instead to the more traditional use of the flowers. Elder is related to honeysuckle and has similar actions. Both plants belong to the Caprifolia-ceae family, which also includes some other important medicinal plants, such as cramp bark and black haw. Compared with honeysuckle, elder flower has a stronger action in resolving the exterior and transforming damp, while honeysuckle has a stronger action in clearing heat and resolving toxicity. *The Divine Husbandman's Materia Medica Classic [Shén Nóng Běn Cǎo]* mentions the flower of another species, *Sambucus japonica (lu ying)*. (Note: This species may not be correct. It is the species listed in the translated version of this book, but no other information can be found about it.) Shen Nong ascribes bitter and cold to the nature of this herb and says it mainly treats various impediments of the bones, hypertonicity and aching pain of the limbs, cold pain in the knees, impotence, shortness of breath, and swollen feet.[1]

Elder bark unblocks the bowels and resolves constipation due to accumulation and stagnation of damp-heat in the stomach and intestines.

Elderberry was official in *The United States Pharmacopoeia* from 1820–1831 and elder flower from 1831–1905. Elder flower was also listed in *The National Formulary (U.S.)* from 1916–1947.

Translation of Source Material

The Chinese use the twigs of one species of elder, *Sambucus williamsii (jiē gǔ mù)*. It is sweet, bitter, and neutral and dispels wind, disinhibits damp, quickens blood, and allays pain. It is used to treat wind-dampness sinew and bone pain, lumbar pain, water swelling, wind-itch, and other related ailments.

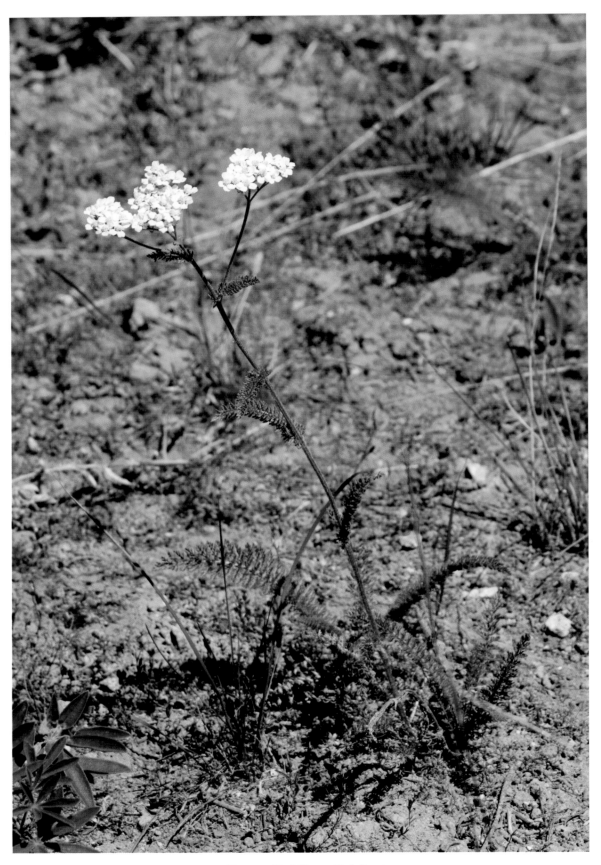

Yarrow (*Achillea millefolium*)

Yarrow

Achillea millefolium

Asteraceae

Achilleae Millefolii folium et flos

Other common names include nosebleed

Flavor and *Qi*: bitter, acrid, slightly cold
Channels Entered: lung, bladder, liver
Actions: anti-inflammatory, antipyretic, diaphoretic, diuretic, hemostatic, hypotensive, mild antispasmodic

Functions and Indications

- ***Resolves the exterior, courses wind, and discharges heat.*** Yarrow is used for the treatment of symptoms such as fever, headache, cough, and sore throat. It is also used to clear heat, scatter wind, and outthrust papules. For papules, an external application of the crushed fresh herb is excellent. If fresh herb is not available, mix dried herb with water to make a plaster. Yarrow's acrid and cooling nature is excellent for resolving the exterior in *tài-yīn* wind-heat patterns. It strongly pushes wind and heat from the fleshy exterior and resolves wind papules. When wind-heat settles into the defense and *qì* aspect, causing binding phlegm in the lungs, yarrow is an excellent choice to clear and dispel heat from the upper burner. Yarrow can also be used for other patterns in which there is phlegm-heat in the lungs, with thick yellow or green sputum, cough, thirst, and fever.

- ***Cools blood and stops bleeding.*** Yarrow is helpful for bleeding in the digestive tract, respiratory tract, or excessive menstrual bleeding due to reckless movement of hot blood. Yarrow's bitter and cooling nature clears heat and effectively stops bleeding. In addition, since bleeding is a form of blood stasis, yarrow's acrid nature helps quicken the blood and therefore stop bleeding. Use fresh plant tincture in small, frequent doses for acute epistaxis. For open wounds, apply dried and powdered leaves to stop the bleeding, relieve heat, and resolve toxins. The powder may be sprinkled on or packed in, depending on the size of the wound. Yarrow is also used for deep-seated macular eruptions associated with blood-heat.

- ***Drains fire from depression and courses liver* qì.** Yarrow is employed to treat such symptoms as dysmenorrhea, hypertension, irritability, headache, and red eyes. Yarrow's bitter and acrid nature effectively drains and courses the liver to help relieve depression, which in itself will undermine the course of fire from depression.

- ***Dispels wind-damp-heat and relaxes the sinews.*** Used to treat hot, painful obstruction of the channels, yarrow is widely applied in rheumatic arthritis and is very effective in combination with other herbs. Its primary function here is to disperse wind and clear heat, helping to reduce stress to the sinews caused by these pathogens. This action indirectly relaxes the sinews in cases of hot, painful obstruction.

- ***Promotes urination and drains heat.*** Yarrow is useful in the treatment of painful and difficult urination, with or without blood in the urine. Yarrow works best as a diuretic when taken as a cold preparation. In the form of a cold infusion, yarrow has a stronger bitter and cooling nature and therefore is more draining. This action is pronounced when yarrow is used to promote urination.

- ***Clears heat and resolves damp.*** Yarrow is applied externally for the treatment of damp-heat rashes and lesions. For this purpose, yarrow is best prepared as a salve or paste. (See the caution below about external use.)

CAUTIONS

This herb is not for use in those with interior cold and should be used cautiously with *qi* vacuity. Do not use during pregnancy. According to some sources, yarrow is contraindicated for use by those with allergies to Asteraceae family plants. It is important to note that people rarely express an allergic response when using yarrow externally.

Yarrow contains the constituent thujone (a chemical known to cause cancer). U.S. regulations require that thujone be removed from any commercial food or beverage containing yarrow, although only trace amounts are present in the plant.

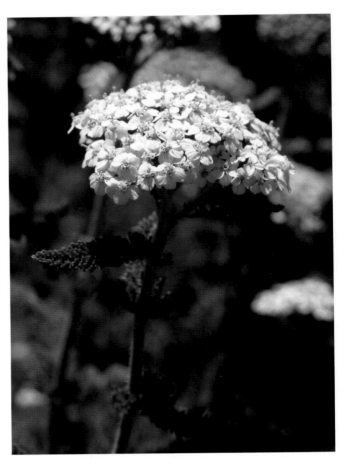

Close-up of yarrow flowers *(A. millefolium)*

Dosage and Preparation

Use 3–9 g in light decoction or infusion; 1–5 ml tincture.

Gather yarrow when the plant is in full bloom, from early summer to midsummer. Bundle and dry it, or make it into a fresh tincture or oil. Good-quality dried herb should be aromatic and contain more flowers than leaves and no large stems. The flowers should be white, not brown, and the foliage should be a bright green.

Yarrow is strongly acrid and bitter and thus has a dispersing and downbearing action. These actions can be modified by method of preparation. The hot infusion is strongly dispersing, while the decoction or cold preparation is relatively more bitter and less acrid and has a pronounced downbearing energy. The fresh tincture has the widest range of actions.

Major Combinations

- Combine as a strong infusion with elder flower and peppermint for external attack of wind-heat with fever, insufficient sweating, sore throat, and rapid floating pulse. Add osha for more severe sore throat, body aches, and headache. Add yerba mansa and encelia for more severe body aches and headaches due to damp evil.

- Combine with Honeysuckle and Forsythia Powder (*yín qiáo sàn*) to strengthen its action. The main action of this formula is to resolve the exterior with acrid and cooling medicinals, diffuse the lungs, and discharge heat. Yarrow acts harmoniously with this formula to strengthen its action.

- Combine with usnea, echinacea, and dandelion leaf for damp-heat in the bladder with predominate heat and symptoms of burning and painful urination, with or without bleeding.

- Combine with fresh tincture of shepherd's purse for heat in the lower burner with bleeding in the urine or stool or excessive menstrual bleeding. Add uva-ursi for more severe pain related to strangury conditions.

- Combine with Chinese skullcap and pleurisy root for phlegm-heat in the lung.

- Combine with yerba mansa and goldenseal or Oregon grape root for external application to damp-heat lesions.

Commentary

Yarrow is often called a warm, stimulating botanical. However, its indications actually contradict this designation. A medicinal that is bitter and acrid can be somewhat stimulating without being warming. Acridity, if sufficient in any plant, can be stimulating, as acridity has a dissipating and moving action. Even a bitter flavor can be stimulating by having a strong draining action. Because it is both acrid and bitter, yarrow is quite stimulating without warming the system; in fact, it cools the system. Dissipating medicinals are *yáng*. However, upon close examination, it is clear that the overall picture of yarrow is cooling due to its overwhelming bitterness and its ability to clear heat and even drain fire.

The genus name, *Achillea*, is derived from Achilleus, the name of the famous hero of the Trojan Wars who gained fame by healing soldiers with herbs. This was the first wild medicinal herb to which I was introduced, and it holds a very special place in my heart. It grows in both low-elevation valleys and high-elevation meadows. There are many cultivated varieties, but the white-flowered yarrow of the wild meadows is the finest medicine. It is a very common plant and is easy to find as well as cultivate in your garden.

This circumboreal plant has been used since antiquity by cultures around the world. The famous botanist Linnaeus says that yarrow was used in Sweden to brew beer, which was said to be more intoxicating than beer brewed with hops. I have tried beer brewed with yarrow and found it difficult to drink due to its flavor; I did not notice any specific intoxicating effect I could attribute to the yarrow.

Yarrow, like chamomile, contains chemicals called azulenes. Azulenes are anti-inflammatory and work both internally and externally to clear heat. Both yarrow and chamomile contain a specific azulene called chamazulene. Chamomile is well known for the blue color of its essential oil, which comes from chamazulene. Yarrow's essential oil is higher than chamomile's in azulenes, also has a deep blue color, and is better at reducing inflammation and clearing heat. The stems of a related yarrow species were used for throwing the sticks of the Book of Changes (I Jing). Another related species from Europe and naturalized in the northern (primarily northeastern) United States and adjacent Canada, *Achillea ptarmica,* is used for loss of appetite, urinary tract infections, rheumatism, diarrhea, and dyspeptic complaints. Several other species are native to Europe and have been used medicinally by local populations, including *A. moschata, A. ageratum, A. nana, A. nobilis,* and *A. atrata.*

Yarrow is a very important herb in the treatment of gynecological conditions and is a favorite of herbalists who follow the Wise Woman tradition. In Susun Weed's book, *Wise Woman Herbal for the Childbearing Year,* Susun recommends combining yarrow with plantain in an ointment for hemorrhoids and cracked nipples. She also recommends an infusion of the herb in a sitz bath for perineal tears.

Yarrow was official in *The United States Pharmacopoeia* from 1863–1882.

Translation of Source Material

In Chinese medicine, several species of *Achillea* are used. *Achillea alpina* and *A. wilsoniana* (*yī zhī hāo*) are acrid, bitter, slightly warm, and toxic, and enter the heart, liver, and lung channels. These herbs quicken the blood, dispel wind, relieve pain, and resolve toxin, and are used to treat knocks and falls, wind-damp pain, lump glomus, swollen welling-abscess, and deep, intractable *yīn* cold disease. They are also applied externally to sores to engender flesh and to treat hemorrhoids.

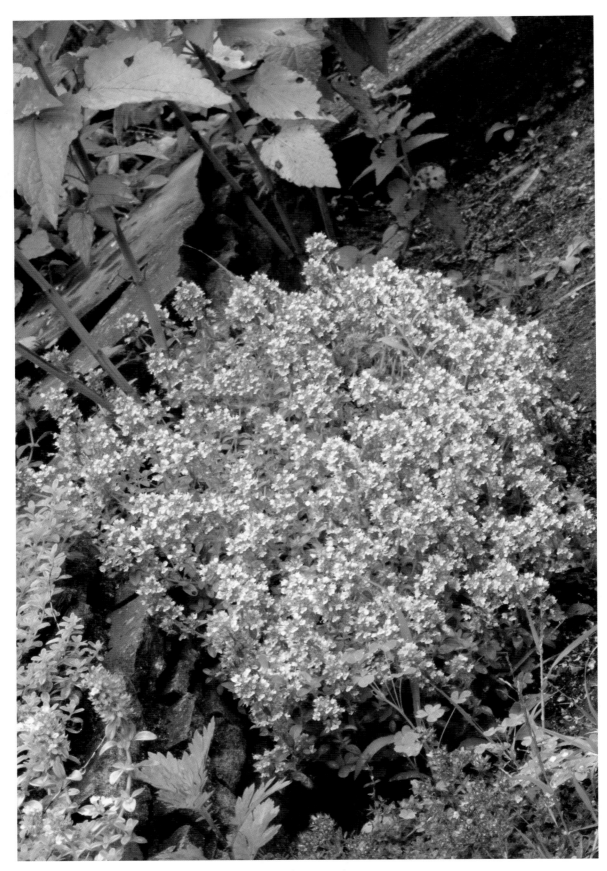

Thyme *(Thymus vulgaris)*

Thyme

Thymus vulgaris

Lamiaceae

Thymi Vulgari folium et flos

Other common names include *shè xiāng cǎo* (Chinese)

Flavor and *Qi*: acrid, slightly bitter, slightly cold
Channels Entered: lung, stomach, liver
Actions: antiseptic, antispasmodic, antitussive, carminative, expectorant

Functions and Indications

- ***Resolves the exterior, courses wind, clears heat, and benefits the throat.*** Thyme is used for the treatment of wind-heat invasion with red, swollen, and sore throat; fever; cough; and headache. This herb is also useful when the pathogen has obstructed the nose with thick yellow mucus. Due to its acrid and cooling nature, thyme effectively courses wind and discharges heat. The nose is the opening of the lung, which belongs to the *tài-yīn* and defense aspect, so is easily attacked by wind-heat causing obstruction of the nasal passageways. Thyme effectively treats defense-aspect wind warmth and is an important medicinal for this stage of disease.

- ***Disperses wind and stops cough.*** Thyme is helpful against wind that has entered the lungs and impaired the lungs' descending function. Although this is a cooling herb, it is very effective in stopping cough, and can be used in both heat and cold conditions when combined with the appropriate herbs. Spasmodic coughs, such as whooping cough, respond very well to this herb.

Because of its safety and effectiveness, thyme is an excellent children's herb, useful for treating colic as well as any of the indications listed above. The essential oil of thyme has been used externally for hot, swollen joints due to wind-heat-damp *bì*.

CAUTIONS

Use thyme with caution in cases of *yīn* vacuity.

Dosage and Preparation

Use 2–6 g in strong infusion; 1–3 ml tincture; 2–8 drops of the essential oil in a syrup. Tincture should be made with fresh leaves and fluidextract from dried leaves.

Gather leaves in late morning, before the sun reaches it highest point, in spring and early summer either just before flowering or when the flowers have opened. Lay the branches on screens or newspaper and allow to dry, out of direct sunlight. Garble (sort and clean) the leaves later to remove major stem material. Good-quality dried herb should contain whole green (generally, dark-green) leaves with few stems and should be aromatic.

Major Combinations

- Combine tincture or strong infusion of thyme with lemon juice and salt as a gargle for sore throat.

- Combine with osha and black sage for sore throat due to external wind-heat invasion.

- Combine with tincture of sundew for spasmodic cough caused by external wind-heat invasion. This is an excellent combination for children with croup or whooping cough.

- Combine with Mulberry Leaf and Chrysanthemum Decoction (*sāng jú yǐn*) for initial stages of wind-heat with sore throat.

- Combine with Stop Coughing Powder (*zhǐ sòu sàn*) for coughing with sore throat due to wind-heat.

Commentary

Thyme is a very useful herb that has long had a place in medicine. One of the many advantages of using this herb is that most people are familiar with the taste and find it agreeable. Thyme originated in the Mediterranean and is cultivated throughout the temperate zones

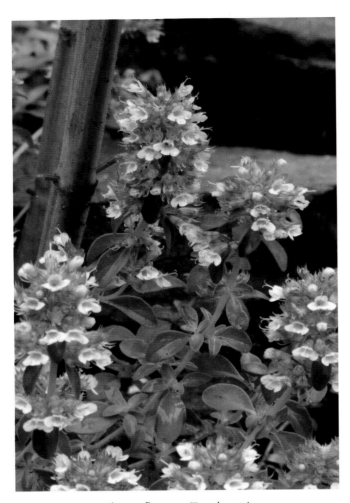

Thyme flowers *(T. vulgaris)*

thyme, is found in the essential oil component of the plant. The German pharmacist Neuman first extracted this chemical from the plant in 1725. Thymol is an excellent antiseptic and antispasmodic and is still used in certain commercial preparations on the market, such as Listerine mouthwash and some brands of toothpaste. The essential oil is commonly used both internally and externally.

Thymus vulgaris leaves are official in the pharmacopoeias of Argentina, Australia, the Czech Republic, France, Germany, Hungary, the Netherlands, Poland, and Romania. It was included in the Nordic pharmacopoeia in 1963 and the Jugoslav pharmacopoeia in 1984. The Swiss pharmacopoeia lists the leaves, flowers, and stalk tips. Both the German and Swiss pharmacopoeias list *T. vulgaris* and *T. zygis* as official.

Translation of Source Material

Chinese medicine uses several species from the *Thymus* genus. *Thymus vulgaris (shè xiāng cǎo)* is used to expel wind, settle cough, and is especially effective in whooping cough, acute bronchitis with laryngitis, and to dispel hookworms. These indications suggest a very recent introduction into Chinese medicine.

Two other species, listed as *dì jiāo* (*Thymus serpyllum* and *T. mongolicus*), are considered acrid, warm, and slightly toxic. They are used to warm the middle and dissipate cold, expel wind, and allay pain. They are also employed to downbear counterflow *qì* in the treatment of vomiting, as well as for abdominal pain, reduced food intake with constipation, wind-cold cough, swollen throat, toothache, and itchiness of the skin.

of the world today. It is an excellent ground- and wall-cover plant in the garden. The leaves are used in many traditional dishes from around the Mediterranean ranging from Spain, France, and Italy to Greece and Turkey. Many varieties of thyme are available; however, I recommend using *T. vulgaris* for medicine.

Thymol, one of the chemical constituents of

Sage

Salvia officinalis

Lamiaceae

Salviae Officinali herba

Also known as garden sage

Flavor and *Qi*: acrid, slightly bitter, slightly cool
Channels Entered: lung, liver, large intestine
Actions: antiseptic, astringent, diaphoretic

Functions and Indications

- ***Clears heat and disperses wind.*** Sage is used to treat sore throat and pain upon speaking. Because it has a recognizable taste, sage is often agreeable to patients as a tea gargled for this purpose. The medicinal's acrid and bitter nature disperses wind and clears heat. Sage is also used traditionally for other types of sore throat, which may include wind-dryness attacking the lung or other lung dryness patterns, as well as lung *yīn* vacuity patterns. Its use in these patterns is explained by its cooling and wind-dispersing action as well as its ability to astringe. The latter function is specific when there is a need to hold in moisture that, if lost, would further injure the system.

- ***Eliminates dampness and stops sweating.*** Sage is very effective for stopping sweating due either to vacuity or repletion patterns including night sweats, spontaneous sweating, and sweating due to damp-heat. For this purpose, the tea should be drunk cool, not hot. Because of its ability to treat damp-heat, sage is helpful for stopping sweating due to damp-heat patterns. Sweating due to damp-heat can be either an internal or external condition. Sage treats both well, although due to its acrid nature it is particularly good for treating externally contracted damp-heat leading to sweating.

- ***Dries dampness and clears heat.*** Sage helps treat damp-heat in the lower burner with itching in the genital area along with malodorous secretions, flatu-

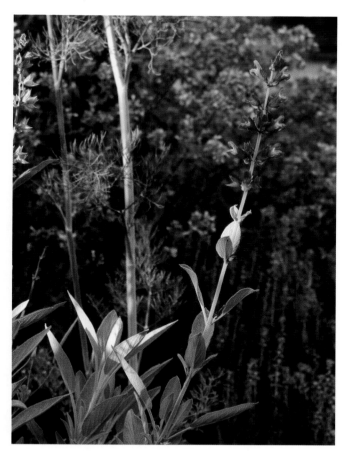

Garden sage *(Salvia officinalis)*

lence, and excretions. Damp-heat has a tendency to settle in the lower burner, which is called damp-heat pouring downward. This is an internal condition arising from various etiologies that lead to damp-heat. Sage dries dampness and cools heat, thus treating this condition. Sage is also used to dry up milk when mothers want to stop breastfeeding.

CAUTIONS

Sage should not be used by nursing mothers.

Dosage and Preparation

Use 3–6 g in light decoction or infusion; 2–5 ml tincture.

Sage tincture should be made with fresh plant material. Gather sage in the late spring and early summer,

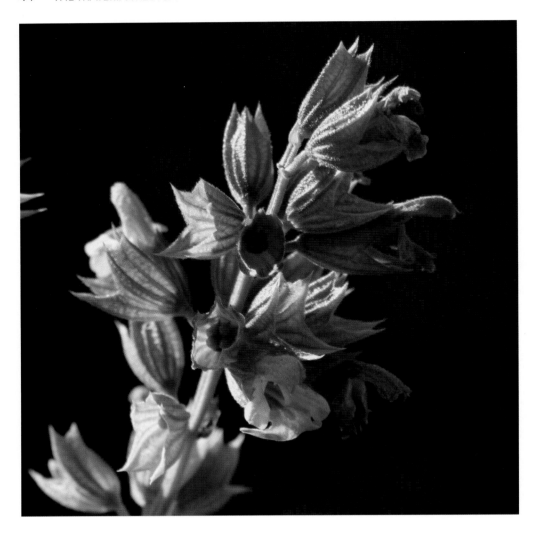

Sage flower inflorescence
(*S. officinalis*)

before the flowers mature. Bundle and dry the herb, and remove the leaves later for storage. Good-quality dried herb should be aromatic, have a gray-green color, and contain no stems.

Major Combinations

- Combine with yerba mansa and goldenseal for damp-heat in the lower burner with a burning sensation or itching in the genitals; vaginal discharge; hemorrhoids; dysenteric disorders; and scanty, burning, malodorous urine.

- Combine with myrrh as a gargle for sore, ulcerated throat.

- Combine with Jade Windscreen Powder (*yù píng fēng săn*) for sweating due to *qi* vacuity with frequent

external invasions. For this, take 20–60 drops of the fresh plant tincture along with Jade Windscreen Powder (*yù píng fēng săn*). This will help stop the sweating more quickly. Discontinue the sage once the sweating has stopped.

Commentary

The Latin name *Salvia* comes from *salvus,* meaning "healthy," which is in turn derived from the Latin verb *salvere,* meaning "to heal." Many plants in the genus *Salvia* are used in medicine. Most of them are used for their aromatic, aboveground parts, rather than their roots. A notable exception is the famous red sage root used in Chinese medicine. While some *Salvia* plants may be used in formulas as a substitute for the sage discussed in this monograph, they are not necessarily analogous.

The *Salvia* species discussed in the following passage are two of the many native sages from the western United States. I have included them here because I use them in significant amounts in clinical practice, but decided not to include them as separate monographs. The comparisons made below are with garden sage *(Salvia officinalis)*.

White sage *(Salvia apiana)* is stronger at clearing dampness and heat and is used for damp-heat in the lower burner with possible *Candida* infection. White sage is also used for damp-heat patterns associated with prostatitis; for this, combine it with nettle root and saw palmetto. It is also better, both internally and externally, for fungal infections. Finally, white sage

has a very long history of use as a ceremonial plant by the native peoples of the western United States, particularly in the southern California region, where the plant is native. The leaves are gathered while fresh, tied in small bundles, and dried. The smoke created when these bundles are burned is renowned as purifying and is therefore used to "clear the air" before a ritual or special event. This is a great way to start and end your day in the clinic. It can even be used between patients, after an especially challenged person has occupied the room.

Black sage *(Salvia mellifera)* is cool and more wind-dispersing; it is better for wind-heat with sore throat but less effective for damp-heat. Black sage is also used

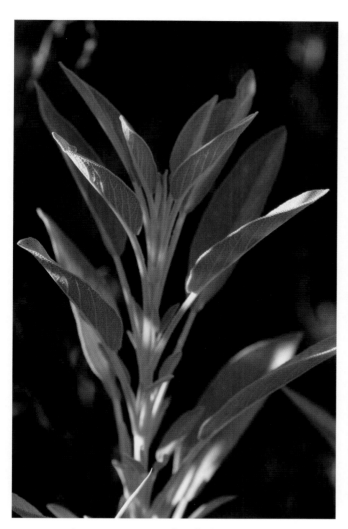

Sage leaves are covered with downy white hairs
(S. officinalis)

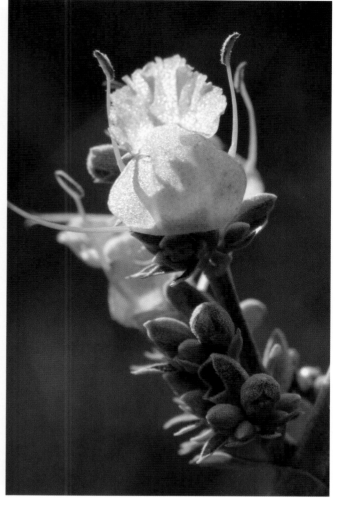

White sage flower (Salvia apiana)

for wind-heat *bì* syndrome with sore and inflamed joints. For this, use the stem along with the leaf.

Salvia officinalis was listed in *The United States Pharmacopoeia,* 1842–1916, and in *The National Formulary (U.S.),* 1936–1950. It is official in the *British Herbal Pharmacopoeia* (1996), the *British Pharmacopoeia* (2002), *Martindale: The Extra Pharmacopoeia* (33rd ed.), and the *European Pharmacopoeia* (2004). It is approved by the German Commission E and the European Scientific Cooperative on Phytotherapy (1999), and is listed in the *PDR for Herbal Medicines* (2nd ed.).

Warm Acrid Medicinals that Resolve the Exterior

The primary action of herbs in this category is resolving exterior cold patterns with symptoms that include chills and aversion to cold with mild heat effusion, headache, generalized pain, absence of sweating, nasal congestion, absence of thirst, tongue with a glossy fur, and floating, tight pulse. Within this category, you will find two very important herbs in the North American materia medica, California spikenard *(Aralia californica)* and osha *(Ligusticum grayi).* While neither is used extensively outside North America, they come from extremely important genera, *Aralia* and *Ligusticum.*

All of the plants discussed here are relatives of plants used in Chinese medicine. Wild ginger *(Asarum caudatum* and others) is closely related to the Chinese species of wild ginger *(xì xīn).* California spikenard is in the ginseng family (Araliaceae) and therefore related to a number of well-known plants in the Chinese materia medica, including ginseng *(rén shēn),* American ginseng *(xī yáng shēn),* notoginseng *(sān qī),* tetrapanax *(tōng cǎo),* and the less-known but more closely related prickly aralia *(hóng sōng mù).* Osha *(Ligusticum* spp.) is very closely related to the famous *Ligusticum chuanxiong (chuān xiōng)* as well as to an herb from the same category, *Ligusticum sinensis (gǎo běn).* The fourth medicinal in this category is American ephedra *(Ephedra viridis* and others), which, although closely related to Chinese ephedra *(má huáng)* botanically, is significantly different from it medicinally.

Osha

Ligusticum grayi, L. porteri

Apiaceae

Ligustici Grayi seu Porteri radix

Also called Gray's osha, oshalla *(L. grayi)*

Flavor and *Qi:* acrid, bitter, aromatic, warm
Channels Entered: lung, bladder, stomach, liver
Actions: antibacterial, antiviral, anodyne, diaphoretic, expectorant

Functions and Indications

- ***Expels wind, resolves the exterior, and stops pain.***
Osha effectively treats wind-heat or wind-cold, with symptoms such as sore throat, fever, nasal congestion, neck pain, cough, headache, and body aches. Osha's strong acridity and affinity for the lung and its respective channel makes it suitable for all attacks from the exterior affecting the upper burner. I use "upper burner" here as a general term, not specific to the triple burner of Warm Disease Theory. I make this distinction because osha can be used for either wind-cold or wind-heat. Osha's acrid and aromatic nature strongly dispels and outthrusts pathogens. When treating wind-cold, its warm and acrid nature scatters cold and, combined with its aromatic nature, outthrusts pathogens. In wind-heat conditions, its acrid and aromatic nature dispels and outthrusts warm pathogens, while its bitter and acrid nature drains heat and relieves pain. Although osha is warm, it can be effective in wind-heat conditions, especially when combined with the appropriate medicinals.

- ***Clears heat and drains fire, especially from the upper burner.*** Sore throat caused by heat damages the blood and channels, thus causing stasis and stagnation. Osha's acrid and aromatic nature quickens the blood, outthrusts pathogenic heat, and assists in the circulation of *qi* to relieve pain. When combined with its bitter nature, its acrid and aromatic nature clears heat and drains the burning fire. Osha has an

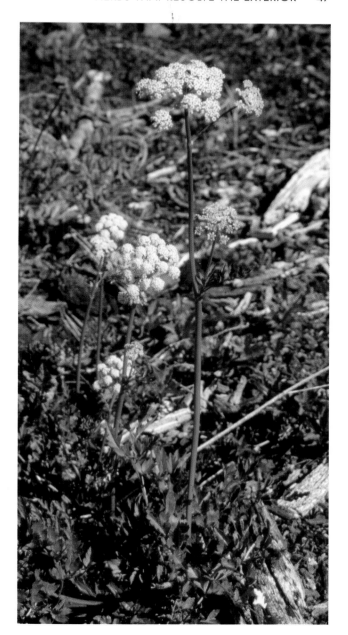

Osha *(Ligusticum grayi)*

affinity for the respiratory tract and is used for symptoms such as fever and cough. It is extremely important for infection in the respiratory tract with yellow sputum, sore throat, and fever, and can also be used for infections affecting the nasal passageways. Osha helps promote expectoration of thick, yellow, sputum that is difficult to expel. To alleviate a sore throat, chew and suck a piece of the root. It has an anodyne quality that relieves the pain, while its antibacterial and antiviral properties help eliminate the pathogen.

● **Dispels wind and dampness.** Osha is used for various types of wind-damp pain such as headache, backache, and joint pain. Wind and dampness lodged in the channels cause the *qi* and blood to stagnate, thus causing pain. Osha's acrid and bitter nature is very good for scattering wind and resolving dampness. If there are pronounced symptoms of cold, cold pathogens causing blood stasis, or severe pain, use the wine mix-fried version of osha.

The wine mix-fried version of the herb will invigorates the blood and *qi* for symptoms of pain caused by blood and *qi* stagnation. Preparing the sliced roots in this manner increases the herb's ability to quicken the blood and resolve *qi* stagnation. Pain that has a sharp and stabbing quality, such as certain types of headaches, angina, trauma, and arthritic pain, responds well to the herb prepared in this manner. It is also helpful for menstrual pain, as well as gynecological disorders including amenorrhea, dysmenorrhea, difficult labor, and lochioschesis.

Dosage and Preparation

Use 1–5 ml fresh plant tincture; 3–12 g in decoction. The fresh tincture is best, but the decoction is also very effective.

Gather the roots in autumn or spring when the aerial portions of the plant have died back for the winter. Slice and dry the roots for storage, or dry them whole. The roots can also be sliced for making fresh plant tincture. Good-quality dried osha root is aromatic and firm, not pithy. Osha is often sold in the form of a whole root. Whole or sliced, it should be free or nearly so of the coarse hairs that grow close to the root crown.

CAUTIONS

Osha should be used with caution during pregnancy. It probably should be avoided completely in the first trimester, as well as by women who have a history of miscarriage or who have a potential to miscarry due to weakness.

Major Combinations

● Combine with thyme and black sage for external attack of wind-heat causing sore, painful throat that is worse with swallowing or talking.

● Combine with pleurisy root for lung heat with thick, yellow sputum. Add marsh mallow for sputum that is more difficult to expectorate. Add to Honeysuckle, Forsythia, and Puffball Powder (*yín qiáo mǎ bó sǎn*) for severe sore throat.

Commentary

This plant is closely related to both *Ligusticum* species used in Chinese medicine, *gǎo běn* and *chuān xiōng*. However, unlike those species, osha is primarily used to clear heat. The taste of this plant is also quite different from that of either Chinese species. I believe osha has both warming and cooling energetics. One only need chew on a piece of the root while suffering from a sore throat to realize just how cooling it can be. This is one of many plants that appear to have both warming and cooling *qi*. Clinically speaking, the difference lies in how the medicinal is used in the formula and whether it is prepared or used raw.

The main plant discussed here is *L. grayi*. It is interchangeable with the more commonly known osha—*L. porteri*—of the Rocky Mountain region of the western United States. I have chosen to focus on *L. grayi* because it is readily available to me and thus the one I use in clinical practice. For many years now I have trekked to the High Sierra and now the Cascade and Siskiyou mountain ranges to pick *L. grayi*. This plant has a large distribution range and is probably more common at this point than the more popular *L. porteri*. Several other species of *Ligusticum* also grow in the western United States; however, none of them are as common as *L. grayi*, and unless they are cultivated, these species should not be used. For many years, *L. porteri* was reported to be very difficult to cultivate, but significant work has been done recently and several people in the United States are now able to cultivate small amounts. I am not aware of any attempts to cultivate *L. grayi*.

California Spikenard

Aralia californica

Araliaceae

Araliae Californicae rhizoma et radix

Also called aralia, elk clover

Flavor and *Qi*: acrid, bitter, slightly sweet, warm
Channels Entered: lung, bladder, kidney, stomach
Actions: expectorant, diaphoretic, stimulant, supplementing

Functions and Indications

- ***Releases the exterior, expels wind, and disperses cold.*** California spikenard is applied in the treatment of wind-cold with symptoms of headache, neck and shoulder tension, and chills. California spikenard is very effective for breaking a fever when there is no sweating. Its strongly acrid nature resolves the exterior and expels wind. The acridity combined with its warm nature make California spikenard a very good medicinal for dispelling wind-cold invasion. It is also useful in wind-cold-damp *bi* syndrome.

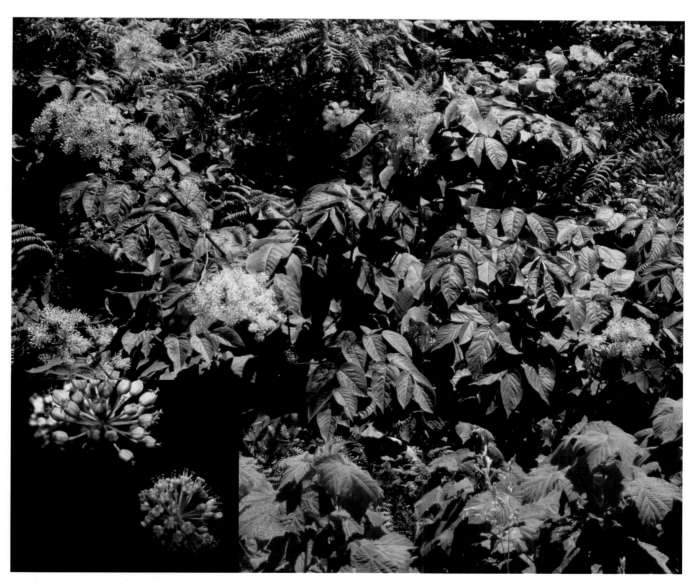

California spikenard *(Aralia californica)* with close-up of flower (inset)

- ***Scatters cold, circulates lung qì, transforms phlegm, and stops cough.*** California spikenard is used to treat cough with copious white or clear sputum; for this function, it is exceptional. It assists with expectoration, transforms phlegm, and benefits the lung *qì*. Its warm and acrid nature scatters cold from the lung and transforms phlegm. Its warm, bitter, and slightly sweet nature also assists lung *qì* circulation. The bitterness and acridity help to downbear and circulate lung *qì*, thus stopping cough.

- ***Supplements lung and spleen qì.*** This herb is helpful in the treatment of *qì* vacuity symptoms such as lethargy, shortness of breath, cough with watery sputum, and a tendency to catch colds. For these indications, I recommend a honey mix-fried version of California spikenard: cooking the medicinal in honey helps to mediate the acridity and strengthen its supplementing action. I use the berries as well as the root and rhizome for this purpose (although the berries need not be mix-fried in honey).

CAUTIONS

Use California spikenard with caution in people with high fever and sweating. Avoid use in those who have *yīn* vacuity with heat signs.

Dosage and Preparation

Use 3–9 g in decoction; 2–4 ml tincture; 1–3 g powdered extract. The same dosages can be utilized for preparations made with the berries.

Gather the roots and rhizomes in late autumn and winter, after the aerial parts have died back. Slice them for drying or to make fresh plant tincture. Good-quality dried root is large and light in weight, with streaks of rust-colored resin through an otherwise cream colored root. It should be aromatic.

Major Combinations

- Combine with osha and elecampane for wind-cold invasion with symptoms of cough accompanied by

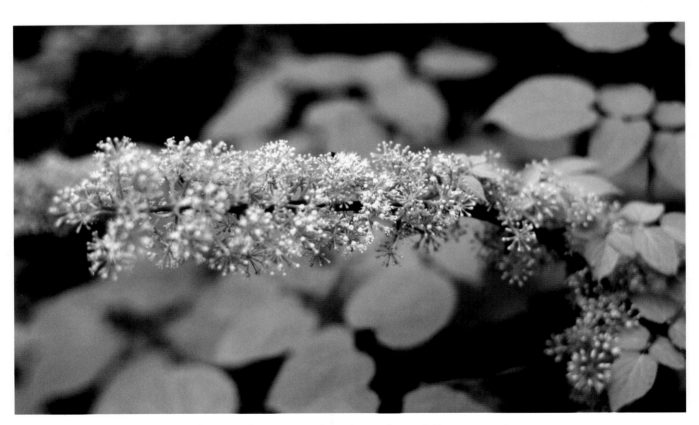

Flower in florescence of another spikenard *(A. racemosa)*

copious white or clear sputum, chills, heat effusion, sore neck, and body aches.

• Combine the honey mix-fried version with Jade Windscreen Powder *(yù píng fēng sǎn)* for pronounced signs of cold and *qi* vacuity in those tending toward phlegm, when wind-cold has disrupted the diffusion of the lung *qi* leading to cough, nasal congestion, and runny nose.

Commentary

California spikenard is a very important plant to me, so much so that I named my first daughter, Aralia, after it. Christopher Hobbs first introduced me to this plant in Fall Creek, a magical spot in the mountains near Santa Cruz, California. I was amazed by its size. This particular plant stood approximately 3.5 meters (approximately 10 feet) tall and easily spread its canopy the same distance, which is enough to make anyone do a double take.

California spikenard is in the ginseng family (Araliaceae) and was used by Native Americans to treat fevers without sweating, consumption, other lung and stomach ailments, and all debilitating diseases. Unfortunately, like so many plants of the western United States, there is little additional information concerning its traditional application in medicine. I believe that with continued experience, we will discover many additional uses for this potentially valuable American medicinal.

The berries of this plant have interesting potential as a supplementing medicinal. While there currently is insufficient evidence for a separate entry, I have talked to several herbalists who have used California spikenard berry with much success in debilitated conditions with frequent external invasions, inability to adjust to changes in the environment, and fatigue.

Several other species of *Aralia* native to North America also are used in medicine. These include the closely related spikenard *(A. racemosa)*, wild sarsaparilla *(A. nudicaulis)*, bristly sarsaparilla *(A. hispida)*, and devil's walking stick or spiny aralia *(A. spinosa)*. All of these species are native to the eastern and central regions of North America, although *A. racemosa* is sometimes listed as occurring in the Four Corners area of the southwestern United States, and *A. nudicaulis* is found as far west as eastern British Columbia south to Colorado.

Although *A. californica* has never been official as medicine in the United States, the closely related *A. racemosa*, which could be analogous, was official in *The National Formulary (U.S.)*, 1916–1965.

Wild Ginger

Asarum caudatum, A. canadense, and others

Aristolochiaceae

Asari rhizoma et radix

Flavor and *Qi:* acrid, bitter, aromatic, hot
Channels Entered: lung, kidney
Actions: anodyne, carminative, diaphoretic, expectorant, stimulant

Functions and Indications

- ***Releases the exterior, expels wind, and disperses cold.*** Wild ginger is excellent when used at the onset of the common cold with symptoms of headache, neck and shoulder tension, and chills. It is especially helpful for sinus congestion due to a cold or allergy, and also when a cold has affected the conjunctiva, causing inflammation with constant lachrymation. The nature of this medicinal is upbearing, and its acridity opens and frees. This makes wild ginger particularly good for diseases of the head and face and especially for bound nasal congestion.

- ***Scatters cold, circulates lung qì, transforms phlegm, and stops cough.*** Wild ginger is employed when cold attacks the lungs, causing pain, or for chronic cough caused by cold. Wild ginger's hot and aromatic

attributes make it a very good penetrating and out-thrusting medicinal for cold evils. This medicinal is especially helpful when chronic cough leads to lung *qi* vacuity and thus spleen *qi* vacuity, causing diarrhea and nausea. It can also be used for external attack of wind-cold-damp in the small intestine with painful diarrhea, as well as for cold evil attacking the stomach with abrupt onset of epigastric pain, aggravation of pain by cold and alleviation by warmth, aversion to cold, and no apparent thirst.

- ***Scatters cold, disperses damp, and subdues pain in the channels and uterus.*** Wild ginger can be effectively used in cases of dysmenorrhea with cold, cutting pain that radiates down the inner thigh (i.e., the liver channel) and into the lower back (i.e., the kidney channel). Such a patient may also present with nervousness and irritability. Wild ginger can also help with amenorrhea due to cold and damp in the uterus. The hot, aromatic, and penetrating nature of this medicinal makes it advantageous in this situation, as it very strongly enters the channels to chase out cold.

Wild ginger is excellent for most pain caused by cold or heat, regardless of the location. I have used it for toothache, trigeminal neuragia, and joint pain in various places in the body. I have also included it in external preparations by incorporating the tincture into a paste to be applied twice daily. Wild ginger's

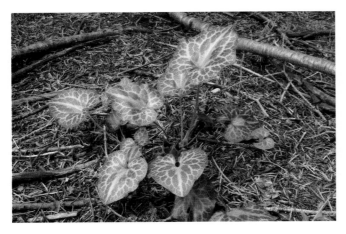

One species of wild ginger *(Asarum marmoratum)*

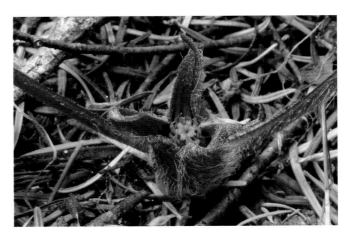

Wild ginger flower *(A. marmoratum)*

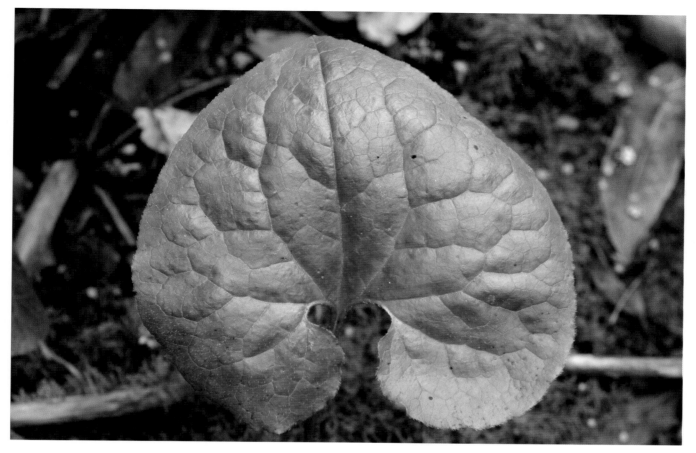

Leaf of the more common wild ginger *(A. caudatum)*

ability to penetrate, open, and free stagnation allows for its use in both cold and heat conditions when treating pain. However, it is important to take its hotness into account and formulate accordingly when using it to treat conditions in which heat is present.

CAUTIONS

Use with caution with extreme fever and excessive sweating. Wild ginger is not appropriate for *yīn* vacuity with heat signs.

Dosage and Preparation

Use 2–6 g in light decoction or strong infusion; 0.5–3 ml tincture.

Note that the essential oils in wild ginger are a large part of its activity and therefore it should not be decocted for long periods of time. Further, an infusion of the herb will be better for relieving the exterior and dispersing wind.

Gather the roots and rhizomes in the autumn or spring, separate from the leaves, and dry out of direct sunlight. Good-quality dried material is light green to whitish in color, lacks leaf material, and has few small rootlets. It should be aromatic and have a bitter, acrid flavor.

Major Combinations

- Combine with California spikenard for cold in the lungs with cough and copious clear or white sputum.

- Combine with valerian, prickly ash, and cramp bark for dysmenorrhea caused by attack of cold and damp with strong, sharp or dull pain before or during menstruation.

- Combine with osha and elecampane for wind-cold sinus congestion with headache and sinus pain.

Commentary

This plant is somewhat different from Chinese wild ginger. The dosage of each is about the same, with a slightly heavier hand used in the West. However, decocting our Western species is not advisable, as the essential oils are considered an important part of the plant's medicinal actions. Based on this, tincture and liquid extract of Western wild ginger species are prescribed most frequently. Furthermore, Western herbalists generally use the rhizome without the leaves, though some use the whole plant.

The growth patterns of the two main North American species *(Asarum caudatum* and *A. canadense)* also are somewhat different from the Chinese species. The Chinese species has definite roots with few rhizomes, in contrast to the Western species, which have mostly rhizomal growth with very few roots, only enough to anchor the plant down. The fresh leaf of our Western species is also considered an emetic, and I have heard firsthand accounts of people getting nauseous after eating it. I have eaten the leaves without experiencing this effect. Note that the species pictured on page 52, which is difficult to differentiate on sight from the two main species except for the mottling of the leaves, has a growth pattern as I have described for the Chinese species above.

The Western species of wild ginger are somewhat delicate, and proper harvesting techniques are essential in order to assure continued availability of this very important herb. The plant loves old-growth forests. Unfortunately, much of its original habitat has been destroyed due to over-cutting in the forest and overall poor forestry practices. I believe this fragile plant could be cultivated very successfully under the proper conditions and that there is potentially a small but solid market for the herb.

Wild ginger is one of several medicinal plants that contains aristolochic acid, known for its excellent medicinal properties as well as its toxicity. Aristolochic acid is anti-inflammatory, antiviral, and stimulates immune system activity. However, it also is infamous for its carcinogenic, genotoxic, and mutagenic properties. In addition to aristolochic acid, wild ginger contains β-asarone, a potentially carcinogenic substance also found in some sweet flag *(chāng pú)* species. Because β-asarone is rapidly broken down in the body, it poses little danger. Unfortunately, unlike β-asarone, traces of aristolochic acid were found in rats nine months after a single dose was administered.[1]

These chemicals have been studied and their potential dangers known since at least the early 1980s. In the mid-1990s, a number of cases of kidney toxicity and several deaths were blamed on aristolochic acid contained in a commercial herbal diet product. It is important to note that these injuries were caused by an adulteration; the product contained *Aristolochia westlandi (guǎng fáng jǐ)*, which was not appropriate for the stated use. Unfortunately, this substitution is a common adulteration in China because the indication for two medicinals—*Stephania tetrandra (hàn fáng jǐ)* and *Aristolochia westlandi (guǎng fáng jǐ)*—are similar, and the plants look similar. However, it is generally understood that these medicinals are not to be used for extended periods of time. Even more unfortunate, some people promote the use of medicinal plants without having a full understanding of what they are promoting.

The people injured by the adulterated diet products were also taking several other drugs at the same time, and the exact cause of the deaths was never confirmed. Nonetheless, Belgium and the United Kingdom have banned the use of plants named *fáng jǐ* and *mù tōng,* irrespective of species. The U.S. Food and Drug Administration has moved to restrict—or perhaps ban—any herb known to contain aristolochic acid or that could be substituted for one that does.

Many plants containing these substances have long histories of use in many cultures, with no known adverse effects when used properly. However, with the preceding cautions in mind, we must seriously reconsider our use of these plants for internal medication. Due to the possible dangers associated with wild ginger species, I do not recommend using them internally, and I strongly warn against using them on a long-term basis.

Wild ginger was official in the *The United States Pharmacopoeia,* 1820–1873, and in *The National Formulary (U.S.),* 1916–1947.

Mormon Tea

Ephedra viridis, E. nevadensis, E. californica, and others

Ephedraceae

Ephedra herba

Flavor and *Qi*: acrid, bitter, warm
Channels Entered: lung, bladder
Actions: astringent, diaphoretic, diuretic

Functions and Indications

- ***Resolves the exterior and stops wheezing.*** Ephedra is used to treat wind-cold with symptoms of wheezing; runny nose with clear, copious mucus; stuffy head; and sneezing. Ephedra's acrid nature resolves the exterior, while its bitter nature downbears lung *qi* to check wheezing. While this is not a strong action, North American ephedra species are a reasonable substitute when *má huáng* is inappropriate due to hypertension or other issues.

- ***Promotes urination.*** Ephedra helps treat edema of any etiology, but particularly edema associated with external pathogens. It is also used for dribbling urinary block or inhibited urination due to kidney vacuity, with symptoms such as urinary frequency, urgency, diminished force of urinary stream, and post-void dribbling. Ephedra's bitter and astringent nature helps to drain and restrain, regulating the flow of urine, which makes this herb especially good for various urinary complaints. Furthermore, its acrid, exterior-resolving nature makes this herb particularly good for external damp conditions.

CAUTIONS

Because of its diuretic and dispersing action, ephedra should be used with caution in *yīn* vacuity patterns.

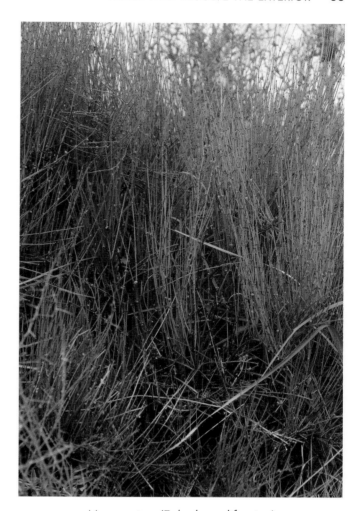

Mormon tea *(Ephedra californica)*

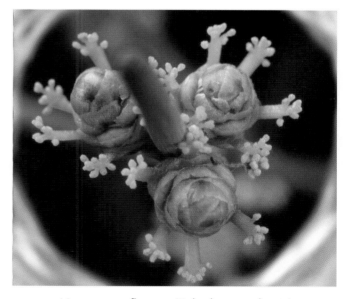

Mormon tea flowers *(Ephedra nevedensis)*

Dosage and Preparation

Use 3–9 g in decoction or strong infusion; 2–4 ml tincture. Note that because of the essential oils ephedra contains, the infusion is a better diaphoretic and will more strongly release the exterior. A decoction of the herb is a stronger diuretic.

Gather ephedra stems at any time of the year, except when the plant is flowering or in seed. Lay them out to dry for storage or processing; alternatively, cut and prepare as a fresh plant tincture. Good-quality dried herb is green to green-gray, whole (not shredded), and has a slight aroma.

Major Combinations

- Combine with yarrow and California spikenard for invasion of wind-cold with cough and wheezing.

- Combine with saw palmetto and aconite for inhibited urination due to kidney *yáng* vacuity.

- Combine with saw palmetto, nettle root, and ginseng for dribbling urinary block due to insufficiency of kidney *qì*.

- Combine with black sage and akebea for externally contracted wind-damp pathogens.

REPRESENTATIVE FORMULA THAT RESOLVES THE EXTERIOR

Yarrow, Elder, and Mint Combination

Source: Unknown; traditional diaphoretic tea

Yarrow	6 g
Elder flower	6 g
Mint	6 g

Preparation: Prepare as an infusion by pouring 1000 ml boiling water over the herb and allow to steep, covered, for 15 to 20 minutes. This infusion should be drunk while hot. For best results, drink a cup of tea, take a hot shower or bath, then drink another cup of tea, wrap up in bed, and sweat it out.

Actions: Disperses wind-heat from the exterior, clears heat, and relieves toxicity.

Indications: Use for initial attack of the exterior by wind-heat. Symptoms include fever with no chills or slight chills, sore throat, headache, cough, slight thirst, and tongue showing no change or having a red tip and/or yellow coating. The pulse should be floating and rapid.

This indication describes a simple case of wind-heat invasion entering through the mouth and nose and affecting the lungs, causing cough, fever, and sore throat. The degree of fever will depend on the strength of the pathogen and the *wèi qì*. The slight chills or lack of chills clearly shows this to be a wind-heat rather than wind-cold pattern. If the pathogen has entered the lungs, then the tongue will have a yellow coat with a red tip. The yellow on the tongue signifies heat, and the red tip shows us that the heat is in the upper burner.

Analysis of the Formula: This is a good example of the simple yet effective style in which Western herbalists generally formulate. Both yarrow and elder flower are bitter, acrid, and cold, and when drunk hot strongly release the exterior, dispersing wind while clearing heat. The assistant, mint, disperses wind, relieves heat, and strengthens the actions of the other herbs in the formula.

Cautions and Contraindications: Use caution for those with *qì* or *yīn* vacuity, as excessive sweating can weaken an already weak patient.

Modifications: Add pleurisy root and apricot seed for more severe cough that is dry and hacking due to strong heat evil.

- Add thyme for spasmodic cough.
- Add osha and thyme for more severe sore throat and headaches.
- Add boneset for more severe fever.
- Add fresh ginger and cayenne for wind-cold.

Commentary

North American ephedra is effective if taken in the early stages of an external condition. It has been reported to be employed by Native Americans to treat asthma in the same manner Chinese ephedra is used; however, I can find no specific reference to substantiate this claim. Apparently, early settlers also used the plant in this manner, but it is unclear where they got the idea. Although the functions and indications of our ephedra are similar to those of Chinese ephedra, ours is much less potent and slower acting. It also lacks some of the chemical constituents that give *má huáng* its stimulating properties.

North American ephedra species are by no means a perfect substitute for Chinese ephedra, but for those with vascular weakness, heart conditions, high blood pressure, or significant *qì* or *yīn* vacuity, this plant will prove to be effective and safe. Many ephedra species are found in the desert region of the western United States, but the species listed here are the ones with which I have had the most experience and find to work in the manner I describe. Some of the other ephedra species that I have used minimally seem to be effective as well, but many have a significant degree of astringency.

The root of the North American species appears to be a perfect substitute for Chinese ephedra root *(má huáng gēn)*. I have used it in place of Chinese ephedra root with excellent results.

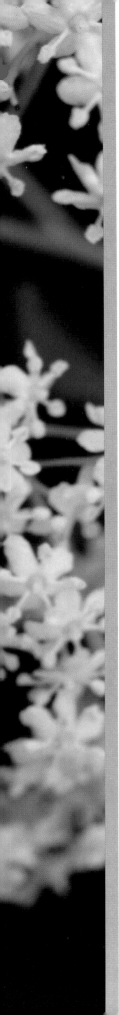

HERBS
THAT CLEAR HEAT

Clearing heat is a generalized term used to describe the action of medicinals that are cool to cold in nature and thus treat repletion-heat patterns. In a Chinese materia medica, this large category of medicinals is often broken into subcategories, which simply represent more specific delineations for individual medicinals. To maintain the tradition, I have chosen to organize this large category in the same manner. It is important to note that many of the medicinals in this group are used across several subcategories. The subcategories are meant only to help organize and identify the main functions of the medicinals.

Clearing heat is a very important category in any materia medica. The idea of clearing heat can be traced back to the *Elementary Questions (sù wèn),* where it says, "Heat is treated with cold." Therefore, the *qì* of the medicinals in this category is cool to cold, and their flavor is nearly always bitter, due to the tendency for bitter to drain. From the Western perspective, heat—as defined by Chinese medicine—is seen in most, if not all, inflammatory conditions.

Aside from the main subcategories of medicinals outlined here, a number of other combinations of actions are associated with clearing heat. These are important to remember, because the herbs listed in the subcategories will not always be effective if used alone. Achieving the desired functions is generally accomplished by combining medicinals, although some of the individual herbs do address one or more of them.

These other major combined actions include:

- Clearing heat and disinhibiting dampness
- Clearing heat and dispelling dampness
- Clearing heat and extinguishing wind (also called draining fire and extinguishing wind)
- Clearing heat and freeing strangury
- Clearing heat and opening the orifices
- Clearing heat and resolving summerheat (often a subcategory in materia medicas, but not in this text)
- Clearing heat and resolving the exterior
- Clearing heat and stanching bleeding
- Clearing heat and transforming dampness
- Clearing heat and transforming phlegm

Herbs that Drain Fire

This subcategory of clearing heat is characterized by the symptomatology that distinguishes fire from heat. Fire is, essentially, an exaggerated form of heat. When fire is a pathogenic factor, the upper portion of the body is nearly always affected, due to the rising nature of fire. Because fire is an exaggerated form of heat, symptoms are often severe, and generally the condition requires swift treatment to resolve the pathogenesis, or at least the most severe symptoms, such as high fever, severe headache, and extreme depletion of fluids. Symptoms such as high fever and redness in the head (including the eyes, face, and tongue) are common due to the rising nature of fire. These symptoms are also generally accompanied by dryness (for example, dry eyes, skin, mouth, or tongue).

However, fire can also affect the middle or lower portions of the body. Symptoms such as scant, reddish urine; pus and blood in the stool; acute diarrhea; and thick, yellow phlegm are all possible signs of fire. Furthermore, fire can cause problems with the blood. Fire can scorch the vessels and force the blood from its course, causing spontaneous bleeding and maculopapular eruptions. The subcategory of herbs that drain fire is often homogenized in modern textbooks with another subcategory, called "clear heat and resolve toxins," which I've treated as a separate category here.

Two medicinals that drain fire are feverfew *(Tanacetum parthenium)* and meadowsweet *(Filipendula ulmaria)*. Feverfew is excellent for downbearing fire and clearing heat; thus it is very effective for symptoms in the upper portion of the body. This is also true for meadowsweet, but to a lesser extent. Meadowsweet is specific for the stomach and more systemic problems arising from fire in the middle and lower burners. In addition, meadowsweet restrains *yīn,* making it valuable for conditions in which fluids are damaged and also for vacuity fire. Its combination of flavors and *qì* make meadowsweet an important addition to the materia medica.

Feverfew

Tanacetum parthenium

Asteraceae

Tanaceti Parthenii herba seu flos

Flavor and *Qi:* bitter, slightly acrid, cold
Channels Entered: liver, stomach
Actions: analgesic, anthelmintic, antirheumatic, febrifuge, stomachic

Functions and Indications

- ***Clears the liver and drains fire.*** Feverfew effectively treats liver-fire flaming upward, with symptoms such as vasodilative migraine headache, red eyes, red face, red ears, agitation, vexation. This herb is also useful for liver-fire invading the lung, with symptoms of cough, difficult breathing, scorching pain in the chest and flanks, and impatience. Feverfew's bitter and cold nature strongly clears heat, downbears liver-fire, and assists *yáng* in returning to its source.

- ***Clears heat, diffuses impediment, and relieves pain.*** This herb is used for the treatment of heat impediment with symptoms of hot, red, swollen, painful joints with or without heat effusion or thirst. Feverfew's bitter, draining, and slightly acrid nature make it useful in the treatment of hot, painful impediment. Its bitter and cold nature effectively drains and cools heat, while its slightly acrid nature helps to disperse stagnation and stasis due to heat damaging the *qi* dynamic and blood.

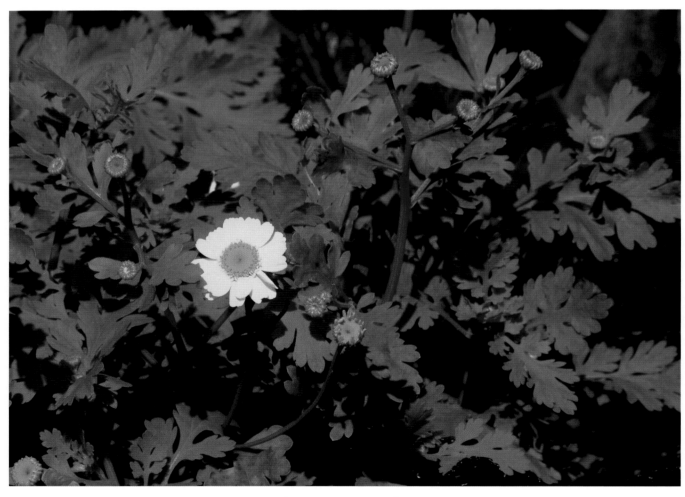

Feverfew *(Tanacetum parthenium)*

• ***Clears the stomach and drains fire.*** Feverfew is employed to treat stomach fire with symptoms of toothache, bleeding gums, epigastric pain, bitter taste in the mouth, and a red tongue with a yellow coat. Feverfew's bitter and cold nature is suitable for directly cooling a hot stomach and for draining fire to resolve symptoms associated with stomach fire.

CAUTIONS

This herb should be applied for patterns of repletion only. Some sensitive individuals may experience a mild to moderate rash, generally in the mouth. Due to its bitter, cold, and downbearing action, feverfew should be used with caution during pregnancy.

Dosage and Preparation

Use 1–7 g in light decoction or infusion; 1–3 ml tincture. The fresh plant tincture is superior to the dry plant tincture.

Good-quality dried herb contains approximately equal parts of flowers and leaves with few stems. The leaves should be green and the flowers white and yellow without browning. There should be a minimum of loose disk flowers floating around in the bag, which might indicate that the flowers were picked past their peak or that they were overdried.

Major Combinations

• Combine with gentian for liver-fire flaming upward with red painful face, red eyes, headache, and other heat signs in the upper body due to the rising of liver-fire. This combination is also effective for headache due to gallbladder heat.

• Combine with echinacea and cayenne for heat entering the blood-construction with symptoms of maculopapular eruptions. In this combination, the bitter, cold, and acrid dispersing and outthrusting actions of echinacea and feverfew treat the symptomatology while moving the pathogenic warmth out of the blood-construction and into the *qi* aspect. Furthermore, the acrid and warming nature of cayenne

helps to disperse and outthrust the eruptions, resolving the main complaint.

Commentary

Feverfew is very popular for the treatment of headaches, including migraine headaches. Unfortunately, it doesn't work for all headaches. In my experience, it works best for headaches associated with heat or fire rising upward, and may actually make headaches associated with cold worse. This is a case in which the mass media has commercialized an herb as a one-size-fits-all remedy. While most practitioners understand how to use feverfew, retailers and magazine articles do not distinguish among appropriate uses of this medicinal. While science struggles to understand why feverfew works for some people and not for others, we, as Chinese herbalists, can clearly see when and why it works by applying the principles of Chinese medicine. A bitter and cold herb will by nature clear heat and downbear *qi*. With this most basic knowledge, it should be clear why feverfew would aggravate conditions associated with cold and *qi* vacuity and benefit those with heat or fire rising upward.

Feverfew's species name, *parthenium,* relates to the Greek word for "virgin" or "virgin goddess," owing to the herb's earlier use in gynecology. Culpeper writes, ". . . [it can] remedy such infirmities as a careless midwife has there caused; if they will be pleased to make use of her herb boiled in white wine, and drink the decoction, it cleanses the womb, expels the afterbirth, and does a woman all the good she can desire of an herb." He recommended an external application of feverfew combined with nutmeg or mace for delayed or painful menstruation. He also recommended bruising and frying the herb in wine and oil and applying it externally for "wind and colic in the lower part of the belly." Interestingly, he notes the herb is "very effectual" when applied externally to the head for headache due to cold causes and vertigo, with a "running or swimming" sensation in the head. This is difficult to reconcile with our current understanding, but one can only surmise that our perception of hot and cold causes and their manifestations in the body are different from Culpeper's. Furthermore, it should be noted that feverfew is used little, if at all, in gynecology today.

Feverfew was made official in *The United States Pharmacopoeia* and *The National Formulary (U.S.)* in 1998. It is also official in the *British Herbal Compendium* (1992), the *British Herbal Pharmacopoeia* (1996), the *British Pharmacopoeia* (2002), *Martindale: The Extra Pharmacopoeia* (33rd ed.), and the *European Pharmacopoeia* (2004), and is listed in *PDR for Herbal Medicine* (2nd ed.) and *Monographs on the Medicinal Uses of Plant Drugs*: *European Scientific Cooperative on Phytotherapy* (1999).

Translation of Source Material

Chinese medicine uses two species of *Tanacetum*. *T. variifolium (tài bái ài)* is acrid, slightly bitter, and neutral. It dispels and settles wind, clears heat, and resolves toxin, and is used to treat child fright-wind, wind-damp numbness, and appendicitis. *T. sibiricum (tù zǐ máo)* is bitter and cool. It clears heat, resolves toxin, and cools the blood, and is employed to treat infectious disease with high fever, clove sore and swollen welling-abscess, and stabbing pain due to blood stasis.

Meadowsweet

Filipendula ulmaria

Rosaceae

Filipendulae Ulmarii herba seu flos

Also known as dropwort

Flavor and *Qi*: bitter, bland, astringent, slightly cold
Channels Entered: stomach, kidney, liver
Actions: anodyne, antacid, anti-inflammatory, anti-rheumatic, antiulcerogenic, astringent, diuretic, mild urinary antiseptic

Functions and Indications

- ***Clears heat and drains fire.*** Meadowsweet is used to treat stomach heat due either to repletion or vacuity, with symptoms such as stomach duct pain, strong appetite, bleeding gums, and bad breath. Meadowsweet is also used for heat-type diarrhea with heat invading the stomach and intestines causing abdominal pain, burning in the anus, thirst with a desire for cold drinks, and voiding of blood-tinged urine. This herb is particularly good for childhood diarrhea as it is safe, relatively gentle, and quick acting. However, do not confuse this herb's gentleness with weakness or ineffectiveness. Meadowsweet's bitter and cold nature strongly clears heat and cools the stomach and intestines. Heat scorches the tissue, vessels, and channels, causing damage, blood stasis (due to blood leaving the vessels), and *qi* stagnation. Meadowsweet's bitter and cold nature, combined with its mildly astringent nature, helps to bring the tissue back to a healthy state, making this medicinal uniquely effective in this type of disorder.

- ***Clears vacuity heat and restrains* yīn.** Meadowsweet is helpful in the treatment of *yīn* vacuity heat with symptoms such as nocturnal emissions, headache, thirst, dull intermittent pain in the joints or muscles, and lower back pain. Meadowsweet is astringent and restrains *yīn*. It is also bitter and cold, draining and cooling heat. The combination of restraining and

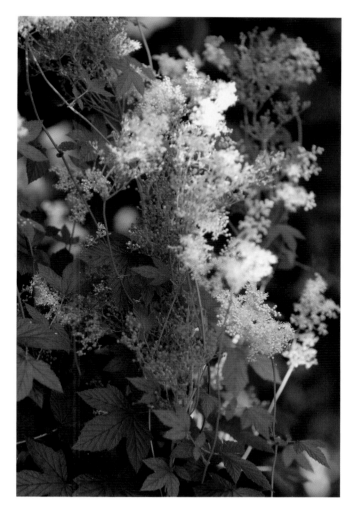

Meadowsweet *(Filipendula ulmaria)*

draining allows for this medicinal to be used in *yīn* vacuity with great effectiveness.

- ***Clear heats and drains damp.*** Meadowsweet is employed to treat bladder damp-heat with symptoms such as frequent, painful, and small voidings of urine. Meadowsweet is bitter and cold and thus clears heat. Although it is astringent, restraining *yīn*, it also drains dampness with blandness. This important combination of astringency and blandness allows draining without damaging *yīn*.

CAUTIONS

Meadowsweet should be used with caution by those who have salicylate sensitivities, including allergies to aspirin.

Dosage and Preparation

Use 3–9 g in decoction; 2–4 ml tincture.

Good-quality dried herb is green with a mix of small amounts of white flowers and 20 to 30 percent stem material.

Major Combinations

- Combine with marsh mallow root for stomach *yīn* vacuity with burning pain in the stomach duct, thirst, and bleeding gums. This combination is an excellent addition to Coptis and Aucklandia Formula *(xiāng lián wán)* for most complaints for which people take antacid drugs.

- Combine with plantain leaf, marsh mallow root, and chamomile for chronic inflammation of the gastrointestinal tract.

- Combine with Oregon grape root bark for *yīn* vacuity heat leading to lower back pain and nocturnal emissions.

- Combine with black cohosh for wind-heat-damp impediment with muscle and joint pain.

- Combine to modify White Tiger Decoction *(bái hǔ tāng)* for *yáng-míng* stage disease to drain fire and protect the stomach from the harsh effects of the formula.

- Combine to modify Major *Qì*-Coordinating Decoction *(dà chéng qì tāng)* to drain fire and protect the stomach and intestines from damage due to heat.

Commentary

Meadowsweet is a very safe and effective herb with a long history of use and extensive modern research. It is particularly helpful for stomach heat due either to repletion or vacuity. Despite its cooling nature, it can be used with little concern of injuring the spleen-stomach *qì*. The combination mentioned above of meadowsweet, marsh mallow root, coptis, and aucklandia, with the addition of a small bit of stevia, has proven to be incredibly effective in the treatment of acid reflux, heartburn, and the like. Eating habits in the West tend to cause people to manifest with stomach heat, whether from vacuity or repletion. I have come to rely on this formula with occasional modifications to treat a great number of the patients I see with common stomach ailments. Priest and Priest recommend meadowsweet with agrimony for stomach pain with excessive acid, but I have no experience with this combination.[1]

Meadowsweet is a simple but effective anti-inflammatory and astringent, which is part of the reason it is so good for the digestive tract. Chronic (and, to a lesser extent, acute) inflammation of the gastric mucosa damages the tissue, which can lead to a variety of problems. In the stomach, the first sign is reddening and edema of the tissue with adherent mucus and, potentially, erosions and bleeding. As the condition becomes chronic, there is atrophy of the glandular epithelium with loss of the parietal and chief cells, leading to decreased production of HCl, pepsin, and intrinsic factor. In such cases, meadowsweet's anti-inflammatory and astringent properties cool the tissue while gently toning with a mild astringent action. Toning the tissue and reducing inflammation results in proper blood and lymphatic flow, thus encouraging healing and correct functioning of the organ.

Culpeper explained the origin of *dropwort*, the herb's now less common name, by saying that it encourages urine that otherwise comes in drops. Gerard spoke very highly of the herb, saying, ". . . it makes the heart marrie," bringing joy and delighting the senses as both an internal medicine and a garden plant. Meadowsweet is in the rose family and is indeed an excellent plant for wet areas in the landscape. It is particularly good situated under or near a window so summer breezes can bring its fresh scent into the house.

Herbs that Cool the Blood

Heat entering the blood or heat entering the blood aspect describes a deep penetration of heat into the body. This pattern of disease is generally associated with toxins and detriment to *yīn* fluids. When heat enters the blood, it can damage the blood and vessels, leading to a frenetic movement of blood. It can also enter the pericardium and affect the heart, leading to symptoms such as agitation, clouded spirit, and mania. A rapid or racing pulse and a crimson tongue are hallmark signs of this syndrome. Blood-heat also is often associated with skin diseases.

Two important medicinals from this subcategory are burdock *(Arctium lappa)* and California figwort *(Scrophularia californica)*. Echinacea, although categorized as an herb for clearing heat and resolving toxins, is another valuable herb to remember when treating this pathological pattern.

Burdock functions in several ways to treat blood-heat. It is an excellent medicinal for clearing heat, but also helps to outthrust, gently nourish *yīn,* and resolve *qi* stagnation caused by scorching fire. California figwort, much like Chinese figwort, clears heat from the blood while enriching *yīn.* Furthermore, California figwort can be used to disperse stagnation and accumulation, making it a very versatile medicinal.

California Figwort
Scrophularia californica, S. lanceolata
Scrophulariaceae
Scrophulariae Californicae herba seu radix et rhizoma

Flavor and *Qi:* bitter, slightly sweet, cold
Channels Entered: kidney, lung, stomach, triple burner, bladder
Actions: alterative, antibacterial, anti-inflammatory, diuretic

Functions and Indications

- ***Clears blood-heat and enriches*** yīn *for vacuity of right with lodged evils.* Figwort root is applied in the treatment of symptoms such as night sweats, sore throat, dry irritation of any mucosa, purple maculopapular eruptions, a peeled crimson tongue, and a rapid, fine pulse. When heat lodges into the construction-blood aspect, it depletes liver and kidney *yīn*, while heat entering the blood stirs and injures the blood and its vessels. Figwort's bitter and cold nature effectively clears heat from both the construction and blood aspects, while its sweet and cold nature enriches and engenders *yīn* to support the right.

- ***Clears heat and drains damp.*** Figwort herb or both herb and root are used to treat various damp-heat patterns such as damp-heat steaming upward, damp-heat pouring downward, and damp-heat mounting, with symptoms including joint pain, lymph congestion,

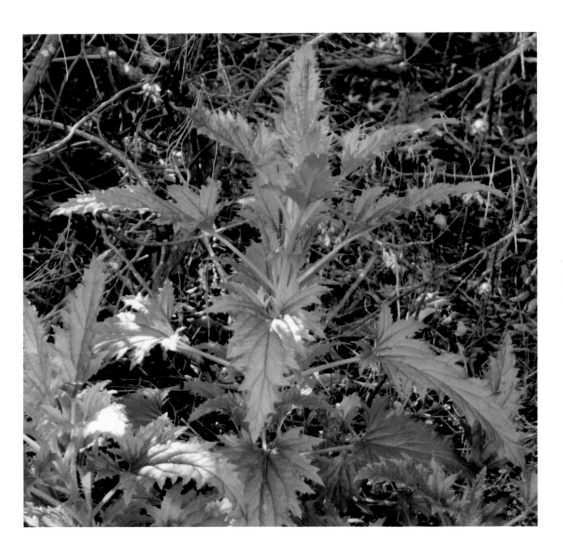

California figwort
*(Scrophularia
californica)*

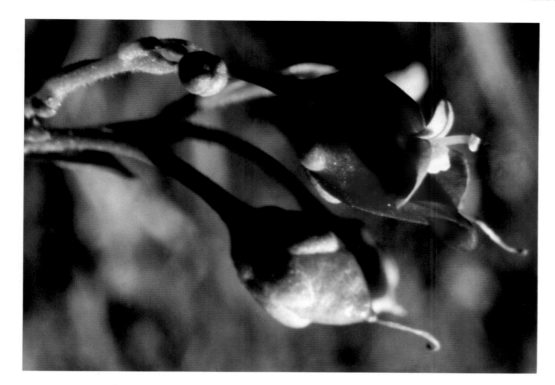

Flower and seedpod
of California figwort
(*Scrophularia
californica*)

skin diseases, hemorrhoids, and strangury. Figwort is a very effective medicinal for damp-heat conditions, as it effectively both drains damp and clears heat. For these patterns, the herbaceous portion of the plant is often used. It is bitter, bland, and cold and drains heat through the urine.

- ***Disperses stagnation and accumulation and clears heat toxin.*** Figwort is helpful for mammary welling-abscess with redness and swelling of the breast, especially around the nipple. A poultice or infused oil made from the herbaceous portion of the plant is a very important remedy for the treatment of this condition, most commonly caused by a blocked milk duct in a nursing mother. Figwort should also be included as part of a formula to be taken internally in such cases. One formula I have used several times with good success is Trichosanthus Powder *(guā lóu săn)* from *Fù Qīng-zhŭ's Gynecology.* Its bitter and cold nature effectively drains and clears heat while dispersing stagnation and accumulation, thus relieving pain and discomfort. Figwort is also used to treat wind-fire scrophula.

CAUTIONS

Avoid use of figwort in those with tachycardia. Use with caution during pregnancy.

Dosage and Preparation

Use 6–15 g in decoction; 2–6 ml tincture; 1–3 g powdered extract.

Bruise fresh leaves and apply to hot glandular swellings. An oil infusion can be prepared for the same purpose. This oil is an important ingredient in salve formulas for various heat conditions throughout the body.

Good-quality dried herb is dark green with sections of somewhat reddish to purple stems. It should have the characteristic—somewhat fetid—"figwort smell." The herb should have no flowers or seedpods. Dried root has a grayish color with signs of blackening due to oxidation; it should have a few small rootlets and be somewhat pliable to hard in texture.

Major Combinations

- Combine with red root and cleavers for damp-heat mounting with symptoms of hemorrhoids and swelling and pain of the scrotum. This combination can also be used for signs of lymph congestion throughout the body. For lymph congestion in the lower burner, add ocotillo.

- Combine with sarsaparilla and coix for joint pain associated with damp-heat.

- Combine with goldenseal, Chinese skullcap, and coix for painful, bloody urination.

- Combine with yellow dock for difficult defecation associated with damp-heat. Add buckthorn bark for constipation.

Commentary

Chinese figwort (xuán shēn) and European figwort (S. nodosa) are the major species commonly used in medicine. The Chinese use only the root of the plant and the Europeans only the herb. American herbalist Michael Moore, the only reliable modern reference for the species, recommends using the whole plant (that is, both root and herbaceous portions). However, while similar, the two plant parts have distinct characteristics. According to the Chinese materia medica, the root of Chinese figwort has heat-clearing and yīn-supplementing qualities. I have found the herb portion to be better for clearing heat and draining damp. For this reason, I tend to use them as two different medicines. Thus, the herb clears heat and drains damp while the root clears heat and supplements yīn. In a case of damp pathogen and extreme or prolonged heat, yīn will be injured, and therefore the choice of herb, root, or both will depend on the duration and severity of the illness as well as the practitioner's formulation preference.

The Costanoan people of the mountain ranges of California's Central Coast used S. californica in various ways. They applied the twigs and leaves as a poultice for swollen sores, boils, sore eyes, and swellings. They used a decoction of the twigs as a disinfectant for sores and the juice of the fresh herb as an eyewash for poor vision. The Kashaya Pomo of the coastal areas of Sonoma County, California, used fresh, warm figwort leaves to bring boils to a head and to draw the pus out of burst boils. The Iroquois of upstate New York and southern Quebec used a decoction of the root of S. lanceolata for various conditions, including hemorrhage and preventing cramps and colds after childbirth. They also used this preparation "for the blood" and for a "sick womb." They used a poultice of figwort root for sunburn, sunstroke, and frostbite.[2]

The name Scrophularia comes from the Latin scrofula, referring to throat glands and their growths. No doubt this relates to figwort's reputation for treating glandular swellings of the throat. This use seems to have been discovered independently for the three main species mentioned here by the cultures associated with each species.

Burdock

Arctium lappa

Asteraceae

Arctii Lappae radix

Other names include lappa; *gobo* **(Japanese for the root);** *niú bang gēn* **(Chinese for the root)**

Flavor and *Qi:* bitter, slightly acrid, cool
Channels Entered: liver, kidney, bladder, stomach
Actions: alterative, antirheumatic, diaphoretic, diuretic, nutritive

Functions and Indications

- *Clears heat, cools the blood, and disperses wind.* Burdock is effective for the treatment of heat in the blood causing skin diseases and rashes such as psoriasis, eczema, and chronic cutaneous eruptions. Burdock is a very important medicinal for the treatment of heat-mediated skin diseases. Because the herb has a gentle action of releasing the exterior, it assists the body in expressing skin conditions, therefore helping to resolve them more quickly. When a warm pathogen enters the body and festers in the lung, it may progress to the construction-blood aspect, and rashes may occur. Burdock has an affinity for the liver and blood and a mild outthrusting action. It directly cools the construction-blood and gently outthrusts the pathogen.

- *Quells fire and clears the liver.* Burdock treats excessive heat in the liver caused by any type of liver disease, including jaundice and hepatitis. Due to burdock's acridity, it gently courses the liver while it directly clears heat, especially heat due to depression and *qi* stagnation. This action is also useful when affect disease leads to stagnation of *qi* and stasis of blood, causing diseases such as mastitis.

- *Clears heat and transforms damp.* Burdock is applied in the treatment of damp heat manifesting

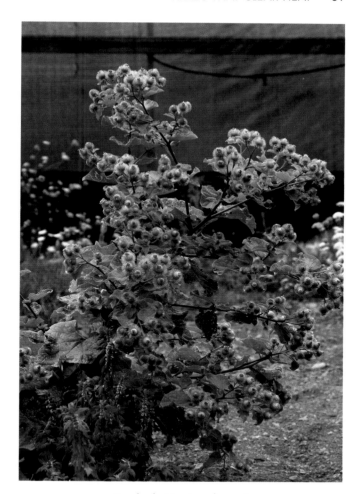

Burdock *(Arctium lappa)*

as damp-heat skin conditions, swollen lymph nodes, lymphedema, strangury, and gout. Burdock's bitter and cool nature clears heat and drains it through the urine. It is very effective at draining heat and dampness and can be used to modify many traditional Chinese formulas.

- *Clears* yīn *vacuity fire.* Burdock is used in the treatment of symptoms associated with *yīn* vacuity fire, including dry stools; scanty, dark urine; blood in urine; mental restlessness; dry throat at night; and a red, peeled tongue. As noted above, burdock enters the construction aspect (i.e., the liver and kidney). Therefore, burdock has a direct action on the liver and kidney and thus can be used to cool these organs. Although viewed as being strong in action, burdock is also considered a food with some nutritive properties. This combination of properties makes it an important medicinal for clearing heat arising from vacuity. However, owing to its overall drying nature, it must be used in formula or it may cause a further decline in *yīn*.

CAUTIONS

Burdock is very safe. However, owing to its gentle outthrusting nature it may, in the short-term, increase the size or number of rashes. This should not be seen as a negative sign, as it only means that the pathogen is being forced out of the body.

Dosage and Preparation

Use 6–15 g in decoction; 2–6 ml tincture; 1–4 g powdered extract.

Tincture of burdock can be made with either fresh or dried material. A decoction is better when treating *yīn* vacuity, as the warming and stimulating alcohol is detrimental to the already vacuous *yīn*.

Good-quality dried root is dark on the outside and whitish on the inside. If you purchase the commonly available cut-and-sifted herb, a small percentage of the material may appear to have webbing, as if infested with bugs. This webbing is the pithy center of the root and is a common "side effect" of the milling process.

Major Combinations

- Combine with dandelion and Oregon grape root for liver-heat or fire. This combination is also excellent for damp-heat in the liver-gallbladder.

- Combine with sarsaparilla and yellow dock for construction-blood-heat with acute rashes or chronic conditions such as psoriasis and eczema.

- Combine with vitex and Oregon grape root for teenage acne.

- Combine with marsh mallow root for *yīn* vacuity heat.

- Combine to modify Mysterious Two Powder (*èr miǎo sàn*) with coix, Chinese skullcap, figwort, and

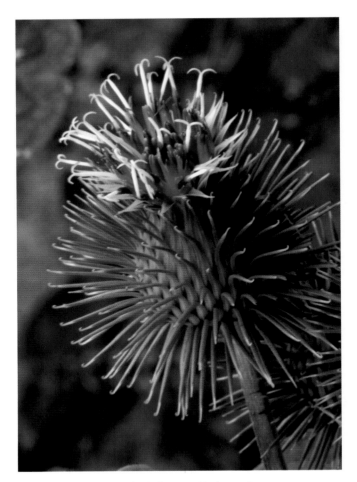

Burdock flower (A. lappa)

ocotillo for damp-heat in the lower burner with swollen lymph nodes; dark, scanty urine; and chronic diarrhea with phlegm in the stool.

Commentary

I've focused here on the therapeutic actions of burdock root only, not the seed. Burdock seed is no longer popular in the West, although it was once found in common use in the United States. Now, it is used primarily by Chinese herbalists. Burdock seed is an excellent remedy for sore throat, fever, and cough. It is also helpful for rashes and other conditions of the skin, especially dry, scratchy, scaly skin. Burdock root, on the other hand, is a famous herb in the West. It is eaten as a food in Japan and also can be purchased in most U.S. natural food stores as such. Burdock is a common weed in localized distribution throughout the United

States. Burdock leaf has a long history of use in Europe as both external and internal medication. Burdock leaf was applied externally to wounds and ulcers, and burdock leaf decoction was taken internally to treat lesions of the gastrointestinal tract. Burdock leaf is strongly antibacterial. To apply fresh leaves externally, beat the leaves to a pulp and apply directly to a wound. Alternately, apply dried, powdered burdock leaf directly to the wound. Culpeper advised using bruised burdock leaf with egg white for the treatment of burns. Culpeper also tells us to beat the root with a little salt and apply it to bites of "serpent" and "mad dogs" to relieve pain.

Various parts of this medicinal are official in the pharmacopoeias of China, France, and Spain. The French pharmacopoeia discusses use of the leaves, and the Chinese pharmacopoeia discusses the seeds and root.

Herbs that Clear Heat and Dry Dampness

Clearing heat and drying dampness refers to the treatment method of drying dampness with cold and bitterness. This category of medicinals is used to treat damp-heat conditions with signs and symptoms such as abdominal pain and distention; thin, hot, putrid-smelling stool; and a yellow tongue coating. Although the herbs in this category do treat dampness, if dampness is a significant portion of the pattern, it may be necessary to combine them with medicinals that treat dampness by disinhibiting or transforming.

This is the most heavily weighted subcategory of heat-clearing medicinals in this text. Goldenseal (*Hydrastis canadensis*) is probably the most famous, and for good reason. Goldenseal is bitter and cold in nature and has a very strong action of both clearing heat and drying dampness. Goldenseal also is good for the treatment of heat evil congestion in the lung, clearing heat and transforming phlegm. Its bitter and cold nature makes it valuable for treating liver-gallbladder damp-heat conditions. Goldenseal is also an important external therapy for various damp-heat conditions.

Oregon grape root (*Mahonia aquifolium* and others) is another important medicinal in this category. Although it is primarily applied in repletion conditions, it can also be used for vacuity heat. Gentian (*Gentiana lutea* and others) is used in essentially the same way as Chinese gentian *(lóng dǎn cǎo),* to clear heat and dry dampness and to treat the liver and gallbladder. Dandelion *(Taraxacum officinale)* is basically analogous to the Chinese dandelion *(pú gōng yīng).* However, since Western herbal medicine generally views dandelion as a treatment for damp-heat conditions, and because this is the way I tend to use the herb, I discuss it here, rather than in the clear-heat and drain-fire subcategory. Like gentian, dandelion is important for treating dampness and heat as well as the liver and gallbladder.

Yellow dock (*Rumex crispus*) has the ability to treat the large intestine in addition to the liver, and thus is useful for the treatment of middle- and lower-burner damp-heat. It also is an important medicinal for the treatment of skin diseases. Globe artichoke (*Cynara scolymus*) is bitter and acrid. Its cold bitterness is very effective for draining damp-heat conditions, especially those associated with the liver and gallbladder. Being acrid, it has a special ability to course stagnant *qì.* Ocotillo *(Fouquieria splendens)* is a lesser known medicinal native to the desert southwest of the United States. Along with clearing heat and drying dampness, it has the special ability to move stagnation, treating both blood stasis and *qì* stagnation.

Goldenseal

Hydrastis canadensis

Ranunculaceae

Hydrastidis Canadensitis rhizoma

Flavor and *Qi:* bitter, cold

Channels Entered: heart, liver, lung, gallbladder, stomach, large intestine

Actions: antibacterial, antifungal, anti-inflammatory, anticatarrhal, astringent, cholagogue

Functions and Indications

- ***Clears heat and dries dampness.*** Goldenseal is used to treat damp-heat dysenteric disorders in the intestines and stomach and damp-heat affecting the intestines, with symptoms such as hemorrhoids, fissured anus, and prolapsed anus with ulcerations. Goldenseal is also used for stomach-heat causing stomach pain, nausea, vomiting, pyorrhea alveolaris, gingivitis with or without bleeding, and malodorous breath. Goldenseal's bitter (draining) and cold (heat-clearing) actions are very strong and make it exceptional for the treatment of damp-heat disorders, especially of the stomach and intestines. This is the most important use of this medicinal, and as such, it can be compared with, combined with, or used as a substitute for Chinese coptis or phellodendron in many cases.

- ***Clears heat and transforms phlegm.*** Goldenseal is employed in the treatment of phlegm-heat obstructing the lungs with symptoms of cough; abundant, malodorous yellow, green, or dark sputum; thick, sticky,

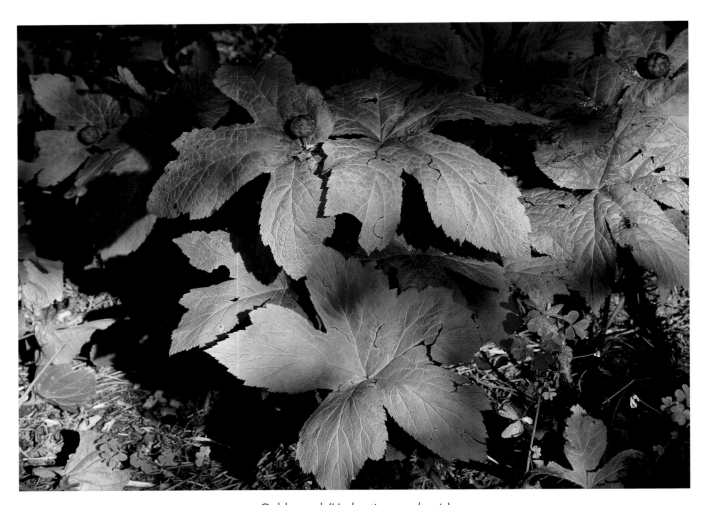

Goldenseal *(Hydrastis canadensis)*

yellow tongue coating; and a rapid, slippery pulse. Goldenseal's strong action of clearing and draining away heat, and its ability to transform phlegm, make it excellent for conditions in which heat is predominate and has scorched the fluids, creating phlegm. It is also useful when phlegm-heat obstructs the nasal passages.

- *Clears damp-heat obstruction of the liver and gall-bladder channels.* Goldenseal is helpful for liver and gallbladder damp-heat with symptoms such as pain in the hypochondriac, flank, and genital areas; jaundice and other damp-heat symptoms such as itching in the genital area; heat or burning in the lower urinary tract or vagina; warmth and pain in the liver area; constipation or diarrhea; and dark, malodorous urine with or without burning. Goldenseal is also useful for heat and dampness lodged in the channels with generalized muscle aches. By strongly clearing heat and draining dampness, goldenseal improves the function of the liver and helps it to rectify the *qi* dynamic when it has been obstructed by the presence of damp-heat.

- *Clears heat and resolves fire-toxin.* Goldenseal is applied externally as a powder, wash, or douche for the treatment of many heat and toxin disorders, including conjunctivitis, bacterial vaginosis, vaginitis, cervicitis, athlete's foot, and abrasions. Goldenseal's bitter and cold nature makes it extremely valuable for external application. Because this medicinal is so valuable as an external application, it can be used in nearly any situation where there is heat, damp-heat, or toxic heat accumulation. Be sure to inform the patient that this herb will stain anything, including skin, a yellow-orange color.

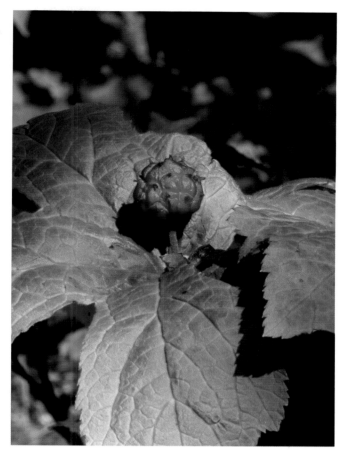

Goldenseal fruit *(H. canadensis)*

CAUTIONS

Goldenseal strongly clears heat and dries damp, so both patterns must be present when using this herb. Do not use goldenseal on a long-term basis. Use with caution for those with spleen *qi* vacuity. This herb is best avoided during pregnancy, especially in the first trimester. Nursing mothers should also avoid use.

Dosage and Preparation

Use 2–6 g in decoction (up to 10 g may be used); 1–4 ml tincture. Goldenseal is best used as a tincture or draft (a simple tea made by putting the powdered medicinal into hot water and drinking the entire cup, powder and all); however, it is effective as a decoction.

Good-quality goldenseal is cultivated. Dried root should be firm to hard and a dark yellow to golden color with few rootlets. The taste of the root is sharply bitter and slightly astringent.

Major Combinations

- Combine with boneset and bupluerum for liver-gallbladder damp-heat with symptoms such as alternating heat effusion and aversion to cold, bitter taste in the mouth, nausea and vomiting, rib or side pain, and dark yellow or reddish urine. This is *shào-yáng* disease, as described in the *Shāng Hán Lùn.*

- Combine with rhubarb for damp-heat in the intestines with abscess, constipation, diarrhea, and/or foul gas.

- Combine with California figwort, red root, and cleavers for phlegm-heat nodules in the neck or inguinal area. Add ocotillo for nodules in the inguinal area.

- Combine with Chinese skullcap and magnolia buds for purulent nasal discharge and blockage of sinuses by phlegm-heat.

- Combine with coptis, aucklandia, and Western sweet cicely for damp-heat patterns, with or without bleeding, of the middle and lower burner, with symptoms of acid regurgitation, diarrhea, vaginal discharge, and scanty yellow urine.

- Combine with gentian for damp-heat patterns in the liver and gallbladder channels with symptoms of jaundice; pain, swelling, or dampness in the genital area; or itchiness in the genital area.

Commentary

Goldenseal was known to white settlers of North America and was exported to England as early as 1759. It was not until 1852, when the herb appeared in the *Eclectic Dispensatory of the United States of America,* that goldenseal was used extensively in professional medicine.

Goldenseal is the "yellow of preference" in Western herbalism. Its medicinal properties can be compared to those of both Chinese skullcap and coptis. Unlike the Chinese yellows, however, goldenseal does not necessarily have a preference for any particular burner and can be used equally in any of the three, as one can see from the functions and indications listed here. Goldenseal is best used as a tincture, as many of the constituents are only slightly or not at all water soluble. Although goldenseal infusions and decoctions have a long history of use in the Native American tradition and are effective, I recommend using a properly prepared tincture.

The Eclectics used goldenseal for boggy, atonic mucous membranes with a tendency to oversecrete, bleed, or develop low-grade infections. This speaks to the Greek and Latin origins of the name *Hydrastis,* meaning to stop the flow of water.

This plant is in serious danger in its wild habitat and has been cultivated only recently. For these reasons, I urge you to use goldenseal only from cultivated sources. Goldenseal's environmental sensitivity was noted as early as 1898 in *King's American Dispensatory,* in which Felter and Lloyd state, "the plant disappears as soon as the ground is disturbed by the settler."

Goldenseal was listed in *The United States Pharmacopoeia* from 1831–1842 and listed there as official from 1863–1936; it was also listed in *The National Formulary (U.S.)* from 1936–1960. Goldenseal is currently official in the pharmacopoeias of Britian, Argentina, Belgium, Brazil, Egypt, France, Mexico, Portugal, Romania, and Spain.

Oregon Grape Root

Mahonia aquifolium and others
(formerly *Berberis* spp.)

Berberidaceae

Mahoniae cortex seu radicis

Flavor and *Qi*: bitter, cool
Channels Entered: liver, gallbladder, kidney, stomach, small intestine, large intestine
Actions: antimicrobial, bitter tonic, liver stimulant

Functions and Indications

- ***Clears heat and drains damp from the middle burner.*** Oregon grape is useful for symptoms such as warmth and pain in the epigastric and hypochondriac areas; reduced appetite; nausea; regurgitation; heartburn; constipation; mild diarrhea (damp-heat invading the spleen); bloating after meals with difficulty digesting fats and protein; conjunctivitis; foul breath with a thick, yellow tongue coating; and a replete, rapid pulse. The herb is also used for damp-heat in the intestines when heat is the predominant sign. This is marked by malodorous diarrhea or constipation; bloody stools; dark, malodorous urine; stuffiness in the epigastric and chest area; abdominal pain; intestinal abscess; fever; mental restlessness or muddled thinking; a red tongue with a sticky, yellow coat; and a rapid, slippery pulse. Oregon grape's bitter and cooling nature effectively drains and cools heat while draining damp from the middle burner.

- ***Clears heat.*** Oregon grape root can be effectively employed to treat heat, either from vacuity or repletion, when the heat has dried up body fluids, causing dry skin, dry mouth, bleeding gums or nose, red eyes, red tongue with or without a yellow coat, and a pulse that is rapid and either thready and weak or full and forceful, depending on the condition. Although Oregon grape root is bitter and cool, effectively treating replete heat, it also is appropriate for vacuity heat. It is enriching and often a first choice when I am

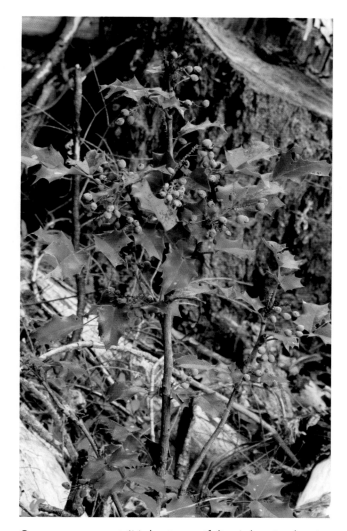

Oregon grape root *(Mahonia aquifolium)* showing berries

treating vacuity heat. I prefer to use the whole root, instead of only the root bark, for this indication. This is not always possible when purchasing the medicinal from a purveyor, but this remains a medicinal that I enjoy harvesting for myself. Furthermore, sometimes "lower quality" material (i.e., whole root) is available when harvesters are too lazy to peel the bark from the root. This could work to your advantage if you wish to use the herb this way.

- ***Clears heat and dries dampness.*** Oregon grape is applied externally as a wash or dusting powder for skin conditions caused by heat or damp-heat. Like many other herbs in this category, Oregon grape root can be used externally to good effect. Prepared

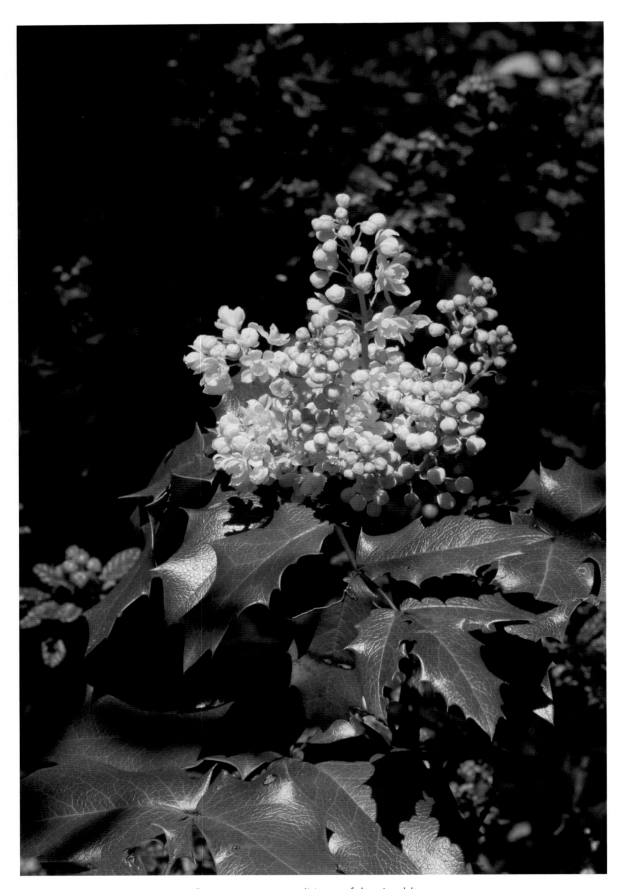

Oregon grape root *(M. aquifolium)* in bloom

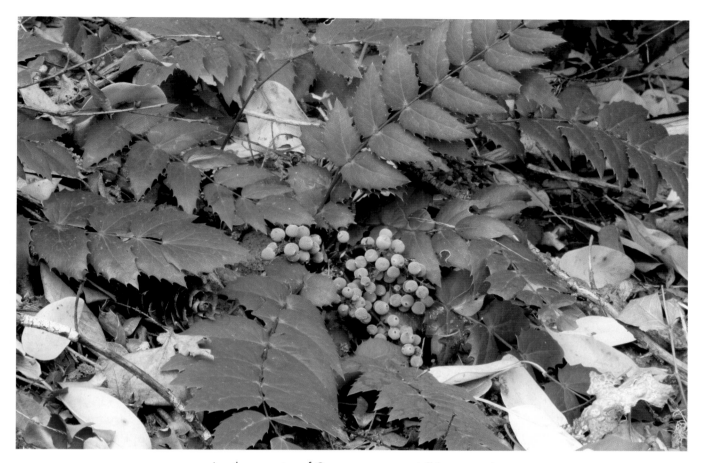

Another species of Oregon grape root (M. nervosa)

as a sitz bath or douche, Oregon grape root is useful for damp-heat vaginal conditions with yellow, malodorous excretions. Prepare Oregon grape leaf as an infused oil and apply externally to clear heat and resolve toxicity for abrasions. This product is cooling and effectively clears heat from the skin on contact.

<hr>

CAUTIONS

Oregon grape root is not for long-term use. Use with caution in weak, vacuous people who have signs of cold.

<hr>

Dosage and Preparation

Use 3–9 g in decoction; 2–4 ml tincture; 0.5–2 ml fluidextract.

Tincture or fluidextract prepared from recently dried root bark is the preferred preparation, although a decoction is best for use in patients who have *yīn* vacu-

ity with dryness. Oregon grape leaf can be prepared as a salve or cream for external use.

Good-quality dried material consists of the root and stem bark only. This should be dark yellow to almost orange. The whole root can be used when the core is yellow. Much of the commercially available Oregon grape root is whole root, often including stem pieces. The most important qualities to examine are the color—the deeper yellow the better—and the bitter flavor.

Major Combinations

- Combine with marsh mallow for stomach heat with symptoms of stomach pain, heartburn, and acid reflux.

- Combine with gentian and lavender for damp-heat in the middle burner with bloating after eating, foul gas and belching, and a thick yellow coating on the tongue.

- Combine with yellow dock, Chinese skullcap, and gardenia for liver-gallbladder damp-heat; add dandelion leaf if damp is the predominate pathogen.

- Combine with burdock for various skin conditions associated with heat, such as acne rosacea, eczema, psoriasis, and simple acne.

Commentary

Although the genus name for Oregon grape was changed from *Berberis* to *Mahonia* some years ago, some confusion persists about this plant's classification. *Berberis* is an ancient Arabic name for barberry. *Mahonia,* with a name given to honor the Irish American botanist Bernard MacMahon, was once considered a group within the *Berberis* genus, but now the two are grouped in separate genera. There are two distinct differences between them. *Mahonia* plants have spiny leaf margins; *Berberis* do not. The fruit of *Berberis* plants contains two to three seeds, while *Mahonia* fruits contain three to nine seeds. Together, the combined genera contain approximately six hundred species.

Oregon grape is a very abundant plant in the Pacific Northwest of the United States. It is a pioneer plant and one of the first to colonize an area after logging companies have raped the acres of forest for timber. The plant's abundance makes it an excellent and sustainable plant for use in herbal medicine. Beyond that, it has a long history of use and appears to be very safe. I have found it dependable and highly recommend it for clearing heat. In addition, I have found it to be safe and effective for clearing *yīn* vacuity heat without damaging the *yīn;* I liken it to Chinese phellodendron for this purpose. Not only does Oregon grape effectively clear vacuity heat, it also assists the construction *qì*, thus building structure within *yīn*.

Native Americans of the Pacific Northwest had other uses for the plant in addition to medicinal applications. They boiled the root to make a yellow dye for basketry and clothing. They collected the ripe fruits and ate them in various preparations, either raw or cooked. The berries were rarely preserved by drying, and some tribes considered them poison. The fruit is quite sour, which may explain why some considered it poisonous. However, the berries can be boiled to make a fine jelly.

Various species of this medicinal were official in *The United States Pharmacopoeia* and *The National Formulary (U.S.)* from the mid-nineteenth through the mid-twentieth centuries. *Mahonia aquifolium* was listed as official in the *British Herbal Pharmacopoeia* (1983). One of the major chemical constituents, berberine, is listed as official in the pharmacopoeias of China, India, and Japan.

Translation of Source Material

Chinese medicine uses a number of species of *Mahonia*, which are divided into three main groups. The first—*shí dà gōng láo yè (M. bealei, M. fortunei, M. japonica)*—is bitter and cool and enters the lung channel. This medicinal clears heat, supplements vacuity, and transforms phlegm. It is used to treat vacuity heat, taxation cough with phlegm and bleeding, steaming bone tidal fever, dizziness and tinnitus, aching lumbus and limp legs, weak knees, heart vexation, red eyes, dizziness, tinnitus, and infestation of worms. One source *(xiàn dài shí yòng zhōng yào)* states the medicinal is "cool and clearing, enriching and strengthening herb, actions are similar to Ligustri fructus, suitable for tidal fever, steaming bone, aching lumbar, weak knees, dizziness, tinnitus, and similar disorders." Other sources attribute functions such as draining fire and reducing fever; treating warm diseases with fever, heart vexation, diarrhea, and red eyes; treating warm heat dysentery; treating red, swollen, and painful eyes; and treating swelling and toxin of welling-abscesses and sores. The wide range of actions given here may be related somewhat to the fact that several species are listed as one medicinal.

Mù huáng lián represents another group of *Mahonia* plants used in Chinese medicine (*M. shenii, M. schochii, M. subimbricata,* and *M. taronensis*). This medicinal is bitter and cold and enters the heart and liver channels. It clears heart and stomach fire and resolves toxin. It is used in the treatment of yellow jaundice, heat dysentery, and red eyes. It is also applied externally for knife wounds, burns, and scalds. The Chinese name literally means "tree coptis," apparently because it has uses similar to those for coptis.

Cì huáng bǎi (M. gracilipes, M. ganpinensis, and *M. fortunei)* is a third group of *Mahonia* plants used in Chinese medicine. *Cì huáng bǎi* is bitter and cool. It clears heat and disperses fire, disperses swelling, and stops pain, and is employed to treat liver-fire, mouth and tongue sores, painful urination, and burns and scalds.

Note: The name *Cì huáng bǎi* is used for three groups of medicinals. The other groups are from the *Berberis* genus, which is closely related to *Mahonia*.

Gentian

Gentiana lutea, G. calycosa, **and others**

Gentianaceae

Gentianae Luteae radix

I dub it *xīlóng dǎn* **or Western gentian**

Flavor and *Qì:* bitter, cold
Channels Entered: liver, gallbladder, stomach
Actions: bitter tonic

Functions and Indications

- *Clears heat and transforms dampness.* Gentian is used in a variety of damp-heat conditions, including damp-heat in the spleen and stomach causing symptoms such as dyspepsia, gastritis, borborygmus, difficulty digesting fats, heartburn, nausea and vomiting; damp-heat brewing in the liver and gallbladder with jaundice, hepatitis and flank pain; damp-heat pouring down into the bladder with frequent, urgent, painful yellow-red urination; damp-heat pouring down into the large intestine with tenesmus and pus in the stool; and also for damp-heat skin problems, such as eczema. Gentian's bitter and cold nature strongly treats damp-heat conditions, especially those associated with the liver-gallbladder system. Whether damp-heat affects the channels or organ systems, gentian enters them and its coldness and bitterness will clear and drain.

- *Clears heat from the gallbladder and restores the downbearing function of the stomach in the treatment of* **shào-yáng** *diseases.* Gentian treats *shào-yáng* disease with symptoms such as nausea, loss of appetite, dull facial expression, and fullness in the costal and hypochondriac regions. These symptoms occur when evil heat enters the gallbladder and impairs the *qì* dynamic. When gallbladder heat rises, the stomach *qì* is not able to downbear. With its bitter and cold nature, gentian clears heat from the gallbladder and, secondarily, the stomach, thus helping to restore the healthy upbearing and downbearing functions of

these organs. This is, of course, only one part of the treatment needed, as this stage of disease calls for harmonization. Therefore, complete resolution of the condition will require combining gentian with herbs that support right *qì*.

CAUTIONS

Do not use gentian in the absence of replete heat. Use with caution in those with spleen-stomach *qì* vacuity.

Dosage and Preparation

Use 3–6 g in decoction; 2–3 ml tincture. When using as a bitter tonic, 5–20 drops are sufficient.

Gather gentian root in the autumn after the aerial parts have died back for the winter. It can be sliced for fresh plant tincture, or sliced, dried, and stored for future use. Good-quality dried material is tan to light brown in color and firm. The flavor in the mouth should be decidedly bitter.

Major Combinations

- Combine with yellow dock, Oregon grape root, and Western sweet cicely for damp-heat in the middle and lower burners with symptoms of poor appetite, constipation, dark urine, and a greasy, yellow tongue coating. For more severe constipation, add buckthorn bark.

- Combine with wild yam for nausea, loss of appetite, dull facial expression, and fullness in the costal and hypochondriac regions associated with *shào-yáng* diseases.

Commentary

Gentiana lutea is analogous to the several species known in Chinese medicine as *lóng dǎn.* It can be substituted in any Chinese formula for *lóng dǎn* and, with organic root available on the Western herb market, it makes good sense to employ this substitution.

Gentian is a classic bitter tonic and, when taken

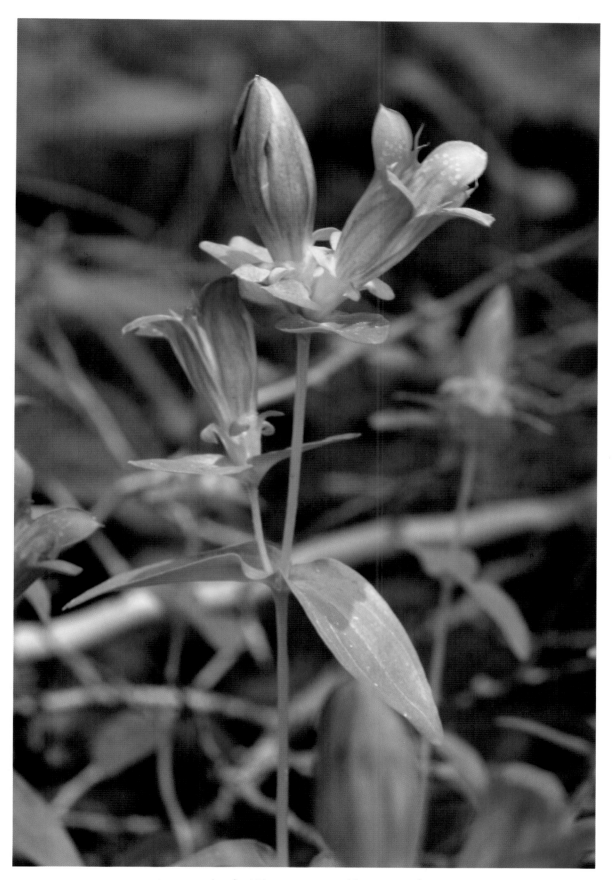

An example of a Western gentian *(Gentiana calycosa)*

in small doses before meals, acts as a stimulant for the digestion. The herb is found in most bitter tonic formulas in the West. The bitter flavor increases appetite and gets the digestive secretions flowing to enhance assimilation of food. This is particularly useful in cases of spleen-liver disharmony as well as spleen dampness and liver depression. When combined with warm herbs such as ginger, cardamom, and others, the bitter flavor remains essential, but the warmth of the formula offsets the coldness of the gentian. This is important, since the pure bitter of gentian can be overstimulating to the digestion and overly cold to the spleen, thus doing more damage than good. Combining it as described makes use of gentian's ability to move damp-heat that can accumulate underneath a vacuity-damp condition. When using gentian as a bitter tonic, be sure to remember that bitter tonics are meant to jump-start the digestive process, not feed it. Thus, such formulas should not be used for vacuity patterns or for extended periods of time.

Several other species of *Gentiana* are used in Western herbal medicine in both Europe and North America. *G. lutea* was official in *The United States Pharmacopoeia* from 1820–1955 and in *The National Formulary (U.S.)* from 1955–1965. An American species, *G. catesbaei,* was official in *The United States Pharmacopoeia* from 1820–1882. *G. lutea* is official in the pharmacopoeias of Argentina, Austria, Britian, the Czech Republic, Egypt, France, Germany, Hungary, Italy, Japan, the Netherlands, Poland, Portugal, Romania, Scandinavia, Spain, and Switzerland. Other species are listed as official in the pharmacopoeias of China, Japan (*G. scabra* only), Austria, the Czech Republic, and Hungary.

Many other species are employed in bioregional practice in the United States and in other parts of the world where any of the three hundred or so species of this genus grows. Many have more or less the same functions and indications. One species I have used and like a great deal is *G. calycosa*, which is native to the northwestern United States. It seems to have all the qualities of the other species mentioned, but is a bit stronger than most of the other species I have used. This may be due in part to the fact that I can get it in a fresher state. Also, I prefer the fresh plant tincture of this species to the tinctures I have made with any other *Gentiana* species, fresh or dried. Would someone please learn to grow it!

Dandelion

Taraxacum officinale

Asteraceae

Taraxaci Officinale planta

Flavor and *Qi*: bitter, cool
Channels Entered: liver, stomach, bladder
Actions: antirheumatic, cholagogue, diuretic, laxative

Functions and Indications

- **Clears heat and drains dampness.** Dandelion is helpful in the treatment of damp-heat jaundice or other damp-heat conditions affecting the middle or lower burner. It is also used for damp-heat rashes. Dandelion is a simple bitter and cool medicinal. Its bitter flavor drains heat and dampness, while its cooling nature makes it an effective herb in the treatment of various damp-heat conditions, especially those associated with the liver and gallbladder.

- **Clears heat, drains dampness, and resolves impediments.** Dandelion treats damp-heat impediment and is employed as an adjunctive treatment for hot, swollen, painful joints. As an adjunctive treatment, dandelion works best when this syndrome presents a specific picture. Things to look for in this case are elevated cholesterol levels, elevated estrogen with PMS symptoms (especially anger), edema, and sugar cravings. As mentioned above, the bitter and cool nature of this medicinal makes it very good at draining and clearing heat from the liver. The liver is in charge of the free flow of *qi*; thus, if overheated, this function is

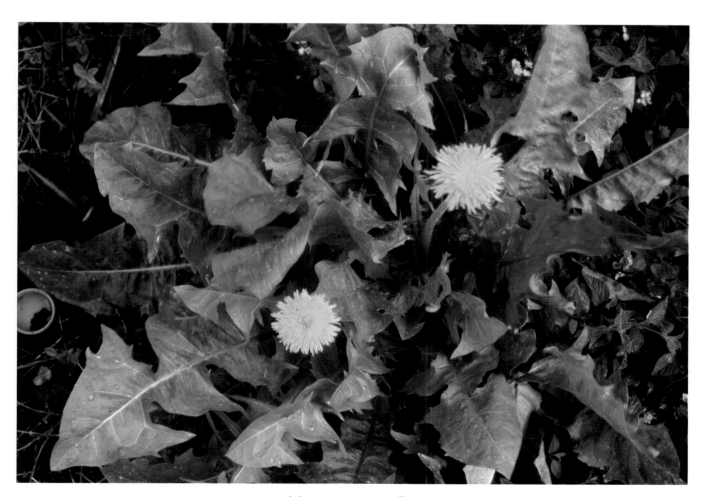

Dandelion *(Taraxacum officinale)*

impaired, leading to stagnation and stasis, which lead to heat accumulation. Furthermore, the liver is in charge of the sinews, which lead to and surround the joints. An overtaxed liver cannot properly nourish the sinews, leading to contracture and pain. Dandelion is well suited for the treatment of such damp-heat impediment.

CAUTIONS

Dandelion is a relatively safe herb, but it should be used with caution by those with *yáng* vacuity.

Dosage and Preparation

Use 3–9 g in decoction; 3–6 ml tincture.

Good-quality dried herb has dark green leaves. The dried root should have a dark, brownish-black coating and be grayish-white on the inside. The root should be firm and hard, not pithy or soft. If the whole plant is used, it should not contain more than 5 percent by weight of flower- or seed heads. Note that the flower generally will mature after it is picked, reducing an otherwise bright yellow flower into a fluffy white mass of pappus.

Major Combinations

- Combine with yellow dock for depressed heat with symptoms such as headache, red eyes, constipation, reddish urine, red tongue with a yellow coat, and rapid, replete pulse.

- Combine with yellow dock and burdock root for damp-heat rashes.

- Combine with corn silk and goldenseal for bladder damp-heat, with or without stones.

- Combine to modify Eight Corrections Powder *(bā zhèng sàn)* to more strongly clear heat and drain dampness with dark, turbid urination.

- Combine to modify Impediment Diffusing Decoction *(xuān bì tāng)* for hot, swollen, red, painful joints.

Commentary

Dandelion is a very important herb for the liver. In fact, Western herbalists perceive this plant as specific for the liver. Chinese herbalists, on the other hand, tend to view this medicinal as useful for clearing heat and toxins without a specific affinity for any organ, even though many texts list liver as a channel entered by this medicinal. In Western herbalism, dandelion is used in almost all liver conditions or conditions associated with the liver. It is considered hepatoprotective and a hepatic trophorestorative.[3]

Dandelion increases bile flow and cools the liver. The plant is diuretic, especially the leaves, and is used for urinary problems associated with inflammatory conditions. Dandelion leaf functions as a potassium-sparing diuretic. This property makes the herb especially valuable for treating edema associated with congestive heart failure, as well as PMS-related water-weight gain.

Fresh dandelion leaves are commonly sold in health food stores as a green vegetable. They traditionally have been eaten as a spring green to cleanse the body after a sedentary winter of heavy eating. The greens have a flavor similar to kale and are an excellent source of nutrients, particularly trace minerals. The roots of dandelion and a relative, chicory *(Cichorium intybus)*, can be roasted and used as a coffee substitute. The two are often combined with other roasted roots to make a pleasant tea for those trying to move away from coffee. Although the roasted root is not as cooling to the liver as raw root, it can help resolve liver *qì* or liver depression, a common problem for those addicted to coffee. The flower, which is high in lutein and beneficial for the eyes, can be made into a traditional wine, a delightful preparation.

A related species, *T. japonicum,* could be a valuable chemopreventive agent against chemical carcinogenesis. In a laboratory study, an extract of the roots of *T. japonicum* showed strong anti-tumor-promoting activities. Furthermore, the extract exhibited anti-tumor-initiating activity on two-stage carcinogenesis.[4] It is likely that our species could be used in the same manner.

Our dandelion and the Chinese species are analogous. The main advantage in using the Western species is the availability of higher quality herb; organically grown *T. officinale* is available.

Dandelion root was official in *The United States Pharmacopoeia* from 1831–1926 and in *The National Formulary (U.S.)* from 1888–1965. *T. officinale* is official in the pharmacopoeias of Austria, Hungary, and Poland. Other species of *Taraxacum* are official in China and the Czech Republic.

Yellow Dock

Rumex crispus

Polygonaceae

Rumex Crispii radix

Other names include curly dock and *niú ěr dà huáng*

Flavor and *Qi:* bitter, slightly cold
Channels Entered: liver, gallbladder, large intestine
Actions: astringent, liver stimulant, mild laxative

Functions and Indications

- *Courses the liver, disinhibits bile, clears heat, and drains dampness.* Yellow dock effectively treats damp-heat brewing in the liver and gallbladder, with symptoms such as epigastric fullness, pain in the chest, constipation, malodorous flatulence, and jaundice. Yellow dock is also used for damp-heat affecting the skin. This is an important herb for the treatment of liver-depression patterns with heat. Its bitter flavor courses the liver and disinhibits bile, thus allowing for a restored liver-gallbladder *qi* dynamic. Its bitter and slightly cold nature effectively clears heat and drains dampness, primarily via the bowels.

- *Clears heat and cools the blood.* Yellow dock is employed in the treatment of heat in the blood causing chronic rashes and other types of chronic skin lesions. Although yellow dock has an action on the blood, its main action is in clearing damp-heat and resolving toxins due to brewing damp-heat. Therefore, it is best for treating wet, oozy skin conditions. When damp-heat brews internally for an extended period of time, the heat can enter the blood and cause skin rashes, nosebleeds, and blood in the urine and stool. Yellow dock's bitter and slightly cold nature enters the blood and effectively clears heat from the blood aspect. As noted, this is not its primary function; however, it is an important medicine when treating blood-heat and should not be forgotten.

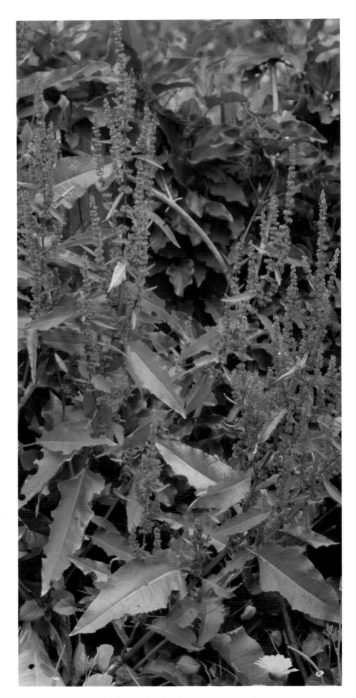

Yellow dock *(Rumex crispus)*

- *Clears heat and drains fire for liver-fire invading the lungs.* Yellow dock is helpful for liver-fire invading the lung with symptoms of coughing up yellow sputum, constipation, and fullness in the chest. Because this medicinal courses the liver and drains fire, it works exceptionally well for this pattern, but is ineffective for other types of cough. It is also employed to

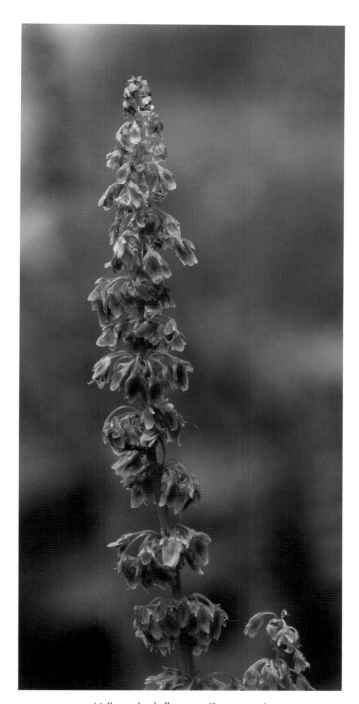

Yellow dock flowers *(R. crispus)*

treat heat-type diarrhea. For this purpose, it should be decocted for a longer period of time.

CAUTIONS

Use yellow dock with caution in *qì* or *yáng* vacuity.

Dosage and Preparation

Use 3–9 g in light decoction; 2–4 ml tincture.

Good-quality dried yellow dock root is dark yellow to orange, firm to hard, and bitter to the taste.

Major Combinations

- Combine with burdock root and *dāng guī* for silver-scale disease *(yín xié bìng)*.[5]

- Combine with *dāng guī* and hemp seed for dry, bound stools due to blood vacuity.

- Combine with mulberry root bark and bamboo shavings for liver-fire invading the lungs with coughing of yellow sputum, constipation, and fullness in the chest.

Commentary

Yellow dock is an extremely common plant and in fact is considered a weed in many places. You may have noticed fields sporting a copper tinge due to the presence of drying yellow dock stems with rust-colored seeds. The stalk stands about 0.5 to 1 meter tall (1.5–3 feet). Yellow dock seeds are generally abundant, and the plant often will pervade an open field.

Yellow dock has a history of use as a source of iron. Midwives commonly use it to treat anemia. In her book, *Wise Woman Herbal for the Childbearing Year,* Susun Weed says, "The yellow roots . . . prepared as a decoction, syrup, or tincture, provide an excellent, fully absorbable, non-constipating source of iron." She goes on to say that the roots "replenish hemoglobin after a hemorrhage."

Along with nettle and dandelion leaves, yellow dock leaves are sometimes incorporated into herbal vinegars high in minerals, particularly potassium and magnesium, as well as vitamin C. These vinegars can be used for cooking and to make salad dressings. Yellow dock leaves are an excellent topical remedy for contact dermatitis *(jiē chù xìng pǐ yán)* caused by nettle sting.[6] Crush the leaves and rub them on the affected area. This will cool the burning sensation and help to relieve the inflammation.

A related dock species sometimes used as medicine is bitter dock *(R. obtusifolius)*. This species is very similar in appearance to yellow dock, but has broader leaves without wavy edges. In addition, the inflorescence is sparser, and the plant's branches leave the main stem at wider angles. The two species do intermingle and cross, so character traits of both species might be seen within a single plant. This does not seem to adversely affect the quality of the medicine in the root. Generally, however, I prefer *R. crispus* as a medicinal, because over the years I have noticed that *R. obtusifolius* root more frequently tends to be pale yellow or even to lack yellow pigment entirely. Such roots are poor-quality medicine and should be discarded.

Yellow dock's species designation, *crispus*, tells us of its curled leaves. The genus name, *Rumex*, likely is derived from the Indo-European word *rumos*, meaning sour or bitter, in reference to its sour leaves and bitter root. Garden sorrel *(R. acetosa)*, a common culinary plant, hails from the same region of the world and is known for its sour and slightly bitter leaves.

At least seven other species of *Rumex* were used by Native Americans for similar purposes. These include the endemic Hawaiian plant *R. giganteus (pāwale)*, which was combined with other herbs to serve as a blood purifier.[7] The related *R. japonicum (yáng tí)* is mentioned in the *Divine Husbandman's Materia Medica Classic*. The author(s) of this ancient text said that the herb was bitter and cold and effective mainly in treating baldness and itchy scabs, eliminating fever, and, in females, healing genital erosion.[8] In Chinese medicine, yellow dock is considered a prominent medicinal in the northwestern regions of the country, but a lesser medicine in the dominant eastern part of the country.

From the time of the ancient Greeks to the present day, yellow dock has held a strong place in Western herbology. *R. obtusifolius* was official in *The United States Pharmacopoeia* (1820–1905); *R. crispus* was official in *The United States Pharmacopoeia* (1863–1905) and in *The National Formulary (U.S.)*, (1916–1936).

Translation of Source Material

Chinese medicine uses several species of *Rumex* in medicine, including the main medicinal described in the above monograph, which is called *niú ěr dà huáng (R. crispus* and *R. nepalensis)*. It is bitter and cold, and enters the heart, liver, and large intestine channels. The medicinal clears heat and cools blood, transforms phlegm and settles cough, frees the stool and kills worms. It is used to treat acute hepatitis, chronic bronchitis, blood ejection, flooding (profuse uterine bleeding), dry bound stool, dysentery, scab and lichen, clove sore, and boils.

Tǔ dà huáng (Rumex madaio) is acrid, bitter, and cool; it clears heat, moves stasis, kills worms, and resolves toxin. It is used to treat coughing with blood, lung welling-abscess, mumps, bound stool, swelling and toxin of welling-abscess, eczema, scab and lichen, pain from knocks and falls, and burns and scalds.

Niú xī xī (Rumex patientia) is bitter, sour, and cold. It clears heat, resolves toxin, quickens the blood, stops bleeding, frees the stool, and kills worms. The medicinal is employed to treat dysentery, chronic enteritis, pain of knocks and falls, internal bleeding, dry bound stool and constipation, scab and lichen, welling-abscess and sore, purulent blister sores, and burns and scalds.

Globe Artichoke

Cynara scolymus

Asteraceae

Cynarae Scolymi folium

Also called common artichoke

Flavor and *Qi:* bitter, acrid, cold
Channels Entered: liver, gallbladder, stomach
Actions: anticholestatic, antiemetic, bitter tonic, cholagogue, choleretic, depurative, diuretic, hepatoprotective, hepatic trophorestorative, hypocholesterolemic

Functions and Indications

- ***Courses the liver, resolves depression, disinhibits bile, clears heat, and transforms dampness.*** Globe artichoke is used to treat liver-gallbladder damp-heat patterns with rib or side pain, nausea, vomiting, sensation of fullness, and abdominal pain. Artichoke is also used for other damp-heat conditions, including spleen-stomach damp-heat and bladder damp-heat. This is an extraordinarily important medicinal for the treatment of liver depression and associated liver-gallbladder damp-heat. Artichoke courses the liver, disinhibiting bile, and transforms dampness with its acridity. It strongly clears and drains heat with its bitter and cold nature.

- ***Harmonizes the* shào-yáng.** Artichoke gently releases the exterior while clearing internal heat, leading the pathogen back out whence it came. Furthermore, artichoke supports the right, and thus is well suited to treat *shào-yáng* disharmony. Pathogens lodged in the *shào-yáng* are neither internal nor external. The pathogen enters the gallbladder through the

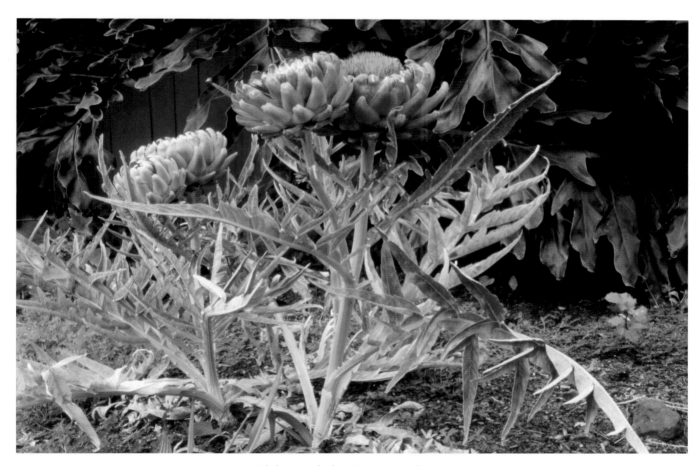

Globe artichoke *(Cynara scolymus)*

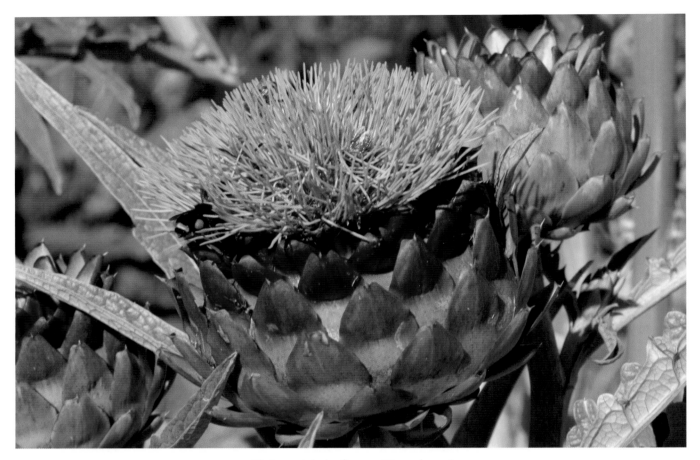

Globe artichoke flower *(C. scolymus)*

interstices, disrupting the *qì* dynamic and causing binding. This calls for harmonization, including outthrusting the pathogen, clearing the interior, regulating the *qì* dynamic, and supporting right *qì*. Artichoke's *qì* is cold; therefore, it also can be applied in a combined *shào-yáng–yáng-míng* pattern.

CAUTIONS

Do not use artichoke if there is obstruction of the bile ducts. Use with caution in patients with gallstones.

Dosage and Preparation

3–9 g in decoction; 1–3 ml tincture; 0.5–2 ml fluidextract.

Tincture made with fresh plant is the preferred preparation, especially for short-term use. A decoction is best for more chronic conditions in which there is a long history of depressed liver and impaired function. Good-quality dried herb is gray-green and hairy and contains little stem. It should be slightly aromatic and strongly acrid and bitter.

Major Combinations

- Combine with gentian and bupleurum for binding depression of liver *qì* with depressive fire.

- Modify Minor Bupleurum Decoction *(xiāo chái hú tāng)* with artichoke for *shào-yáng* disorders, especially when there is replete heat or concurrent damp-heat.

- Modify Major Bupleurum Decoction *(dà chái hú tāng)* with artichoke for combined *shào-yáng–yáng-míng* disorders.

- Combine with curcuma *(yù jīn)* and cyperus for binding depression of liver *qì* with depressive heat and symptoms such as rib or side pain, vexation and pain in the chest, exaggerated emotional responses, and a wiry pulse.

Commentary

Artichoke is used primarily for damp-heat conditions; it can also be used for heat without dampness. Because it is both bitter and acrid, artichoke clears heat and drains damp as well as courses liver *qi*. These qualities make it an important herb for treating brewing damp-heat that obstructs the *qi* dynamic. This is likely why artichoke is one of the most popular bitter tonics in Europe. However, most bitter tonics do not have the liver-coursing action of artichoke leaf. (For more information on bitter tonics, please see the commentary for gentian.) Artichoke's *qi* is cold. Its effectiveness as a liver-coursing medicinal makes it particularly useful in many conditions in which the liver *qi* is depressed, leading to heat or even fire.

Globe artichoke has been a revered vegetable since ancient times. In the fourth century BCE, Theophrastus described it as "a plant whose head is a particular pleasant food, both boiled and raw, but especially when it is in blossom." Like milk thistle, the water extracts of the leaf and root promote regeneration of the liver. The root has shown promise as a supplementing medicinal, but I do not have enough experience with it yet to offer valid clinical information.

Artichoke is listed as official in the pharmacopoeias of Brazil, France, Romania; the *British Herbal Pharmacopoeia* (1996); and *Martindale: The Extra Pharmacopoeia* (33rd ed.); and is approved by the German Commission E. It is also listed in *PDR for Herbal Medicines* (2nd ed.).

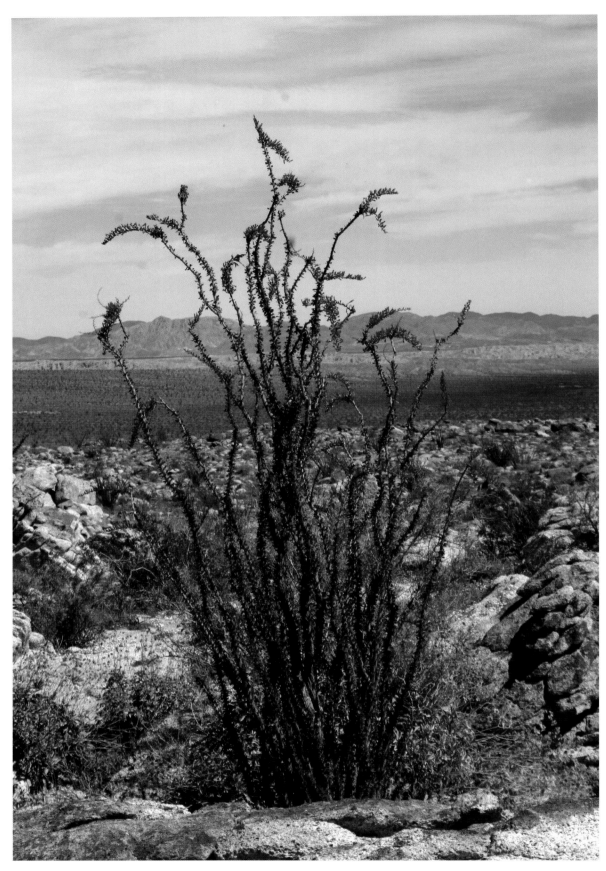

Ocotillo *(Fouquieria splendens)*

Ocotillo

Fouquieria splendens

Fouquieriaceae

Fouquieriae Splendins cortex

Other names include candlewood, couchwhip, and boojum

Flavor and *Qi:* bitter, acrid, cool
Channels Entered: liver, spleen, triple burner
Actions: Lymphatic

Functions and Indications

- ***Clears heat and transforms dampness.*** Ocotillo is used in the treatment of damp-heat brewing internally, with symptoms such as fullness in the lower abdomen, frequent short voiding of urine with dull ache, vaginal discharge, hemorrhoids, and itching and redness on the inner thighs. This herb can be used when damp-heat affects both the wood (liver-gallbladder) and earth (spleen-stomach) phases. When damp-heat encumbers the earth phase, signs will include lack of appetite, thirst with no desire to drink, and sticky stool or even constipation if heat is predominant. When damp-heat brews in the wood phase, there will be alternating heat effusion and aversion to cold, a bitter taste in the mouth, and rib or side pain.

- ***Quickens the blood and resolves stagnation.*** Ocotillo treats blood stasis and *qi* stagnation in the lower burner, with symptoms such as hemorrhoids, leg varicosities, and concretions and conglomerations. Ocotillo's acrid nature resolves stasis and stagnation; its bitter nature clears heat associated with accumulation of *qi* and blood. Together, ocotillo's acrid and bitter natures are effective for blood stasis and associated *qi* stagnation.

CAUTIONS

Use ocotillo with caution in those with *qi* vacuity.

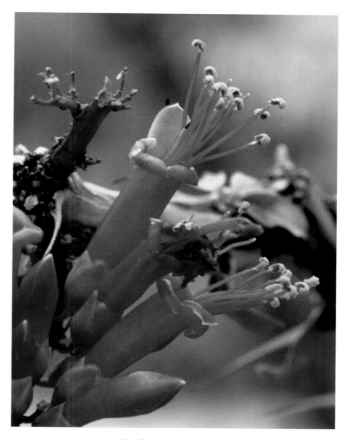

Ocotillo flowers *(F. splendens)*

Dosage and Preparation

Use 3–9 g in light decoction; 2–4 ml tincture.

Good-quality dried material is a light tan inner bark with a forest-green skin covered by a dry, scaly outer bark; it should have the sharp, fetid odor characteristic of ocotillo. The flowers should be immature and maintain their rich, deep, red color.

Major Combinations

- Combine with red root and cleavers for lower-burner damp-heat, welling-abscess, and damp-heat mounting. This combination also can be used for concretions and conglomerations. Although these are not generally seen as a damp-heat issue in Chinese medicine, the combination of these medicinals in tincture form is very useful for treating various types of concretions and conglomerations associated with gynecological pathologies, such as fibroid cysts and inflammatory masses.

- Combine with red root and horse chestnut for blood stasis with or without lower-burner damp-heat for symptoms such as hemorrhoids, leg varicosities, and endometriosis.

Commentary

Ocotillo is a very safe and effective herb. A common plant in the desert southwest of the United States, ocotillo is significantly underused relative to its efficacy and safety. Its action is not swift, but definite. The flowers are sweet, sour, bitter, and neutral; they soothe the heart and liver and are used for dry eyes with blurred vision, vexing heat in the five hearts, and night sweating.

The Mahuna Indians of the Southwest United States considered this medicinal specific for treating the blood, using it as a blood purifier and tonic.[9] Many native peoples prepared the flowers and seeds as food or drink. The most interesting of these food uses comes from the Papago Indians, who pressed out the blossoms, hardened the juice like rock candy, and chewed it as a delicacy.[10]

Ocotillo is not commercially available, and the plant is protected in the state of Arizona. Thus, if you're going to gather it, pick in California, Utah, New Mexico, Texas, or Mexico, or, if you live in Arizona, on your own private property. One large branch of this plant will provide you with one to three kilograms of dried bark.

Herbs that Clear Heat and Resolve Toxicity

Heat toxin is a category of repletion disease in Chinese medicine characterized by scorching heat *(zhuó rè)*, heat effusion, swelling and distention, pain, suppuration, and putrefaction. The medicinals in this category are closely aligned with what Western herbalists would deem antibacterial, antifungal, or antiviral medicinals. According to biomedical theory, bacterial, fungal, or viral pathogens are the ones that lead to the signs and symptoms associated with this category of medicinals in Chinese medicine.

Four medicinals in this subcategory of heat clearing are discussed here. The most important and also the most versatile is echinacea *(Echinacea* spp.). Echinacea may be the most important addition yet to the Chinese materia medica from the Western materia medica. In fact, when I was at the Beijing Medicinal Botanical Gardens, I saw echinacea growing alongside the Chinese medicinals. It was the only American species I saw in the entire garden.

Echinacea is bitter and acrid, clearing heat and draining fire while resolving toxins, transforming dampness and phlegm, and scattering the blood to stop the frenetic movement of it caused by heat or fire. Usnea *(sōng luó)* is a medicinal with more specific uses, but is no less valuable within its range of action. Usnea *(Usnea barbata* and others) combines the flavors of bitter and bland to create a downward and disinhibiting action. Its main focus is on the lung and bladder, thus making it helpful for conditions such as pulmonary welling-abscess and strangury. Sarsaparilla *(Smilax* spp.), closely related to the Chinese species *(tǔ fú ling)*, is a very important medicinal for treating heat toxin associated with dampness and impediment syndromes. Red clover *(Trifolium pratense)* is often used in Western herbalism, especially folk medicine, and is considered weaker in action than many other medicinals in this category. However, red clover does have a definitive heat-clearing, toxin-resolving action, as well as an ability to vitalize the blood by quickening and nourishing it.

Echinacea

Echinacea spp.

Asteraceae

Echinaceae herba seu flos cum radice cum semen

Numerous common names include purple coneflower, narrow leaf purple coneflower, pale coneflower, *sōng guŏ jú*

Flavor and *Qi*: acrid, bitter, cool
Channels Entered: lung, liver, bladder
Actions: alterative, anti-inflammatory, immunomodulator, lymphatic, vulnerary

Functions and Indications

- ***Clears heat, resolves toxins, and dispels wind.*** Echinacea is helpful in any form of heat or fire toxicity due either to external pathogens or internal derangement, including wind-heat throat impediment, wind-fire scrofula, wind-heat invading the lung, eczema, and psoriasis. This herb is very effective in the beginning stages of a heat (or cold) disease (i.e., *wèi* of the Four Aspects or *tài-yáng* of the Six Stages). However, don't overlook echinacea in later stages of disease, which is, perhaps, the most appropriate time for its use (e.g., *yíng* and *xuè* of the Four Aspects or *jué-yīn* of the Six Stages). Echinacea's acrid and bitter flavors have a powerful action. When treating external invasion of wind and heat, its acrid nature dispels wind and outthrusts pathogens, while its bitter and cool nature clears heat. When treating later-stage disease, echinacea's acridity enters and disperses the pathogenic *qì*, while its bitter flavor drains it. This action, combined with the cool nature of this herb, gives echinacea a strong and unique ability to clear heat or fire and resolve toxins.

- ***Clears heat and transforms phlegm.*** Echinacea is employed in the treatment of phlegm-heat obstructing the lungs, with symptoms of cough and heat effusion with thick yellow or green sputum that is

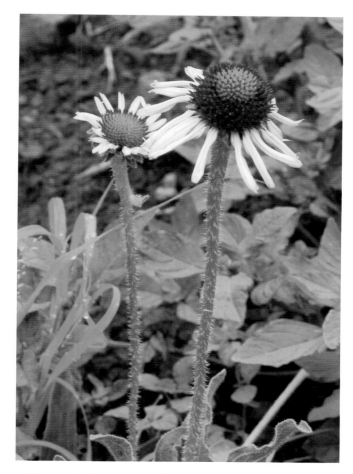

Narrow leaf purple coneflower *(Echinacea angustifolia)*

difficult to expectorate. This herb is also effective when heat has been allowed to penetrate the lungs, causing abscess and bleeding with purulent expectoration. Echinacea's acrid nature transforms phlegm while its bitter and cool nature clears heat.

- ***Clears heat and cools the blood.*** Echinacea is used to treat symptoms associated with stings and bites of any poisonous animal. The herb is famous for its ability to enter the blood to treat such toxins. Its acrid and bitter nature attacks evil *qì* and drains heat toxin. When treating these types of conditions, I often give a tincture of echinacea separately and tell the patient to take 30 to 60 drops every 30 to 90 minutes, depending on the severity of the condition. I believe that a tincture allows the medicinal to more swiftly enter the blood, attack the evil *qì*, and resolve heat toxins.

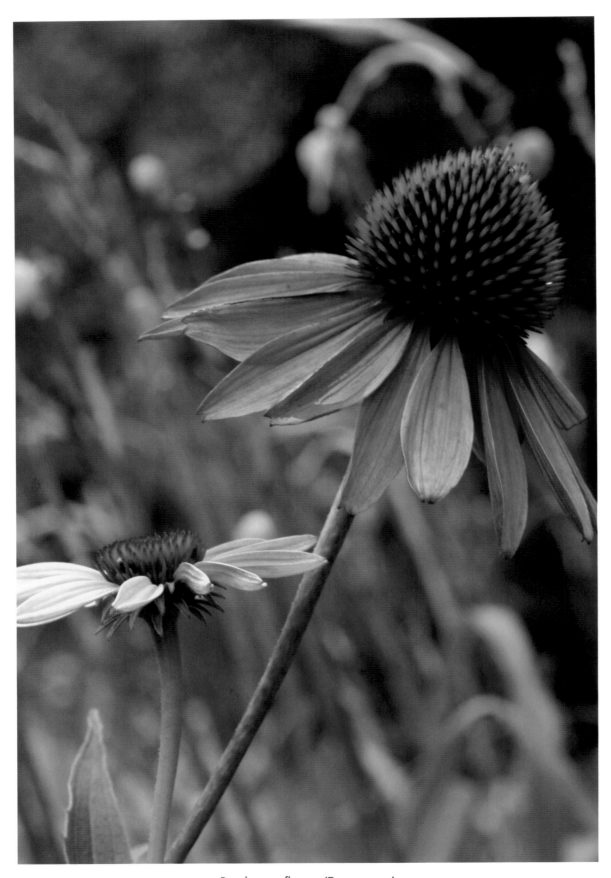

Purple coneflower *(E. purpurea)*

- *Clears heat, drains fire, and stops bleeding.* Echinacea treats extreme heat and fire that has damaged the network vessels causing bleeding, such as repletion lung-fire, heat vomiting, and heat strangury. As noted, echinacea is very good at clearing heat and draining fire. In patterns such as those described here, its acrid nature enters the *qi* of the blood and assists the blood in staying within the vessels.

- *Clears heat and resolves toxins.* Echinacea is applied to treat symptoms associated with either damp-heat or damp-toxin, with symptoms such as boils, carbuncles, lymphatic swelling, sore throat, otitis media, sinusitis, strangury, blood in the stool, or vomiting of blood. Echinacea is commonly used externally for clearing heat and resolving toxins in open wounds, boils, carbuncles, and sores. For external use, the tincture can be combined with green clay to make a paste to apply to unexpressed boils and venomous bites. For open wounds, combine with freshly powered goldenseal and a small amount of green clay to make a paste. Apply this paste and change the dressing twice a day, keeping the wound clean and clear of debris. Echinacea is also used for red papules, macules, boils, and carbuncles due to or associated with blood-heat, and for bleeding due to blood-heat in conditions like red turbidity (urinary) and repletion hemorrhoids.

CAUTIONS

Because echinacea stimulates the activity of the immune system, there is much debate about whether or not it is appropriate for those with autoimmune diseases. Some sources report that it is contraindicated; others state that it is indicated. I choose to not use echinacea in people with autoimmune conditions, unless I feel it is indicated for a specific acute pattern. Because of its acrid flavor, echinacea's coolness does not damage the spleen, so those with spleen *qi* vacuity can use it safely. Conversely, prolonged use of an herb with this nature could injure the *yīn* and blood humors; therefore, use caution in extended therapy.

Dosage and Preparation

Use 3–9 g in decoction (up to 30 g in acute illness); 2–4 ml tincture; 1–2 ml fluidextract; 1–3 g powdered extract.

Note: For maximum effectiveness in severe, acute disease, use frequent, moderate-to-large doses of echinacea. For less severe acute or more chronic cases, standard dosing is sufficient. During acute infections, I recommend dispensing this herb in addition to the prescribed formula as a simple tincture or other preparation to be taken hourly or at some other regular interval throughout the day. Generally, I suggest that the patient take a large dose immediately (4–8 ml) then take 1–3 ml every 30 to 60 minutes, depending on the severity of the illness.

Good-quality dried echinacea herb should be green to dark green with little stem material. The flowers should have most of their purple rays attached, with heads intact. The seeds should be brown, ranging from light to dark, and not soft. The root dries to a blackish gray color. The sliced root has dark radiating lines. All parts should be numbing to the mouth and throat upon chewing.

Major Combinations

- Combine with fringetree bark for *shào-yáng* disorders, or add to Minor Bupleurum Decoction *(xiǎo chái hú tāng)*.

- Combine with goldenseal and usnea for phlegm-heat in the lungs with thick, yellow, purulent sputum. This combination is also useful for urinary turbidity due to damp heat.

- Combine with trichosanthus fruit and fritillaria for phlegm-heat coughing with thick yellow or green sputum.

- Combine with isatis and leopard lily for febrile disease with painful or swollen sore throat due to fire, fire toxin, or phlegm-fire patterns. It can also be combined with usnea and California figwort for the same patterns.

- Combine with coptis and plantain ground into a powder to make a paste for application to external wounds.

- Combine with Jade Windscreen Formula *(yù píng fēng săn)* for prophylactic use when there is a threat of contracting an illness from family or a patient.

- Combine with Honeysuckle and Forsythia Powder *(yín qiáo sàn)* to strengthen its ability to clear heat and resolve toxins. This is an effective and potent addition to an already valuable formula. This combination is available as a patent remedy.

Commentary

I find echinacea invaluable in clinical practice. Its ability to clear heat in a number of heat patterns can be nearly druglike in its swiftness. Because of its strength in clearing heat in a variety of heat patterns (including damp-heat, wind-heat, heat-phlegm, heat-toxin, and heat-bind), echinacea is included in a multitude of formulas in Western herbalism to perform the function of what Chinese herbalists would call "clearing heat." With this in mind, we Chinese herbalists can incorporate the herb into many of our traditional formulas to increase their effectiveness. The two common formulas listed under Combinations are just examples; many other formulas might also benefit from the addition of echinacea. Although the entire plant (including seeds) is often included in bulk formulas, I often use only the root. There is not necessarily any therapeutic reason for this; rather, it is a matter of ease when working in a busy clinic. However, when preparing echinacea as a tincture, I combine all the parts of the plant.

Echinacea is one of the most popular herbs in America. Unfortunately, because of this popularity, many species are in danger in their native habitat. Therefore, we should use only cultivated plant mate-

rial. *E. purpurea,* a common garden flower, is easy to cultivate, readily available in commerce, and can be grown in almost any garden. In the proper climate, other species, such as *E. angustifolia,* also will grow well. However, for cultivation purposes, *E. purpurea* is most desirable; unlike its relatives *E. angustifolia, E. pallida,* and others, it does not have a tap root, but instead holds the earth with a thick growth of smaller but more prolific roots.

Most Native American peoples had several uses in common for at least three species of echinacea. They chewed the plant (primarily the root) or gargled a tea for sore throat, toothache, and mouth sores. They applied a poultice or wash as a local anodyne for burns, septic disease, wounds, poisonous bites, sores, and rheumatic swellings. They used echincea as internal medication for poisons, toxins, and associated swellings in the body. The Cheyenne combined echinacea root with puffball mushroom spores and skunk oil for external application for boils.[11]

The Eclectic physicians of the late nineteenth and early twentieth centuries favored the plant heavily. In 1898, Felter and Lloyd wrote, "Conspicuous among the remedies introduced within recent years, echinacea undoubtedly takes the first rank." Ellingwood stated in 1919, "It is the remedy for blood poisoning, if there is one in the Materia Medica." In *Physio-Medical Therapeutics, Materia Medica and Pharmacy,* published in 1897, Lyle says to use echinacea for a black tongue as well as septicemia.

Echinacea is official in many countries. It is listed in the *British Herbal Pharmacopoeia* (1996), the French Pharmacopoeia (1988), the Commission E Monographs, and the *WHO Monographs on Selected Medicinal Plants* (1999). Both *E. angustifolia* and *E. pallida* were official in *The National Formulary (U.S.),* 1916–1950.

Usnea

Usnea barbata and others

Usneaceae

Usneae thallus

Also called old man's beard

Flavor and *Qi*: bitter, bland, cold
Channels Entered: lung, bladder
Actions: antibiotic, antiviral, cardiotonic, diuretic, expectorant, febrifuge

Functions and Indications

- **Clears heat, resolves toxicity, and disinhibits dampness.** Usnea is used to treat heat and toxicity affecting the lungs and bladder, including heat evil invading the lung, phlegm-heat obstructing the lungs, bladder damp-heat, and other types of strangury associated with heat. Usnea's bitter and cold nature clears heat and resolves toxins, while its bitter and bland flavor disinhibits dampness. These properties make usnea extremely helpful in the treatment of damp-heat in the lower burner—as well as in lung ailments in which the *qi* dynamic of the lung has been disrupted due to dampness, phlegm, or heat. The lungs are the "upper source of water." Chapter 21 of the *Sù Wèn* states, ". . . the lungs who, regulating the water passages, send it [fluid] down to the bladder." By disinhibiting dampness, usnea helps to promote the free movement of fluids in the body.

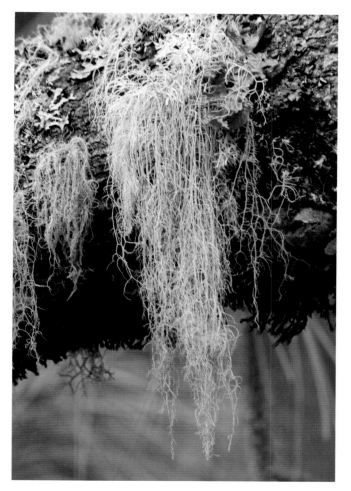

Usnea, also known as old man's beard (*Usnea* sp.)

CAUTIONS

Usnea is sometimes used as a prophylactic remedy against colds, influenza, and other infections, and is sold as such in health food stores across America. This is inadvisable. Because the nature of this medicinal is cold, overuse could damage spleen *qi*.

Dosage and Preparation

Use 3–6 ml tincture; 6–15 g in decoction.

Usnea is a type of lichen. Lichens consist of a symbiotic relationship between a fungus and an alga. In this case, the fungus is the white "cord" on the inside, which is coated by the gray-green alga on the outside. Most authorities have suggested that the primary medicine comes from the alga that covers the fungus, but separating them is neither necessary nor practical.

The herb is administered primarily in tincture form in the West, rarely as a decoction. The tincture is best prepared using hot alcohol, but due to the extreme volatility of this solvent, I don't recommend you try this. There is a special extractor for this purpose, called a Soxlet extractor. Therefore, I recommend that you purchase commercially produced tincture of this medicinal from a reputable manufacturer.

The strong heat-clearing medicine comes from the gray-green alga that covers the white, elastic fungal

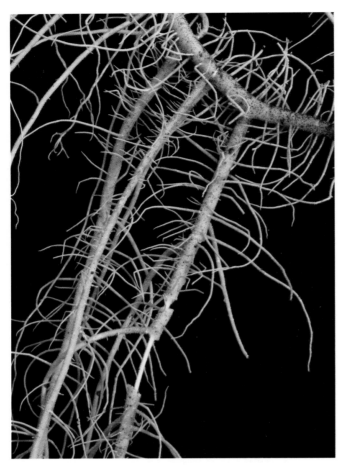

A close-up of usnea showing the the inner white fungal cord coated by the outer gray-green alga (*Usnea* sp.)

host. I have heard that some commercial preparations are made using only that portion of the herb. These would be stronger products, at least theoretically, but there is no available data comparing them; I do not have any experience comparing them and thus cannot offer an opinion at this time.

Good-quality dried material is light (bright) gray-green and pliable. There must be a white cord with an elastic quality under the gray-green cortex (i.e., if there is no white cord or there is one but it does not have an elastic quality, the material is not usnea). It is acceptable for the cortex to be somewhat brittle, but the interior cord should be elastic.

Major Combinations

- Combine with Oregon grape root, dandelion, and uva-ursi for damp-heat strangury.

- Combine with Chinese skullcap and elecampane for phlegm-heat in the lungs.

- Combine with goldenseal and elecampane for treating amoebic (epidemic) dysentery.

Commentary

Usnea is a common lichen that grows on trees and bushes all over the world. The herb is readily available in tincture form, but rarely is found in bulk in health food stores. However, some herb shops do carry it. Many commercial products containing usnea are available, including several from Germany and the United Kingdom.

Usnea is mainly used for infections of the respiratory and urinary tracts. It is strong, effective, and relatively abundant. It will reduce fever and clear infection as well as any herb. While it is not used widely among the general public, this is an oversight. There is some concern about commercial harvesting due to usnea's sensitivity to pollution; it is one of the first organisms to die from air pollution. Usnea also collects toxins from air pollution, so harvesting it near cities or highways could potentially expose the patient to these toxins. However, there are uncountable acres of usnea growing in clean forests around the world. In most places where there is sufficient rain, it may grow up to 1 meter (about 3 feet) in length in one season. In drier climates, it may only grow a couple of centimeters (perhaps up to 1 inch). With these factors in mind, it is important for practitioners to demand that suppliers keep close tabs on the source of the herb to ensure that it is clean and safe to use.

Translation of Source Material

Two species of *Usnea* are used in Chinese medicine, *U. longissima* and *U. diffracta (sōng luó)*. The medicinal is bitter, sweet, and neutral (one source says bland, slightly bitter, and cool). It clears the liver, transforms phlegm, stanches bleeding, and resolves toxin. It is used to treat headache, red eyes, coughing with profuse sputum, malaria, scrophula, white vaginal discharge, flooding and spotting, excessive bleeding due to external injury, swollen welling-abscess, and poisonous snakebite.

Sarsaparilla

Smilax officinalis and others
Liliaceae
Smilax radix et rhizoma
Also called greenbrier and *tŭ fú líng*

Flavor and *Qi:* bitter, slightly acrid, slightly cold
Channels Entered: liver, lung, spleen, stomach
Actions: alterative, anti-inflammatory, antipruritic, antiseptic

Functions and Indications

- ***Resolves toxicity and drains dampness.*** Sarsaparilla is used to treat damp-toxin in the skin with hot, red lesions with or without suppuration, including eczema and psoriasis. Sarsaparilla's bitter and slightly cold nature drains and resolves toxicity, while its bitter and slightly acrid nature drains damp and scatters toxins.

Due to its slightly acrid and slightly cold nature, sarsaparilla can also be used for wind-heat skin diseases. Also, owing to its *qi* and flavor, sarsaparilla is sometimes incorporated as an assistant in formulas to treat heat entering the construction-blood aspect.

- ***Clears heat, dispels damp, diffuses impediment, and relieves pain.*** Sarsaparilla is helpful in the treatment of all types of heat impediment, no matter the etiology, including impediments of the skin, joints, and flesh.

CAUTIONS

None noted.

Dosage and Preparation

Use 3–9 g in decoction; 2–4 ml tincture.

Good-quality dried material is slightly reddish in color.

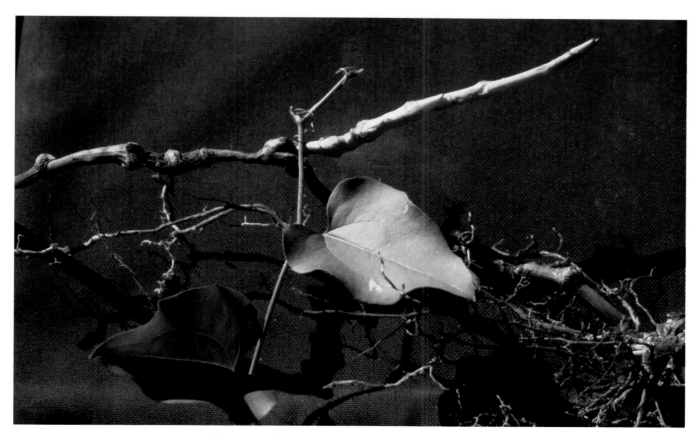

A sarsaparilla species from the western United States *(Smilax californica)*

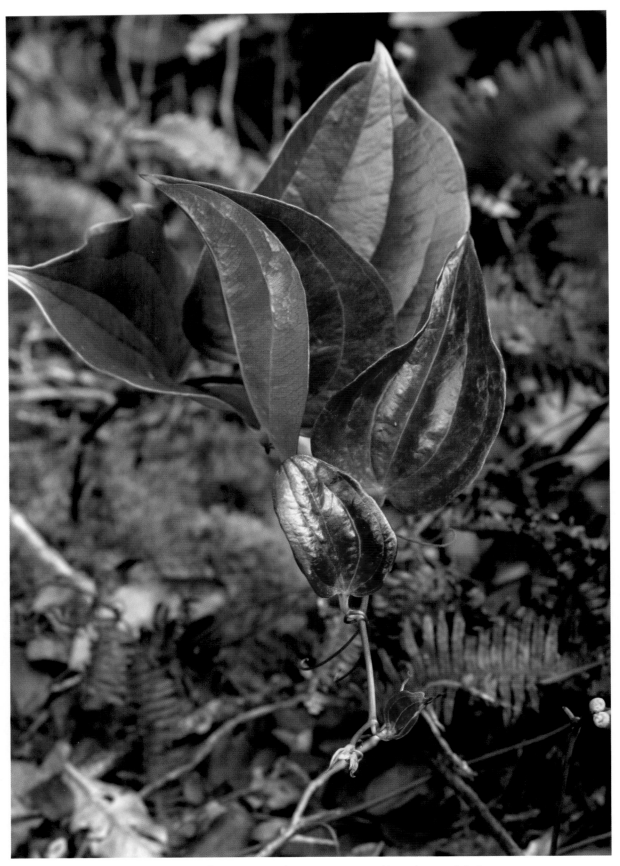

A sarsaparilla species endemic to Hawai'i *(S. melastomifolia)*

Major Combinations

- Combine with echinacea, Oregon grape root, California figwort, and burdock for damp-toxin in the skin with hot, red lesions and suppuration.

- Combine with echinacea and Four-Valiant Decoction for Well-Being *(sì miào yǒng ān tāng)* to strengthen the formula.

- Combine with Impediment-Diffusing Decoction *(xuān bì tāng)* to assist the formula. I generally give this formula as a tea pill with the sarsaparilla as a separate tea (usually with a little licorice) to be taken when the patient takes the tea pills.

Commentary

There are about three hundred species of *Smilax* worldwide. They come from Jamaica, North and South America (including Mexico and the southern, eastern, and western regions of the United States), Central America, and China. There is even a species endemic to Hawai'i—*S. melastomifolia.* Significant differences exist among the species, although some are very similar. Michael Moore states he prefers the *Smilax* species from the western United States (found in California and southern Oregon)—which he calls "groovy stuff."[12] This species, *S. californica,* is very abundant in my area and I find myself using it more and more often. Unfortunately, it is not available in commerce.

My friend and colleague David Winston employs sarsaparilla as part of a larger protocol for Lyme disease. Sarsaparilla binds endotoxins and heals gut mucosa, making it an important part of a protocol for leaky gut syndrome. He also uses it for certain autoimmune conditions, including rheumatoid arthritis, scleroderma, and psoriatic arthritis. The Cherokee of western North Carolina and northwestern Georgia used several species of *Smilax.* They made decoctions to treat rheumatism and stomach troubles and to aid expulsion of the afterbirth.[13] The Iroquois of upstate New York and southern Quebec used *S. herbacea* in a compound decoction as an external steam and wash for rheumatism, and in a different compound decoction for "loss of senses during menses." They also used *Smilax* root in decoction for elderly people with stomach troubles.[14]

Smilax officinalis is very similar to the species used in Chinese medicine and can be used as an analogue to *S. glabra (tǔ fú líng).* The advantage of using *S. officinalis* is that the quality is generally far superior to that of the Chinese product sold in the United States.

Although the etymology of the genus name is unclear, one source states that it could come from the Greek word *smil,* meaning "a carving tool." The common name comes from the Spanish *sarza,* meaning bramble or thorny bush, and *parilla,* meaning "tendril" or "vine."

Sarsaparilla (from several species of *Smilax*) was official in *The United States Pharmacopoeia* from 1820–1955 and in *The National Formulary (U.S.)* from 1955–1965. The pharmacopoeias of Belgium and Portugal list several species of *Smilax,* while the pharmacopoeias of China and Japan specify *S. glabra* as the official medicinal.

Red Clover

Trifolium pratense

Fabaceae

Trifolii Pratense flos

Flavor and *Qi*: bitter, slightly sweet, cold
Channels Entered: liver, heart, lungs
Actions: alterative, expectorant, lymph tonic

Functions and Indications

- *Clears heat, resolves fire toxicity, quickens blood, and reduces swelling.* Red clover is helpful for toxic swellings that manifest both externally and internally. Red clover is also extensively used for concretions, conglomerations, accumulations, and gatherings. It is bitter and cold in nature, and its slightly sweet flavor stimulates the body to invite it deep into the construction and blood aspects. Although its bitter and cold nature clears heat and resolves fire toxicity, this action is not swift, and the medicinal must be used in large doses. Nevertheless, it is an important part of therapy when treating concretions, conglomerations, accumulations, and gatherings, especially concretions and accumulations. Red clover is also applied in the treatment of rashes and other skin diseases, such as eczema and psoriasis.

- *Nourishes and quickens the blood.* Red clover is employed to treat a variety of conditions associated with vacuous, static blood. This is a very mild action, although very popular in the Western herbal tradition. There is a strong tradition of using this herb to treat various conditions in which blood vacuity has led to blood stasis or there are concur-

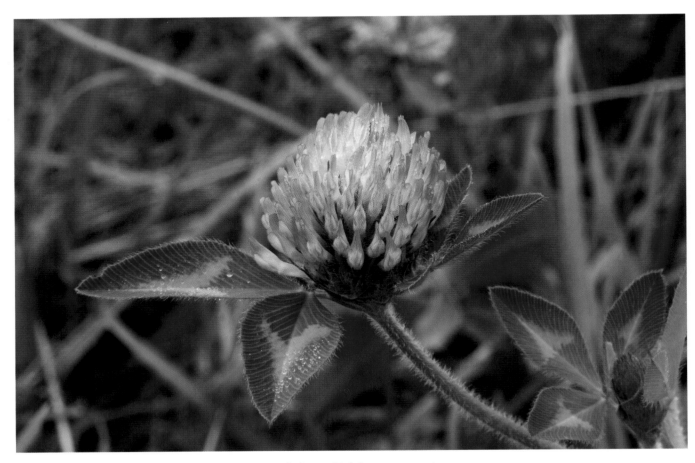

Red clover *(Trifolium pratense)*

rent pathologies. When used in this manner, red clover can be an effective part of treatment for concretions, accumulations, and aggregations, with or without signs of heat. Due to the cold nature of this medicinal, proper formulation is essential when using it for this purpose.

CAUTIONS

Use caution with this herb for anyone on blood-thinning medication, as red clover may have the potential to further thin the blood and cause spontaneous bleeding. If improperly dried and allowed to ferment, the coumarins contained in red clover become dicoumarol, which has blood-thinning effects. Properly dried red clover is unlikely to cause such effects. However, unless you are absolutely sure of your supplier, observe caution.

Dosage and Preparation

Use 3–9 g in light decoction or infusion (up to 30 g may be used); 2–4 ml tincture.

Good-quality dried flowers are whole and purple without brown discoloration; the herb should contain no more than 15 percent leaf, which should be bright to slightly dark green.

Major Combinations

- Combine with sarsaparilla and sassafras for various skin diseases due to heat entering the blood and to wind.

- Combine with grindelia and fritillaria for cough due to heat in the lungs, with thick yellow sputum containing blood.

- Combine with goldenseal, honeysuckle, and forsythia for toxic, suppurating swellings.

- Combine with astragalus and plantain for slow-healing abscesses.

Commentary

The genus name of this plant, *Trifolium*, is a simple compound Latin term denoting the three *(tri)* leaflets of each compound leaf *(folium)*. Red clover grows as a weed in northern latitudes throughout much of the world. Because of its use as a cover crop and fodder, it can be found nearly anywhere farming has taken place. Red clover is widely used in commercial formulas and available in bulk (flowers or whole herb with flowers). Although whole herb is commonly used today and less expensive, the flower heads are the traditional medicine, and I prefer them.

Red clover is mild and gentle, but its combined nourishing and quickening effects on the blood give it an interesting and important place in the materia medica. Although it is effective for the indications described in the monograph above, red clover is a relatively gentle herb. Thus, it should always be used as a part of a larger protocol and at an appropriate dosage. Used properly, it does clear heat and makes a significant difference when added to formulas. Red clover also contains a rich mineral complex that is widely perceived as having blood-nourishing properties, and many Western herbalists recommend it as a nourishing tonic in small doses. In addition, red clover very gently quickens the blood, an action that may be increased by allowing the herb to ferment partially during drying. This action has the potential to benefit many people in today's world of sedentary lifestyles.

Translation of Source Material

In Chinese medicine, red clover *(sān xiāo cǎo)* is neutral and slightly sweet. It clears heat, cools the blood, and is used to treat withdrawal disease.

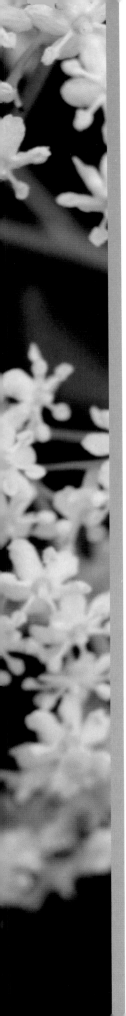

HERBS
THAT PRECIPITATE

This is a very important category in the materia medica, but one that must be applied carefully. Medicinals from this category are used when evils have accumulated in the interior to cause a binding of *qì*. This binding will eventually lead to heat, which dries fluids and can cause the stool to slow or bind; binding may also be directly caused by heat. As heat can rise, the precipitating method is sometimes used to treat heat or fire in the upper part of the body, particularly conditions associated with the lung or its channel pathway, owing to the relationship between the large intestine and the lung *(yáng-míng)*. The patterns treated with this category of medicinals are patterns of repletion. Repletion of this nature is generally treated agressively; thus, this method of treatment (one of the eight methods) is an attacking method. Depending on the medicinals prescribed, this method can be applied to treat blood stasis, phlegm, food accumulation, and parasites.

Buckthorn bark (*Rhamnus* spp.) is the lone representative for this category in this text. It effectively treats bound stool due to heat accumulation. Buckthorn also clears heat and can be used for liver-fire scorching the lungs. It also drains heat impediment to relieve pain.

Buckthorn Bark

Rhamnus californica, R. cathartica,
R. purshiana, R. frangula

Rhamnaceae

Rhamni fructus seu cortex

Common names include California coffee berry *(R. californica),* cascara sagrada *(R. purshiana),* and alder buckthorn *(R. frangula)*

Flavor and *Qi:* bitter, cold
Channels Entered: large intestine, stomach
Actions: diuretic, laxative

Functions and Indications

- ***Drains heat and purges accumulation.*** Buckthorn is employed to treat all forms of repletion constipation in which heat is involved, with symptoms of heat effusion; abdominal distension that dislikes pressure; a thick, slimy, yellow tongue coating; and a surging pulse. Buckthorn is bitter and cold and is a draining precipitation medicinal. Very similar in action to Chinese rhubarb, buckthorn is extremely useful for the treatment of *qi* aspect and *yáng-míng* stage heat accumulation.

- ***Clears heat, drains fire, and resovles phlegm accumulation.*** Buckthorn is used in the treatment of liver-fire invading the lung (also known as wood-fire

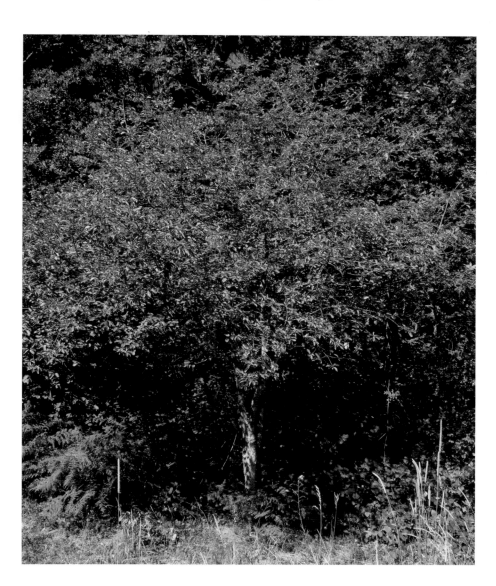

Buckthorn tree *(Rhamnus purshiana)*

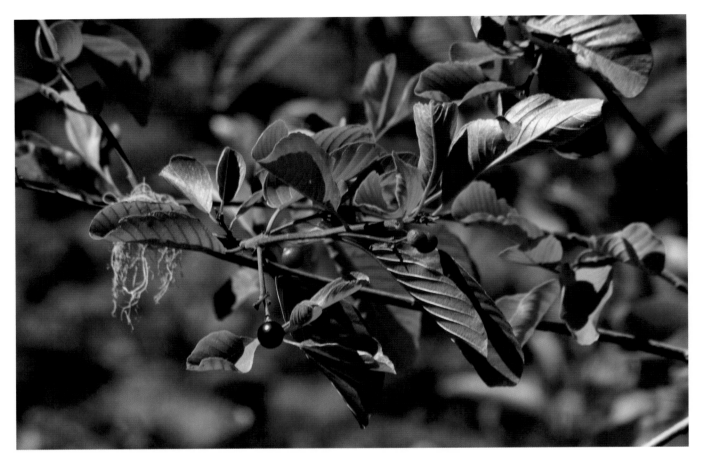

Buckthorn leaves and berries *(R. purshiana)*

tormenting metal) with sinus congestion; constipation or sluggish, dry, or mucousy stools; and difficult and scant-dark urination. There may be other symptoms associated with fire flaring upward, such as red eyes, hot pain in the chest, headache, impatience, and bitter taste in the mouth. Bitter and cold in nature, buckthorn drains fire from the liver, precipitates stool, and assists the lungs' depurative, downbearing functions, thus draining phlegm from the sinuses and lungs.

- *Clears heat, dispels dampness, diffuses impediment, and relieves pain of heat impediment.* When decocted for longer periods of time (i.e., along with the rest of the formula), buckthorn's ability to precipitate stool will be reduced, but it will still be useful for treating heat impediment. Its cold and bitter nature clears heat, drains dampness, and relieves pain caused by impediment.

CAUTIONS

Buckthorn should not be used for extended periods of time or during pregnancy. Buckthorn is a particularly strong purgative, but when used at an appropriate dosage is safe and very effective. Use caution for patients with insufficient original *qi*.

Dosage and Preparation

Use 1–6 g of bark in cold infusion or decoction; 1–3 ml tincture (bark or berries).

For a stronger precipitating effect, a short decoction or cold infusion is best. When using this medicinal for clearing heat and treating impediment syndromes, a longer decoction time may be appropriate to reduce its precipitating action.

Good-quality bark is brown on the outside and golden-yellow inside. The berries should be shiny, black, and plump if fresh and firm if dried.

Major Combinations

- Combine with bitter orange and ginger for constipation with cramping; for more severe cramping, add wild yam and licorice.
- Combine with California figwort, black cohosh, and yerba mansa for hot, red, swollen joints and pain due to arthritis or gout.

Commentary

The genus name *Rhamnus* is likely derived from the Greek work *rhabnos,* meaning "cane" or "rod." The species name *cathartica* is derived from the Greek *kathartikos* and *karthos,* meaning "cleansing" and "pure," respectively.

Buckthorn bark is used primarily as a laxative. In fact, it is almost never used for anything else. It is helpful when there is sluggish movement of stool. For this, only a small dosage is needed. Because of its diuretic effects, it also is very useful when constipation is accompanied by urinary problems or vice versa—a sort of Eight Corrections Powder *(bā zhèng sàn)* idea, except with a stronger focus on the bowels than the bladder.

It is interesting to note that the original pattern for *bā zhèng sàn* is Heart channel heat and, according to one source, *R. californica* was used by the Yokia of Northern California for mania.[1] Parkinson recommended a decoction of buckthorn berries for inflammation of the joints and gout. Since the bark and berries contain nearly the same medicine, it is reasonable to assume the bark might also have this function. My experience so far using buckthorn bark for this purpose has been quite positive. The anthraquinones the plant contains, which are responsible for the laxative and downbearing properties, are destroyed or transformed in the boiling process, so these actions are lessened substantially, but the anti-inflammatory, heat-clearing action is not. Furthermore, the boiling process helps direct the action to the joints. To strengthen this action, take buckthorn with a small amount of wine or alcohol.

Since the mid 1990s, I have used only *R. californica.* I find it to be just as effective as more commonly used species, but without the cramping that can accompany their use. This could be related to improper aging of commercially available bark. Non-aged bark is harsh and may cause severe griping with explosive precipitation. Aged buckthorn bark creates a medicine that is not only effective, but also gentler and less painful to use.

Although *R. californica* has never been listed as official, *R. purshiana* and *R. frangula* are listed across most of Europe as official. *R. carthartica* is listed as official in the pharmacopoeias of Argentina, Russia, and Spain.

Translation of Source Material

Chinese medicine recognizes several species of *Rhamnus. Nǚ ér chá (R. heterophylla)* is acrid, slightly bitter, and cool. The medicinal clears heat, cools blood, and stops bleeding. It is used to treat blood ejection, flooding and spotting, irregular menstruation, dysentery, and bleeding hemorrhoids.

Dòng lǜ cì (R. globosus) is bitter, astringent, and slightly cold. It kills worms, downbears *qì,* expels phlegm, and disperses food.

Jiàng lí mù zǐ (R. leptophylla) is bitter, cold, and slightly toxic. It disperses food, moves water, and frees the stool. It is used to treat food accumulation and bloating, water swelling and drum distention, and binding constipation in the large intestine. The leaf of this plant *(jiàng lí mù yè)* is administered for food accumulation and bloating. The root of the plant *(jiàng lí mù gēn)* is bitter and cold. It disperses food, moves water, and eliminates stasis. It is employed to treat food accumulation and bloating, water swelling and drum distention, and menstrual block.

Lù tí gēn (R. utilis) is bitter and cold. It clears heat, cools the blood, and resolves toxin. It is used in the treatment of scab, dampness papules, sand distention, and knocks and falls.

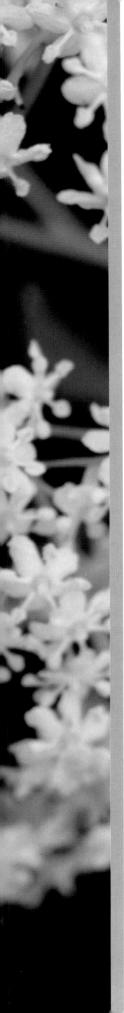

HERBS THAT DRAIN DAMPNESS

The concept of draining or disinhibiting dampness relates to encouraging the flow of pathogenic dampness through the urine. Dampness is one of the *six excesses* and can cause myriad problems throughout the body. By nature, dampness is viscous and lingering, and diseases complicated by dampness are often difficult to treat. Dampness slows movement and promotes stagnation, leading to an accumulation which in turn can lead to heat and transform into phlegm. Dampness can also cause *qi* stagnation and blood stasis. The spleen is the most likely viscus to be damaged by dampness, and this may be associated with many digestive disorders, including low appetite and thirst; abdominal distention; glomus and oppression in the stomach duct and chest; nausea and vomiting; and a thick, slimy tongue coating and a soggy, moderate pulse. Accumulated dampness may also be evidenced by vaginal discharge, swelling in the lower body, or weeping skin diseases.

Three medicinals from this category are represented in this text. Cleavers *(Galium aparine)* is a particularly important medicinal in this category. It is bitter, salty, and cold; thus it treats dampness, heat, and phlegm accumulations. Plantain *(Plantago* spp.) is the leafy portion of a plant that provides a seed with which most Chinese herbalists are familiar, *chē qián zǐ*. Although the herbaceous portion is used in Chinese medicine, it is lesser known there than in the West. Plantain is cooling and bland, percolating and draining dampness and heat. Plantain is also useful because of its ability to generate flesh. This is a very important quality when treating either external or internal lesions. Nettle *(Urtica dioica)* has a wide range of actions, but it is first a cool, bland, dampness-percolating medicinal.

Cleavers

Galium aparine

Rubiaceae

Galii Aparine herba

Other common names include clives, clivers, bedstraw

Flavor and *Qi*: bitter, salty, cold
Channels Entered: kidney, bladder, spleen, lung
Actions: alterative, aperient, diuretic

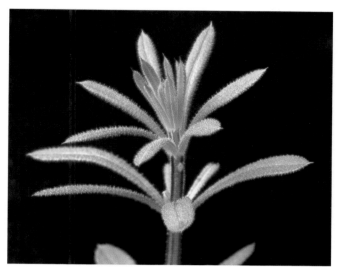

Cleavers *(Galium aparine)*

Functions and Indications

- ***Disinhibits dampness and clears heat.*** Employed for any damp-heat condition, especially in the lower burner, cleavers is excellent both for draining dampness and clearing heat. It can be used for a variety of conditions, but should be reserved for those in which dampness is the primary evil. Because of its ability to drain dampness, this herb is valuable in a plethora of damp conditions, both hot or cold, when combined with other appropriate medicinals. Cleavers disinhibits dampness with its bitter flavor and cold nature, at the same time effectively clearing heat. Cleavers has a distinct affinity for the lower burner, and its salty flavor is important when there is clumping of heat and dampness leading to hot swelling.

- ***Drains dampness, clears heat, resolves toxins, and dissipates hot swellings.*** Cleavers is helpful for treating skin eruptions that ooze. The herb also can be used for damp-heat skin conditions such as psoriasis. Cleavers's dependable effectiveness in this indication is linked to its bitter flavor and cold nature. Although bitter and cold, cleavers does not easily damage the spleen, making it helpful for patients with weak righteous *qi*.

- ***Softens hardness and transforms phlegm.*** Cleavers is employed in the treatment of phlegm nodes and scrophula. The herb can be used for phlegm nodes in which no heat is associated with the ailment, or for scrophula in which heat, specifically vacuity heat, is a prime factor. Cleavers's bitter and salty flavor soft-

ens hardness and transforms phlegm, while its cold nature clears heat due to depression associated with phlegm nodulation. Sometimes called a "lymphatic" in Western herbal medicine, cleavers is very effective for swollen, hot lymph nodes.

- ***Clears heat and drains dampness.*** Cleavers drains dampness through the small intestine for heart-heat or heart-fire patterns with insomnia, irritability, mouth sores, rapid pulse, and a yellow tongue coating. The herb's bitter flavor enters the fire phase to drain heat and dampness. This is not a primary action for cleavers, but I have found it to be a valuable adjunct in formulas that address this pattern.

CAUTIONS

Due to its draining action, use cleavers with caution in cases of *yīn* vacuity.

Dosage and Preparation

Use 5–15 g in decoction or infusion; 3–6 ml tincture.

Fresh juice, prepared by juicing with a commercially available juicer, is another excellent method of administration. Give fresh juice at a dosage of 15–30 ml. Although freshly prepared juice is significantly superior to a preserved product, juice may be preserved

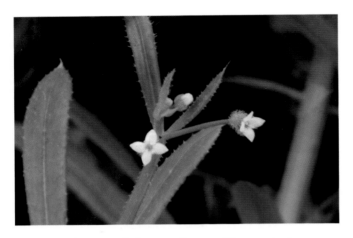

Close-up of cleavers flowers *(G. aparine)*

for later use by adding alcohol or glycerin. Good-quality dried material is clean and bright green and may contain flowers, but should be without fruits or roots.

Major Combinations

- Combine with red root, ocotillo, and buckthorn for damp-heat mounting.

- Combine with California figwort, red root, and echinacea for scrophula with hot, painful nodes in the neck, armpits, or groin.

- Combine with yellow dock and burdock for damp-heat affecting the skin in recalcitrant skin conditions, such as psoriasis and eczema.

- Combine with water plantain root, poria, and phellodendron for damp-heat pouring downward into the bladder, with dark, difficult urination.

Commentary

Cleavers is extraordinarily common throughout the Western Hemisphere. It can be found growing in almost every part of the United States, as it can colonize even the small patches of ground found in large cities. The herb is tender, and should be stored in glass and away from any sunlight (even indirect), lest its properties diminish too quickly.

The name *Galium* comes from the Greek root *galion,* meaning "bedstraw," owing to the plant's growth formation. The name *Galium* has the Greek root *gala,* meaning "milk," because some species have been used in cheese production as a rennet substitute to curdle milk. The species name comes from the Greek *apairein,* meaning "to seize," probably in reference to the plant's hooked hairs, which readily stick to surfaces such as clothing and hair (including hairy legs).

Cleavers has been known since antiquity as a remedy for many diseases. Greco-Roman healers applied it internally for snake and spider bites and externally for earache and glandular swellings. Later, cleavers was considered beneficial for dropsy, liver and skin diseases, goiter, and scrofula. During the nineteenth century the herb was recommended for cancer, and references to its use in various cancers are still sometimes seen. The following is the opening sentence from the monograph for cleavers in *King's American Dispensatory:* "A most valuable refrigerant and diuretic, and will be found very beneficial in many diseases of the urinary organs, as suppression of urine, calculous affections, inflammation of the kidneys and bladder, and in scalding of urine in gonorrhœa." This statement clearly demonstrates the plant's significance in what is widely considered the most important materia medica written in North America.

The Mi'kmaq Indians of Nova Scotia, Prince Edward Island, and surrounding coastal areas; the Ojibwa of the upper Midwest and southern Ontario; and the Penobscot of northern New England and Canada's maritime provinces all used cleavers for "kidney troubles." The Ojibwa also used cleavers for "gravel, urine stoppage, and allied ailments."[1]

Translation of Source Material

In Chinese medicine, *bā xiān cǎo (Galium aparine, G. asperifolium)* is bitter, acrid, and cold and enters the *shao-yīn* and *tài-yīn* channels. The medicinal clears damp-heat, dissipates stasis, disperses swelling, and resolves toxin. It is used to treat strangury-turbidity, bloody urine, knocks and falls, intestinal welling-abscess, swollen boils, and middle ear infection.

Plantain

Plantago major, P. lanceolata

Plantaginaceae

Plantaginis herba

Other common names include ribwort, common plantain, English plantain, lance-leaf plantain, *dà chē qìán (P. major)*

Flavor and *Qi:* sweet, bland, cold
Channels Entered: bladder, spleen, stomach
Actions: anti-inflammatory, demulcent, diuretic, vulnerary

Functions and Indications

- ***Clears heat and drains dampness.*** Plaintain is used to treat *lín* syndrome with painful, scanty, dark yellow urine. The herb also helps clear heat and drain downward for phlegm-heat in the lungs. Plantain has a sweet and bland flavor and is cold in nature. It percolates and drains dampness with its blandness and effectively clears heat with its cold nature. While primarily used internally for the lower burner, it is also valuable for the lungs due to its draining and heat-clearing actions. Furthermore, plantain's sweet flavor provides a *yīn* nourishing quality. Because *yīn* can be easily damaged either by *lín* syndrome or the medicinals used to treat it, this makes plantain a particularly important medicinal in this category.

- ***Clears heat and stops bleeding.*** Plantain is an excellent medicinal for clearing heat and stopping bleeding due to heat damaging the vessels, with symptoms of coughing blood, blood in the urine, and blood in the stool.

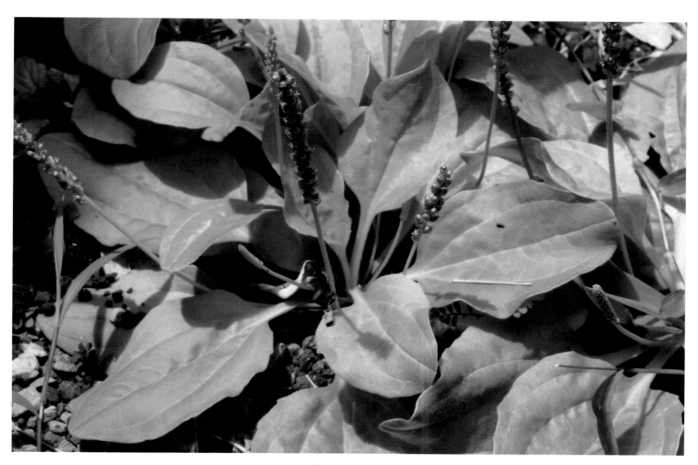

Common plantain *(Plantago major)*

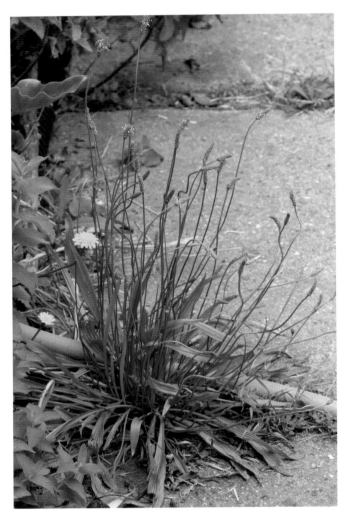

English plantain *(P. lanceolata)*

- *Clears heat and generates flesh for healing of lesions, either internal or external.* Plantain is sweet and cold and invaluable in the treatment of flesh wounds, whether internal or external. This medicinal is one of the superior botanicals for healing flesh and is critical for sores, cuts, abscesses, or any other condition in which the flesh must heal. Apply it externally in the form of a poultice, or incorporate it as an ingredient in a salve or ointment. An infusion or decoction is best for internal use.

CAUTIONS

Use caution when administering plantain internally for those with spleen *qi* vacuity.

Dosage and Preparation

Use 5–15 g in decoction or infusion; 3–6 ml tincture.

Prepare plantain for external application either by crushing the fresh leaves and applying them directly to the affected area or infusing them in oil to make an infused oil or salve. Good-quality dried herb is light to dark green and whole. There should be no odor; however, when tasting the leaf, one should experience a slightly slimy sensation after holding it in the mouth for a couple of minutes.

Major Combinations

- Substitute this medicinal for Chinese plantain seed in Eight Corrections Powder *(bā zhèng sàn)* to help support the right and treat damage caused by heat in the bladder. This is especially useful when there is blood in the urine.

- Combine with goldenseal, gardenia, arnebia, and Chinese angelica as an external application for heat-toxin welling-abscess.

Commentary

The genus name *Plantago* comes from the Latin *planta,* meaning sole of the foot, referring to the leaf of *P. major,* which looks similar to the bottom of a human foot. A common plant around the world, plantain leaves are used in the West, while the seeds (and, to a lesser extent, the leaves) are used in Chinese medicine. Although different species are used in China and the West, there is little difference among their properties and they can be used interchangeably.

Because of its cooling and healing properties, I have used plantain with great success in the form of a fresh juice as an enema for ulcerative colitis. All patients reported relief of the pain and burning sensation and further stated that relative to any other treatment, this treatment gave them the most immediate relief. Plantain juice may also be administered internally for stomach ulcers, corrosion of the esophagus due to acid regurgitation, and similar conditions.

This plant contains baicalin, one of the same con-

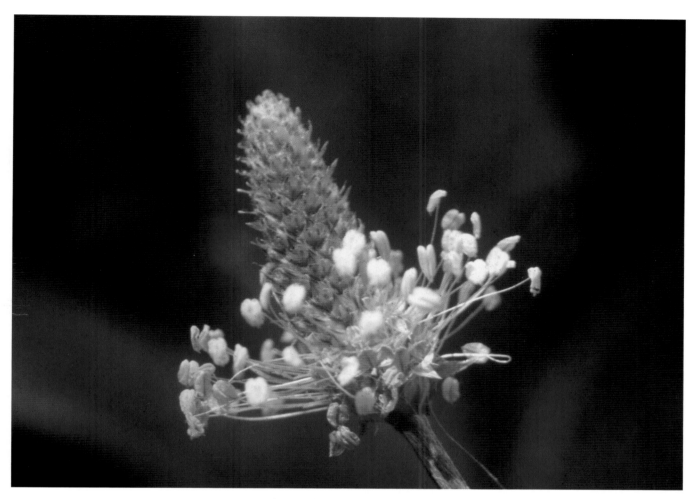

Plantain flower *(P. lanceolata)*

stituents found in Chinese skullcap, which has shown anti-inflammatory and anti-allergic properties. Plantain has been employed as medicine since antiquity and is mentioned in many of the oldest texts. Salmon says taking the liquid juice of plantain in doses of three to eight spoonfuls for several days "helps distillation of rheum upon the throat, glands, lungs, etc."[2] According to Native American ethnobotanical literature, many tribes used plantain for all the indications listed in this entry, perhaps an example of European settlers teaching native peoples about a plant they brought with them across the Atlantic.

Translation of Source Material

Most practitioners are aware of *chē qián zĭ*—Chinese plantain seed—a major component in many diuretic formulas. The leaf is known as *chē qián yè,* a name that encompasses three species *(P. asiatica, P. depressa, P. major).* This medicinal is sweet and cold. It disinhibits water, clears heat, brightens the eyes, and dispels phlegm. It is used to treat urinary stoppage, strangury-turbidity, vaginal discharge, bloody urine, jaundice, water swelling [edema], heat dysentery, diarrhea, nosebleed, red swollen eyes, throat impediment nipple moth [acute tonsillitis], cough, and ulcerating sores on the skin.

Nettle

Urtica dioica, U. urens, **and others**

Urticaceae

Urticae Dioicae herba

Other common names include stinging nettle, dwarf nettle, *qiàn má* **(Chinese)**

Flavor and *Qi:* salty, bland, slightly acrid, sweet, cool
Channels Entered: liver, lung, bladder
Actions: antirheumatic, astringent, diuretic, tonic

Functions and Indications

- ***Promotes urination, clears heat, and leaches out dampness.*** Nettle effectively treats accumulation of dampness anywhere in the body, with symptoms such as premenstrual water retention, urinary difficulty, edema, and joint stiffness. Nettle is also used for phlegm-damp obstructing the nasal passages. The herb disinhibits water through bland percolation and its cool nature clears heat. Its slightly acrid nature helps to disperse damp accumulation and address phlegm-damp obstructing the nasal passages.

- ***Expels wind-dampness and wind-heat.*** Nettle is used to treat obstruction of the channels by dampness causing pain and poor mobility of the joints. Nettle also expels wind-heat from the skin for rashes that are damp and hot in character. Nettle has a slightly acrid flavor and is cool in nature. It enters the channels and expels wind-dampness impediment. Due to its coolness, it is especially appropriate for hot conditions, but it can be employed in cold conditions with the appropriate formulation.

- ***Cools and nourishes the blood.*** The herb is helpful for treating excessive menstrual bleeding or mid-cycle spotting, coughing of blood, nosebleeds, or blood in the stool. Sweet in flavor and cool in nature, nettle enters the blood, gently cooling, nourishing, and helping to stop bleeding syndromes due to blood vacuity or heat entering the blood.

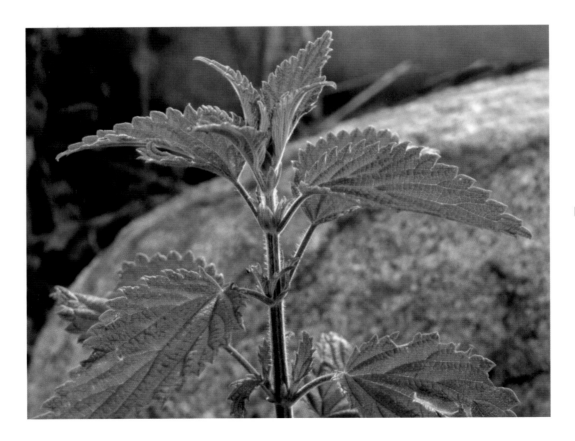

Nettle *(Urtica dioica)*

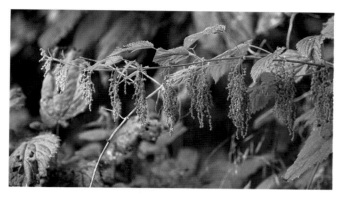

Nettle flowers *(U. dioica)*

- **Softens hardness.** Nettle is applied in the treatment of nodes and stones, including scrofula, urinary calculi, and gallstones. Although not much used for this application today, the herb does have a long history of use for such conditions. Because nettle is salty and slightly acrid in flavor as well as cool in nature, it softens hardness, and I frequently include it as an adjunct for swollen, hard lymph nodes.

CAUTIONS

If nettle is consumed with only scant amounts of water, it will be less effective as a diuretic. The German Commission E warns against using nettle as a diuretic when fluid retention is caused by cardiac or renal failure.

Dosage and Preparation

Use 9–30 g in decoction or infusion; 4–9 ml tincture; 3–6 g powdered extract.

Good-quality dried herb is dark green in color and should be as whole as possible. The herb should contain little stem (less than 10 percent), and no large, fibrous stems should be present.

Major Combinations

- Combine with plantain and uva-ursi for hot, painful urinary tract disorders.

- Combine with yerba santa when phlegm fluids obstruct the nasal passages.

- Combine with Sichuan fritillaria, scented Solomon's seal, and grindelia for blood vacuity with blood-streaked sputum.

- Combine with yerba mansa and Chinese angelica for wind-damp impediment with pain, especially in the knees and elbows.

- Combine with California figwort, red root, and Chinese skullcap for swollen, hard lymph nodes. If there is considerable redness or fever, add echinacea, honeysuckle, and forsythia.

Commentary

The genus name *Urtica* comes from the Latin *urere*, meaning "to burn," from the sensation one gets from rubbing against the plant. The species name, *dioica*, refers to the plant's dioecious ("two-housed") nature, meaning that both male and female plants exist and are needed for reproduction. It has been speculated that the common name nettle comes from the Anglo-Saxon word *noedl*, meaning "needle" or possibly from the Latin *nere*, meaning "to sew."

Nettle leaf is commonly eaten as a nutritious spring vegetable. It is rich is many nutrients, mainly minerals. Because of its high mineral content, it is good for those with anemia. However, although the herb is commonly employed as a nourishing tonic in the Western tradition, this practice should be undertaken with care. There is a danger of damaging *yīn* if large quantities of nettle tea are consumed and there is a significant diuretic effect.

Nettle is found in the writings of many famous masters of our past, including Dioscorides, Hippocrates, Hildegard von Bingen, and Paracelsus. Among these authors, Dioscorides seemed to favor the plant most, listing in his writings numerous applications, including suppressed menstruation, cancerous ulcers, burns, furuncles, growths, swollen glands, sprains, nosebleeds, spleen complaints, pleurisy, pneumonia, asthma, facial ringworm, and oral diseases; he also described diuretic, antiflatulent, and softening effects.

Many Native American tribes had medicinal uses

for nettle, most of which echo what I've included in the main description for this herb. However, I am including a few interesting additional applications to provide a historical context for the importance of this medicine. The Iroquois of upstate New York and southern Quebec used the plant with dried snake blood for "witching medicine."[3] When treating pain, the Hesquiaht of coastal British Columbia rubbed the fresh plant on the affected area, stinging the skin and causing counter-irritation. For swelling and arthritis, they steamed the leaves and roots to apply as a poultice. The Hesquiaht were not the only tribe to use the plant as a counter-irritant; others include (but are not limited to) the Kwakiutl (chest pains), Nitinaht (arthritis), Okanagan-Colville (arthritis), Northern Paiute (arthritis), Thompson (arthritis), Carrier (arthritis), Chehalis (arthritis), Cowlitz (paralysis), S'Klallam (soreness and stiffness), Kashaya Pomo (rheumatism and other such pains), Quileute (rheumatism), and Quinault (paralysis).

The far-reaching uses of nettle are not all medicinal. Native peoples have made rope, twine, fine thread, fishing nets, bowstrings, clothing, and other items from nettle stem fibers. Many tribes employed the plant in ceremonies. The Okanagan-Colville of the Northwest made a nettle tea to be drunk while "sweathousing" and washed their skin and hair with it in order to cleanse the body. They also bathed in a nettle decoction to protect against witchcraft.[4]

Nettle seeds and root also have significant medicinal properties, which are not discussed here. Both the seed and root have nourishing properties, especially the seed, and potentially can be used as a supplementing medicinal. The root is used medicinally in a similar way to the herb, as explained above.

Nettle herb, leaf, and root are medicines approved by the German Commission E.

Translation of Source Material

Chinese medicine recognizes four species of *Urtica (U. cannabina, U. angustifolia, U. fissa, U. laetevirens),* all known as *qián má.* The medicinal is acrid, bitter, cold, and slightly toxic. It is used to treat wind-damp pain, postpartum tugging wind, childhood fright-wind, and nettle rash.

HERBS THAT DISPEL WIND AND DAMPNESS

Medicinals for dispelling wind and eliminating dampness comprise a special category sometimes erroneously called "antirheumatics" in the West. The function of these herbs is to remove the pathogenic factors of wind and dampness from the channels, network vessels, flesh, and joints. When wind and dampness penetrate these areas of the body, they produce pain, and due to the nature of wind, this is usually a wandering pain.

Four medicinals are represented in this text that dispel wind and eliminate dampness. Angelica is likely a familiar sight in this category of Chinese medicinals, which is typified by angelica duhou. The angelica described in this text is different enough that I cannot call it analogous to the Chinese species; however, it is used for the same types of patterns.

Yerba mansa *(Anemopsis californica)* is another classic example of a medicinal in this category. It is acrid, bitter, warm, and especially good for the treatment of dampness, particularly stagnant dampness, accumulated dampness that has gathered to form phlegm, and damp toxin. Sassafras *(Sassafras albidum)* is helpful for treating wind-dampness and cold, but has the added benefit of quickening the blood, which is static in chronic conditions. Wintergreen *(Gaultheria procumbens),* another valuable herb in this category, also treats lower burner damp-heat conditions, such as strangury.

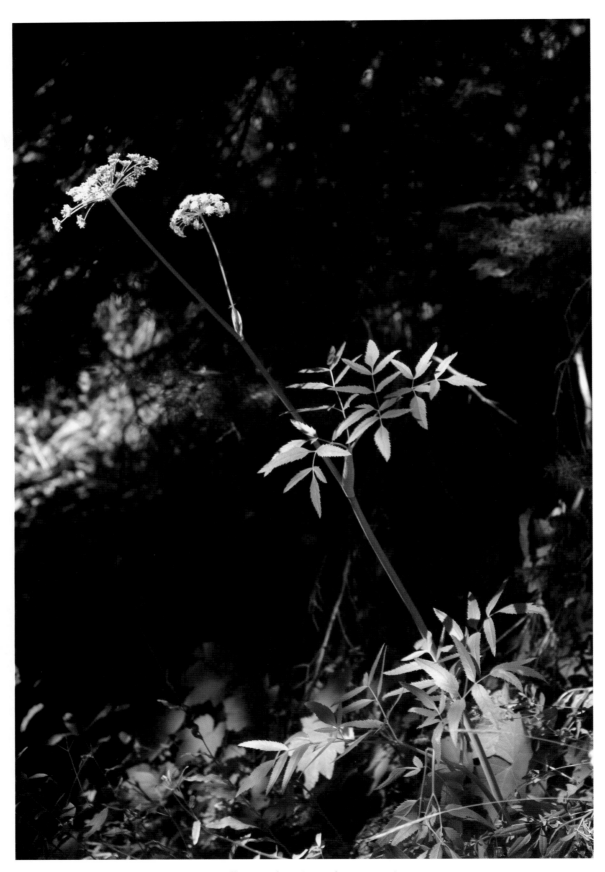

Lyall's angelica *(Angelica arguta)*

Angelica

Angelica breweri, A. arguta,
A. hendersonnii

Apiaceae

Angelicae Breweri seu Argutae
radix

Also known as Brewer's angelica, Lyall's angelica, Henderson's angelica

Flavor and *Qi*: acrid, bitter, warm
Channels Entered: kidney, lung, bladder
Actions: anti-inflammatory, antirheumatic, diuretic

Functions and Indications

- ***Dispels wind-dampness and scatters cold.*** Angelica is used in the treatment of wind-cold-damp impediment with symptoms such as pain and stiffness in the joints (especially the joints of the upper body) and a sense of heaviness. Angelica is acrid and warm and effectively expels wind, dampness, and cold. When these influences enter the channels, the *qi* stagnates and the blood becomes static. This leads to pain; thus the term "impediment." Angelica's warmth and acridity also activate the *qi* and blood within the channels, relieving pain.

- ***Releases the exterior, expels wind, and disperses cold.*** Angelica treats wind-cold with symptoms of headache, neck and shoulder tension, and chills. Angelica's warm and acrid nature expels wind and disperses cold, resolving the exterior and effectively treating external attacks of wind-cold.

- ***Courses* qi, *quickens blood, and relieves pain.*** Angelica is an excellent medicinal for pain due to *qi* stagnation and blood stasis associated either with wind and cold or traumatic injuries. Use internally as described below, or prepare as a liniment for external application to treat joint pain, muscle soreness, or traumatic injury.

CAUTIONS

Use angelica with caution for *yīn* vacuity with heat signs, as well as for individuals with sensitive stomachs or a history of acid reflux. Avoid use during pregnancy.

Dosage and Preparation

Use 3–9 g in decoction; 2–4 ml tincture.

Angelica decoction is the preferred preparation, as the tincture is very acrid and difficult to mask, even when added to a large formula. Prepare tincture for internal use from dried plant material. For external preparations, fresh plant tincture is preferred. Good-quality dried material is firm, aromatic, and resinous. There should be significant resin marbling the inner parts of the roots.

Major Combinations

- Combine with yerba mansa and turmeric for wind-damp-cold impediment of the shoulders, elbows, or wrists. This combination is also excellent when applied externally as a liniment or plaster.

- Combine with osha for wind-cold invading the exterior with symptoms of stiff neck, sore throat, chills, slight fever, and headache. This combination is also good for wind-dampness invasions.

Commentary

Although the two main Western species of angelica I've discussed here *(Angelica breweri* and *A. arguta)* have only limited commercial availability, they are both abundant, and their availability could change with demand. I have been using *A. breweri* since before I began to practice professionally. The plant is native to the north and central high Sierra and high Cascade Mountains of California and Oregon. Although not available to me until recently, the ethnobotanical literature strongly supports the applications I've listed here, which encouraged me to include the plant in this book.

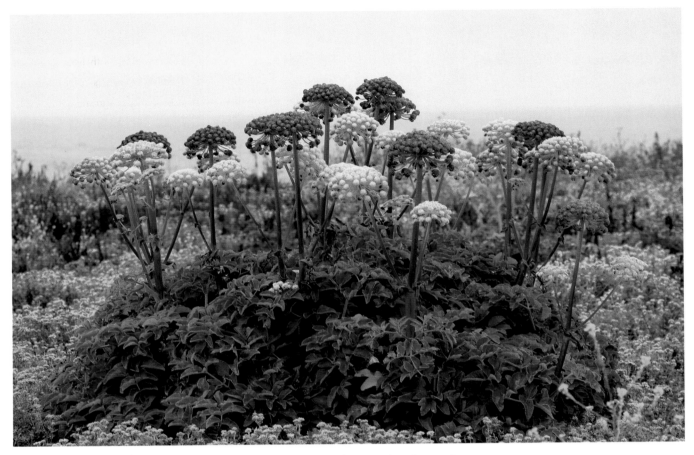

Henderson's angelica (A. hendersonii)

The second species listed here, *A. arguta,* has a larger range and is more widely employed by herbalists in the western United States. Several small wildcrafting companies supply *A. arguta.* The root is significantly smaller, but still large enough to be a viable commercial product. I have only limited experience with this plant, but botanically it is very similar to *A. breweri,* and medicines prepared from the two are nearly indistinguishable.

The Miwok of the Sierra Nevada range and western foothills chewed the root of *A. breweri* for headaches and colds. The Paiute of Nevada's Great Basin prepared the same plant as a decoction for colds, chest ailments, and kidney problems. They also chewed the root for sore throat and coughs and incorporated the mashed root in a salve for cuts and sores. The Shoshoni had, perhaps, a more developed sense of this plant and included it as a minister in formulations to amplify the effects of other medicinals.

Yerba Mansa

Anemopsis californica

Saururaceae

Anemopsi Californicae radix et rhizoma

Other common names include yerba del manso, manso, lizard tail

Flavor and *Qi*: acrid, bitter, warm, aromatic
Channels Entered: lung, bladder, spleen
Actions: antibacterial, antifungal, anti-inflammatory, antirheumatic, astringent

Functions and Indications

- ***Dispels wind and dampness.*** Yerba mansa is employed in the treatment of wind-damp impediment, especially when associated with cold, with symptoms of joint pain, swelling of the joints, and joint pain made worse by cold, damp weather. Yerba mansa also can be used to treat phlegm lodged in the channels. The herb is acrid and warm in nature, aptly dispelling wind and dampness and resolving impediment due to external invasion of wind-dampness. Due to its warm nature, it is especially helpful for wind-dampness associated with cold. However, its bitter nature gives it a distinct drying action, making it most applicable in dampness conditions; with appropriate formulation, this herb can be included with good effect in formulas for either wind-damp-cold or wind-damp-heat. The mashed leaves make a very good plaster for these conditions, although I use the roots primarily, due to better availability. When prolonged dampness conditions go untreated, dampness will gather in the channels. Over time, it will congeal into phlegm. When phlegm collects and stagnates in the channels, *qi* and blood cease to flow normally, and impediment and pain ensue. Yerba mansa's acrid, bitter, and warm nature transforms phlegm in the channels, quickens the blood, invigorates the *qi*, and resolves pain and impediment.

- ***Dispels wind and scatters cold.*** Yerba mansa is helpful for invasion of wind-cold evil with symptoms of heat effusion, aversion to cold, cough, headache, generalized

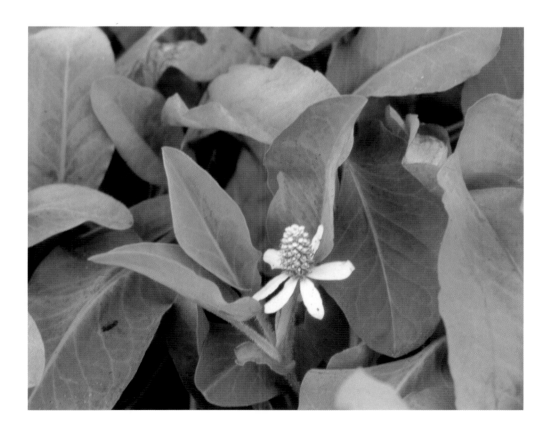

Yerba mansa *(Anemopsis californica)*

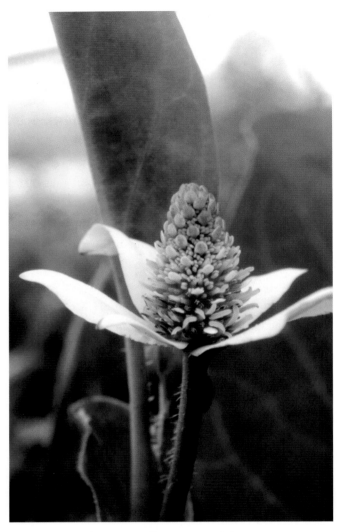

Yerba mansa flower (A. californica)

origin. Because this herb very strongly dries dampness, it can be combined with appropriate herbs to treat toxic swellings of a damp-heat nature. Yerba mansa is bitter and warm and effectively drains dampness and scatters cold. It is also acrid and warm, dispersing stagnation and transforming stagnant dampness.

CAUTIONS

Yerba mansa is relatively safe, but because of its dispelling and drying qualities, it is best avoided during pregnancy. Use caution with patients who have *qì* or *yīn* vacuity due to the herb's strong moving and drying properties. Although yerba mansa is warm in nature, it is commonly used in heat and heat-toxin conditions. This may seem counterintuitive to some; however, this is one of the exceptions in which herbs with warm *qì* can be used to treat warm diseases.

Dosage and Preparation

Use 3–9 g in decoction; 2–4 ml tincture.

The fresh plant tincture is best, although tincture made with dry plant material will suffice. The decoction works very well, but the taste can be quite challenging. The leaves (or root) can be prepared as a wash or made into an ointment for external application. The leaves also make an excellent bath for joint or muscle impediment. Good-quality dried root is rusty colored with an aromatic odor. It should be acrid, bitter, and somewhat numbing to the taste.

Major Combinations

- Combine with black cohosh, California figwort, and willow bark for stiff, hot, painful joints. For severe, acute conditions, add small doses of yucca root.

- Combine with ambrosia, magnolia buds, and yerba santa for sinus congestion with clear or white phlegm. This can be administered for phlegm that is either copious and runny or difficult to discharge. For yellow or green phlegm, add echinacea, goldenseal, and Chinese skullcap.

aches and pains, absence of sweating, nasal congestion, and runny nose with clear, thin phlegm. Yerba mansa's acrid and warm nature dispels wind, scatters cold, and effectively outthrusts external invasion of wind-cold pathogens. The herb has an affinity for the head and face and is specific for external invasion of wind-cold affecting the sinuses. Its bitter flavor and tendency to be drying effectively drain and dry sinus congestion. This use can extend to phlegm-heat in the sinus with thick, sticky, yellow snivel.

- *Dries damp, scatters cold, and assists slow-healing sores.* Yerba mansa is effective against slow-healing sores and toxic swellings (such as innominate toxin swelling) in which the etiology is of a damp and cold

• Combine with goldenseal, Chinese skullcap, and echinacea for damp-heat toxic swellings and sores. Apply both externally and internally, combining with licorice and ginger for internal use. Add *dāng guī* and astragalus for slow-healing sores.

Commentary

Yerba mansa challenges goldenseal as a strong antibacterial, although it is not a substitute for that herb. Goldenseal is cold in nature and yerba mansa is warm, an important distinction that should not be overlooked. As an antibacterial, yerba mansa works best when the origin of infection and inflammation is a cold-induced disorder. Disorders such as influenza and pneumonia that begin as *tài-yáng* disease patterns are those indicated here. In *tài-yáng* disease, if the external evil is unresolved, it can fall inward and become congested in the lung, giving rise to heat. This can manifest as upper respiratory infection, which would include the lung and sinus. This is a perfect situation for yerba mansa. The herb is bitter, acrid, and warm, creating an upbearing and outthrusting action that assists the lungs in restoring proper *qì* diffusion while eliminating congested evils.

In wind-warmth patterns when the pathogen is attacking the lung defense with symptoms such as sore throat, fever, thirst, cough, red-tipped tongue, and a floating and rapid pulse, this herb may not be so effective as a simple. However, combined with other appropriate herbs, yerba mansa can be incorporated into a formula for its wind-dispelling and dampness-drying properties, as long as we keep in mind its warming energy. As an example, combining yerba mansa with Lonicera and Forsythia Powder (*yín qiào sǎn*) for the aforementioned wind-warmth pattern can be an excellent choice, especially with coughing of yellow sputum and excretion of yellow snivel. Yerba mansa is known for its antibacterial and antifungal properties, which may be serviceable in these conditions. Although there is no data to support such a claim, yerba mansa is also likely an antiviral.

Yerba mansa is very effective in wind conditions. It affects the upper part of the body most profoundly and thus may be effectively employed for rhinitis and sinusitis. Yerba mansa scatters wind and transforms dampness. It can be used in both chronic and acute stages of disease and is particularly helpful when the condition is associated with headache.

For millennia, the Native Americans of the southwestern United States and central Mexico have treated rheumatism and arthritis with yerba mansa. It is most helpful in cases in which the condition is made worse by damp and cold conditions. The plant has anti-inflammatory actions, but remember that it is warm in nature, so it functions as an anti-inflammatory via moving (and, to a certain extent, astringing) effects, not cooling. Thus, it is especially helpful when the inflammation is caused by stagnation resulting from a cold and damp condition. When the stagnation is broken and the *qì* and blood are allowed to move through the area, the inflammation will subside. Yerba mansa combines well with California figwort, California peony, angelica, and wild ginger for such conditions. If the condition is caused by heat, reduce the angelica and wild ginger and add black cohosh and large gentian root. Yerba mansa also can be made into an external anti-inflammatory preparation to apply to the affected area.

In addition to the applications listed above, Native Americans used this medicinal to treat stomach ulcers, colds, chest congestion, and menstrual cramps, and as a general pain reliever. They made it into an external wash for open wounds and sores, and mashed the leaves to apply to swellings.

Yerba mansa's antibacterial and antifungal properties are very strong, and this herb is indispensable in the pharmacy. Used externally, it shows significant potential for the treatment of various conditions, including fungal infections of the foot, vaginal infections, and nail fungus.

Sassafras

Sassafras albidum

Lauraceae

Sassafras Albidi cortex radicis

Flavor and *Qi:* acrid, bitter, warm, aromatic
Channels Entered: lung, liver, stomach
Actions: alterative, antirheumatic, antiseptic, carminative, diaphoretic, diuretic

Functions and Indications

- ***Scatters cold, transforms dampness, and dispels wind.*** Sassafras is used to treat wind-damp-cold impediment. Sassafras is acrid and aromatic, mobile and penetrating. Thus, it is an important medicinal for outthrusting external wind-damp attacks. While its aromatic and acrid nature makes sassafras particularly good for wind and damp conditions, it is important to note that these qualities also quicken blood and stimulate the movement of *qi*. Although warm in nature and able to scatter cold, sassafras is often used for heat conditions. Heat in impediment syndromes is generally caused by stagnation and stasis. Thus, resolving stagnation and stasis can clear heat. This is likely how and why sassafras can be effectively used for impediment syndromes with associated heat. Sassafras is also helpful for wind-damp affecting the skin with itching. For this indication, sassafras may be used in either heat or cold conditions.

- ***Quickens the blood and transforms stasis.*** Sassafras treats blood stasis from a variety of etiologies, including trauma, impediment syndromes, and blocked menstruation. Sassafras can be administered either internally or externally for blood stasis. The herb is

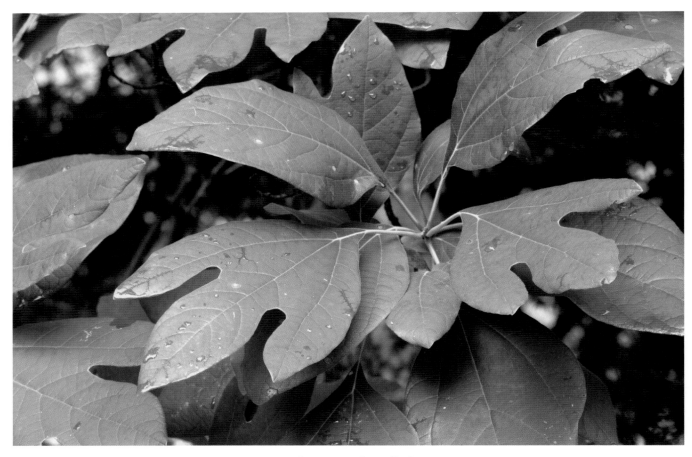

Sassafras *(Sassafras albidum)*

acrid, bitter, aromatic, and warm. It is mobile and penetrating. It moves *qi* and quickens blood, penetrating into the channels to open and free them while quickening the network vessels.

CAUTIONS

Safrole, a constituent found in significant quantities in sassafras (and in smaller amounts in cinnamon, nutmeg, and camphor), has been found to be carcinogenic in animals. The U.S. Food and Drug Adminstration and Health Canada have both banned food products containing safrole.[1] Furthermore, since sassafras root bark can be used to synthesize some popular recreational drugs, such as MDMA (ecstasy) and MDA, the sale of this product is monitored by the U.S. Drug Enforcement Agency. For these reasons, many people have shunned sassafras, but its correct use at proper dosages has never, to the author's knowledge, caused cancer in humans. McGuffin et al. state that the herb is not for long-term use and that the recommended dosage (which they list as 10 g of root powder and 2–4 ml of liquid extract of root bark) should not be exceeded.[2] Do not use sassafras for long periods of time and do not use the essential oil internally.

Dosage and Preparation

Use 3–6 g in infusion or light decoction; 1–2 ml tincture.

Good-quality dried root bark is rusty colored and strongly aromatic. It is common for the product to be "dusty" after being processed.

Major Combinations

• Combine with Oregon grape root, sarsaparilla, and red clover for stubborn skin conditions from various etiologies associated with heat.

• Combine with California figwort, Oregon grape root, and burdock for wind-damp-heat impediment.

• Combine with wintergreen, yerba mansa, and angelica for wind-damp-cold impediment.

Commentary

Sassafras is a common tree of the eastern United States that gives us a delightful, aromatic bark. The bark is employed as a demulcent and warming carminative to soothe and invigorate the digestive process when gas and bloating are prevalent. It moves *qi* and clears heat from the joints in rheumatic conditions, reducing pain and increasing mobility. It is commonly used in eruptive skin conditions as well as eczema and psoriasis. It is a good herb to add to a formula for chronic urinary troubles.

Europeans first learned about sassafras in the sixteenth century when French and Spanish explorers found their way to the East Coast of the United States. The first tree sprouts were planted in Britain in 1612. This medicinal was quite popular in Europe from the seventeenth through the nineteenth centuries to treat syphilis and as a general blood purifier.

The Latin *Sassafras* is likely from the Latin word *saxifragus,* meaning "to break stones," owing to the plant's historical use for treating kidney stones. The species name *albidum* comes from the Latin *albus,* for "white." This tree is common in my hometown in Massachusetts and is found throughout the eastern part of the United States. It is available in health food stores and herb shops in bulk, tincture, and many formulas.

Sassafras was or is official in the *Deutsches Arzneibuch 6 Ed.* (1926) and *Martindale: The Extra Pharmacopoeia* (31st ed., 1996). Oil of sassafras is listed as official in the pharmacopoeias of Portugal and Spain.

Wintergreen

Gaultheria procumbens

Ericaceae

Gaultheriae Procumbens folium

Flavor and *Qi*: acrid, bitter, cool, aromatic
Channels Entered: liver, kidney, bladder, stomach
Actions: anti-inflammatory, antirheumatic, diuretic

Functions and Indications

- ***Dispels wind-dampness and clears heat.*** Wintergreen is helpful for treating wind-damp impediment when wind-cold-damp has transformed into a heat impediment, presenting with symptoms of hot, swollen, painful joints and joint pain made worse by windy, damp, or hot weather. Because of its ability to dispel dampness, this herb is effective for acute syndromes in which dampness has lodged in the muscles, causing muscle aches and stiffness. The plant is also applied externally for these conditions. Wintergreen essential oil is the main preparation used externally and is found in many liniments (including Chinese formulations). Wintergreen is acrid and cool and thus an excellent herb for dispersing wind and clearing heat in chronic or acute inflammatory conditions. It is helpful in conditions related to external attack of heat or to other factors that have been left untreated and have thus transformed to heat.

- ***Drains damp and clears heat in the lower burner.*** Wintergreen is useful in damp-heat *lin* syndrome, with symptoms of painful urination, obstructed urination, blood in the urine, pain due to benign prostatic hypertrophy, and pain in the anatomical kidneys due to inflammation. Wintergreen is bitter and cool. Bitter drains, and cool clears heat, making the herb effective for damp-heat conditions. Furthermore, wintergreen has an affinity for the anatomical kidneys and the rest of the lower burner. Thus it is very helpful for treating biomedically defined kidney inflammation as well as disorders associated with

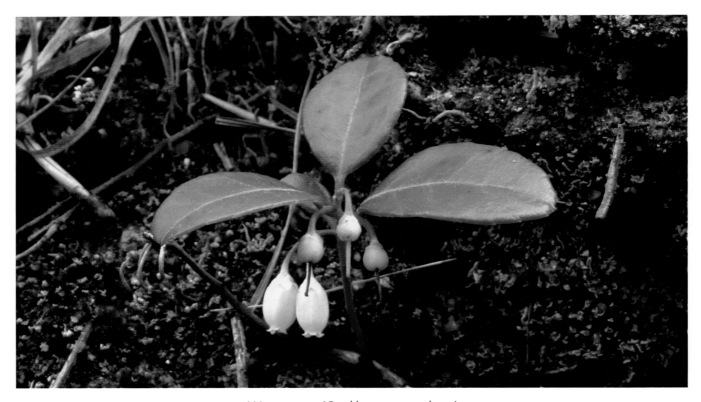

Wintergreen *(Gaultheria procumbens)*

either repletion or vacuity heat syndromes of the water phase. It may also be used to clear heat from kidney *yīn* vacuity with symptoms of increased sexual desire and spermatorrhea.

- ***Penetrates the channels and mobilizes* qì *and blood.*** Wintergreen is employed to treat patterns of *qì* stagnation and blood stasis that have transformed into heat, such as dysmenorrhea, amenorrhea, colic, pain in the epigastrium or abdomen, and toothache. Depression of *qì* and blood lead to depressive heat. Wintergreen is bitter and strongly aromatic. It is mobile and penetrating and opens depression, making it an important medicinal for various types of depressive heat.

CAUTIONS

Because the salicylates contained in wintergreen may interact with some drugs, causing bleeding and other side effects, exercise caution with patients taking abortifacients, anticoagulants, anti-emetics, anti-epileptics, cytotoxics, diuretics, NSAIDs, or uricosuric drugs. It should be noted that natural salicylates are less active than aspirin; therefore less caution is required.[3] Wintergreen essential oil is for external use only.

Dosage and Preparation

Use 2–6 g in infusion (hot or cold); 0.5–3 ml tincture.

For lower burner damp-heat, a cold infusion is best. Wintergreen essential oil should be used externally only. This oil is combined with other ingredients to prepare pastes, plasters, liniments, and oils for treating trauma. Good-quality dried herb is green, aromatic, and contains no stems.

Major Combinations

- Combine with cleavers and usnea for damp-heat *lín* syndrome with scanty, dark yellow urine, with or without pain and blood in the urine.

- For external use, combine with yerba mansa and cayenne to make a paste for joint pain. For this purpose I prefer the essential oil, mixing it thoroughly into the paste. Wintergreen also combines well with St. John's wort, arnica, and cayenne in liniments or oils for external application.

Commentary

Although wintergreen is cooling in nature, it is mobile and penetrating. These qualities make it particularly useful clinically, since many medicinals that have these qualities are warming. The berries are sweet, slightly acrid, and warm and can be used to nourish the kidney *yáng*.

I grew up eating wintergreen berries. The plant is an abundant forest-floor dweller in the northeastern United States. Many native peoples ate the berries, either raw or prepared as cakes that were dried and stored for the future. The Iroquois made them into a sauce or relish to be served with corn bread.[4]

Salal (*Gaultheria shallon*), a related species growing in the northwestern United States and western Canada, has very similar applications. The Quinault of the southwestern coast of the Olympic Peninsula used salal medicinally to treat diarrhea, colic, and heartburn, and as food made into cakes and dipped in whale or seal oil.[5]

While wintergreen is not official in any country, methyl salicylate (a component of the oil from wintergreen leaves) is listed in many pharmacopoeias around the world. Some of these pharmacopoeias state that the product must be synthetic, while others allow it to come from the plant source. The source must be indicated on the label.

Translation of Source Material

Chinese medicine uses two species of *Gaultheria*. Dà tòu gǔ xiāo (*G. forrestii*) is bitter, acrid, and warm. It dispels wind, eliminates dampness, and is used to treat wind-damp paralysis and frostbite.

Tòu gǔ xiāng (*G. yunnanensis*) is acrid and warm. It dispels wind and eliminates dampness, quickens the blood and frees the network vessels, and is employed in the treatment of wind-damp joint pain, water drum distention, knocks and falls, toothache, and dampness papules.

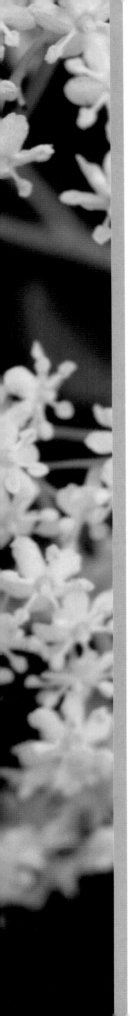

HERBS THAT TRANSFORM PHLEGM AND STOP COUGHING

This category is divided into two or even three categories in many materia medicas in order to distinguish the medicinals as warm, cooling, or having the ability to stop coughing. I have combined them here because I am not presenting very many plants. However, one should not assume that the three medicinals discussed in this chapter are used only for phlegm in the lungs. Transforming phlegm implies a relatively gentle process of eliminating phlegm. Stopping cough, on the other hand, requires downbearing *qì* and restoring the depurative function of the lung.

Pleurisy root *(Asclepias tuberosa),* an important medicinal in this category and the whole materia medica, has a wide range of actions. This herb is bitter, acrid, and cold in nature, and is very effective for diffusing lung *qì* and circulating the *qì* of the chest. Thus it helps with a wide variety of ailments in the chest, including cough, major chest bind, and asthma. Yerba santa *(Eriodictyon californicum)* is likely the most famous of native California herbs. Unlike pleurisy root, yerba santa is warm and is useful for transforming phlegm in the lung and spleen. Yerba santa also has the extra benefit of warming spleen *yáng* and resolving rheum. Both pleurisy root and yerba santa resolve the exterior, but their actions are different. Grindelia *(Grindelia* spp.) is bitter, acrid, and cool in nature and valuable for diffusing and downbearing the lung *qì*. Grindelia also treats the lower burner with cool and bitterness, clearing heat in the kidney and bladder.

Yerba Santa

Eriodictyon californicum, E. tricocalyx,
E. angustifolium, **and others**

Hydrophyllaceae

Eriodictyonis Californicus folium

Also called mountain balm

Flavor and *Qì:* acrid, bitter, sweet, warm
Channels Entered: lung, spleen
Actions: anti-inflammatory, decongestant, digestive, expectorant

Functions and Indications

- ***Transforms phlegm and downbears lung* qì.** Yerba santa is used in patterns such as phlegm-damp obstructing the lung with coughing of copious white sputum, chest oppression, and difficult breathing. Yerba santa is also helpful for phlegm glomus. The herb's warmth and acridity penetrate deeply to transform phlegm, while its bitterness downbears lung *qì.* It is very effective for the treatment of phlegm, especially cold phlegm and phlegm-damp.

- ***Warms* yáng *and transforms rheum.*** Yerba santa is employed to treat symptoms such as loss of appetite, chronic cough, panting, fullness of the chest, phlegm in the stool (with or without diarrhea), and expectoration of copious white, possibly frothy, sputum. Yerba santa's sweet nature further addresses phlegm by reaching to the source—the spleen—warming spleen *yáng* and improving recalcitrant phlegm-damp conditions.

- ***Courses the exterior, dissipates wind, and diffuses lung* qì.** Yerba santa is helpful in the treatment of

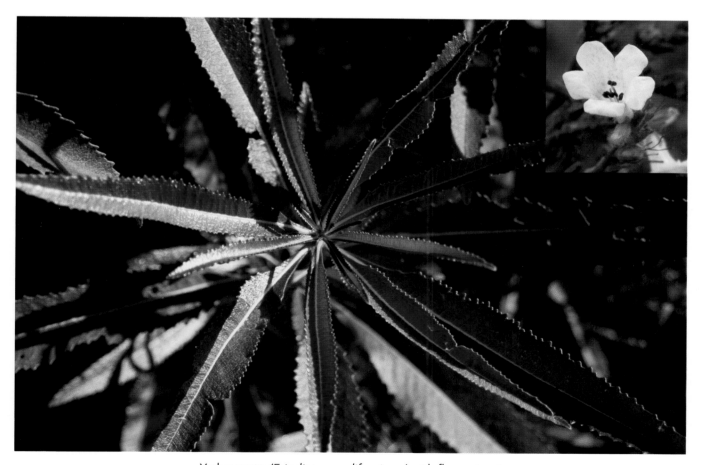

Yerba santa *(Eriodictyon californicum)* with flower inset

runny nose of any etiology, with clear or white phlegm, watery eyes, and sneezing. Yerba santa is an effective medicinal for allergies and hay fever, especially when the allergies are mediated by food. When added to an appropriate formula, this herb can be valuable in heat conditions affecting the sinuses. Yerba santa's acridity is the main flavor responsible for this action. Acridity courses the exterior, dissipates wind, and diffuses lung *qi*. The acrid and bitter flavor helps to address the source of nasal mucus, the lung. Wind impairs the function of the lung, thus disrupting its downbearing action on fluids in the body and creating accumulation of fluids in the lungs. These fluids will then transform into phlegm within the channel and orifices associated with that system. Furthermore, the lung governs *qi*, and any disruption of the lung can lead to *qi* vacuity. *Qi* vacuity in the spleen can lead to production of phlegm. Thus, sweet and acrid flavors address the "ultimate" source of phlegm, the spleen. Yerba santa warms and boosts the spleen while transforming phlegm, fully addressing the source of this condition.

CAUTIONS

Use yerba santa with caution in those with *yīn* vacuity.

Dosage and Preparation

Use 3–9 g in decoction; 2–4 ml tincture.

Yerba santa is useful as a tea or tincture, but I prefer the fresh plant tincture, which has a warmer nature and is better for transforming phlegm and rheum.

Yerba santa leaves can be gathered nearly any time of year, but new growth gathered in spring or early summer yields the best-quality herb. The leaves are quite resinous and tend to stick together. When drying, they should be spread out to encourage even drying. Good-quality dried herb is dark green and resinous, free of stems and flowers, and should have a somewhat sweet smell.

Major Combinations

- Combine with grindelia for cough with panting and asthma. This combination is also good externally for rashes due to poison oak or poison ivy.

- Combine with Chinese angelica, wild ginger, and yerba mansa for runny nose with copious, clear mucous secretions.

- Combine with elecampane for cough with loss of appetite, weak limbs, and lethargy.

Commentary

The name *Eriodictyon* comes from the Greek *erion,* meaning "wool," in reference to the woolly underside of the leaf. The species name *californicum* is a reference to the fact that, other than southwestern Oregon, this species is endemic to California.

Yerba santa is one of the few native California herbs enjoying international acclaim. This plant is an excellent decongestant, and, secondarily, functions well as an expectorant for conditions involving either heat or cold, depending upon the other herbs in the formula. The herb is exceptionally helpful for congestion in the lungs and nasal passages with feelings of heaviness in the head and fullness in the chest. It is especially good when the sputum is copious and runny (cold).

Yerba santa increases salivation and acts as a digestive stimulant. The Native Americans of Mendocino County rolled yerba santa leaves into a ball to make a chew that was said to make a person sweet inside.[1] The initial taste is bitter, but this flavor gives way to a peculiar sweetness. The initial bitterness stimulates the flow of bile, the spicy sweet flavor increases saliva production, and the combination of these two flavors generally stimulates the digestive process.

Most of the native peoples within the plant's range had multiple uses for yerba santa. According to one source, the Miwok of the western Sierra Nevada range used the plant for colds, cough, and rheumatism both internally and externally, and as a dermatological, gastrointestinal, and orthopedic aid.

Professor John Michael Maisch introduced yerba santa into the medicine of North American white settlers at a meeting of the Philadelphia College of Pharmacy in March 1875. Later that year, Dr. J. H. Bundy of California published an article in *The Eclectic Medical Journal,* and, with Professor John Scudder's publication of the botanical name in the same journal in 1876, the plant became widely known and a part of common practice. Parke-Davis was the first pharmaceutical company to market the extract, and to this day yerba santa is included as an ingredient in some pharmaceutical preparations for its ability to moisten the mucous membranes of the mouth and throat.

Yerba santa was official in *The United States Pharmacopoeia* from 1894–1905 and 1916–1947, and has been listed in *The National Formulary (U.S.)* since 1947.

Pleurisy Root

Asclepias tuberosa

Asclepiadaceae

Also called butterfly weed, wind root

Flavor and *Qì*: bitter, acrid, cold
Channels Entered: lung, large intestine
Actions: anticatarrhal, antitussive, diaphoretic, expectorant

Functions and Indications

- **Clears heat, diffuses the lung qì, and transforms phlegm.** Pleurisy root is valuable for lung-heat with symptoms of pain in the chest, fever, and cough, with difficult or no expectoration. Pleurisy root has a bitter and acrid flavor and is cold in nature. Its bitter and acrid flavors transform phlegm and drain the lung of repletion heat while diffusing the lung *qì*. Its cold nature strongly clears heat. Together these flavors and nature combine to transform phlegm, clear heat, and assist the lung *qì* in its depurating and diffusing action. Pleurisy root also resolves the exterior, helping the body push out any pathogens that may have entered from the exterior.

- **Circulates the qì of the chest, relieves pain, and harmonizes the upper burner.** This herb is very effective for major chest bind *(dà jié xiōng)* caused by chronic heat and phlegm, in which heat is predominant and the pulse is tight and rapid. Pleurisy root has an acrid and bitter flavor. Acridity outthrusts, while bitter downbears. This combination of flavors creates a har-

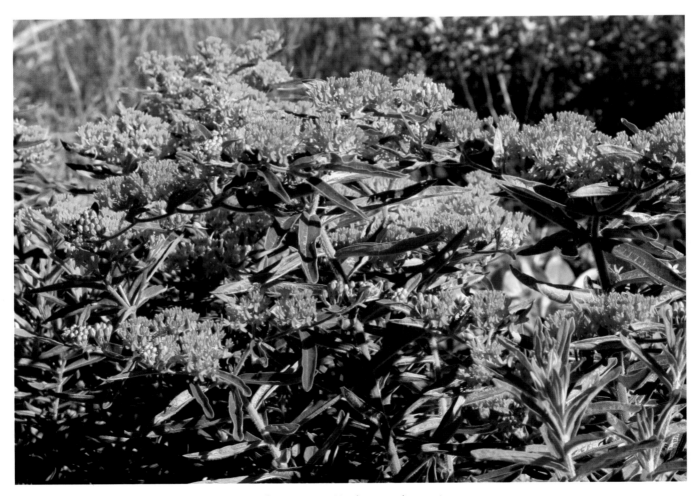

Pleurisy root *(Asclepias tuberosa)*

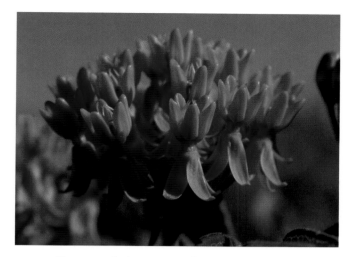

Close-up of pleurisy root flower (A. tuberosa)

monizing action in the chest, where this medicinal has an affinity. Owing to its acridity and cold nature, pleurisy root circulates the *qì* in the chest, transforms phlegm, and clears heat, thus relieving pain and effectively resolving chest bind. Pleurisy root also helps with hot asthma accompanied by chest pain and difficult breathing. The herb is effective for any type of heat in the chest, but because of its cold nature should be combined with warming medicinals for extremely deficient patients.

- **Resolves the exterior and expels wind.** Pleurisy root is used to treat external wind-heat invasion with sweating that is not complete, cough, fever, sore throat, and a floating and rapid pulse. Pleurisy root is acrid and cold, outthrusting wind and heat. This is a major application for this medicinal and occupies a significant portion of the literature detailing the historical use of the plant.

- **Clears heat and cools the blood.** Pleurisy root treats fever with dry skin, a red tongue, and a rapid and replete pulse. Heat entering the blood at the blood aspect causes serious illness, and pleurisy root is an important medicinal for this pattern. Pleurisy root has a bitter flavor and is cold in nature, a combination that is essential for the treatment of heat at the blood aspect. Furthermore, this medicinal is acrid in nature, which activates the *qì* and, secondarily,

quickens the blood. This secondary action is beneficial to the overall action of the herb, as stasis and stagnation are common confounding factors when heat enters the blood aspect. Pleurisy root also helps with skin rashes for which blood-heat is part of the pattern.

CAUTIONS

Pleurisy root is cold in nature and should be used with caution by those with spleen *qì* vacuity or internal cold. Avoid use of pleurisy root during pregnancy.

Dosage and Preparation

Use 2–6 g in strong infusion or decoction; 2.5–5 ml tincture.

The fresh plant tincture of pleurisy root is superior to the dry preparation. Gather pleurisy root in autumn, after the plant has withered, or in early spring. The root is either prepared fresh or sliced and dried for storage. Good-quality dried root is grayish white and firm. It is quite fibrous, so cut-and-sifted root will contain significant amounts of fibrous material.

Major Combinations

- Combine with American ginseng and sweet flag for phlegm-heat in the lung. Adjust the dosages of the medicinals to fit the clinical picture.

- Combine with grindelia and Fritillaria and Anemarrhena Powder (*èr mǔ sǎn*) for severe dry cough with thick, yellow, difficult-to-expectorate sputum.

- Combine with lobelia for hot, spasmodic cough with difficult expectoration.

- Combine with black cohosh for acute rheumatic fever with arthritic pain that is worse with motion, abdominal pain, and high fever.

- Combine with bugleweed for chest pain due to heat stagnation (with or without cough) with blood streaked sputum.

Commentary

Pleurisy root is exceptional for treating lung-heat, especially when phlegm is a confounding factor. Further, pleurisy root is a very effective medicinal for major chest bind *(dà jié xiōng)*. The following quote from an Eclectic physician, Grover Coe, in 1858 illustrates its value:

> In fact we [can] think of no pathological condition that would be aggravated by its employment. It expels wind, relieves pain, relaxes spasm, induces and promotes perspiration, equalizes the circulation, harmonizes the action of the nervous system, and accomplishes its work without excitement; neither increasing the force or the frequency of the pulse, nor raising the temperature of the body.

The genus name *Asclepias* comes from that of the ancient Greek god of medicine, Asklepios. The species name *tuberosa* refers to the plant's enlarged root system. This genus is endemic to North America. Fibers from *Asclepias* have been found in Ohio in textiles dating back as far as 700 BCE. The Cherokee used the plant for pain in the breast, stomach, and intestines.[2] In addition, most Native Americans within its range used it for lung diseases.

Under the heading "Acute bronchitis," modern herbalists Mills and Bone state, "Diaphoretic herbs are indicated during the febrile phase, particularly *Asclepias tuberosa* [pleurisy root] which is almost a specific for acute lower respiratory tract infections. It is often combined with *Zingiber* to enhance its effectiveness."[3]

Pleurisy root was official in *The United States Pharmacopoeia* from 1820–1905 and in *The National Formulary (U.S.)* from 1916–1936. It is listed in the *British Herbal Pharmacopoeia* (1983), *Martindale: The Extra Pharmacopoeia* (33rd ed.), and *PDR for Herbal Medicine* (2nd ed.).

Grindelia

Grindelia spp.

Asteraceae

Grindeliae flos immaturus et folium

Also called gum weed, tarweed

Flavor and Qì: bitter, acrid, cool
Channels Entered: lung, kidney, bladder
Actions: anti-inflammatory, antispasmodic, expectorant

Functions and Indications

- **Diffuses and downbears lung qì and expels phlegm.** Grindelia is used to treat cough and panting of many different etiologies. Although this herb is cooling in nature, grindelia can be used for a variety of conditions, either hot or cold, when combined with other appropriate medicinals. Grindelia's acridity diffuses lung *qì* and its bitterness downbears it. By supporting the lung's depurative, downbearing function, grindelia supports the body's *qì*, helping to make expectoration more complete. Furthermore, the herb has a slightly moistening and cooling action and thins the phlegm so it is easier to expectorate.

- **Transforms phlegm.** Grindelia is helpful in a variety of phlegmatic conditions (both substantial and insubstantial), with symptoms of headache; dizziness; lassitude of spirit; dull, stagnant complexion; and oppression in the chest. Grindelia is an important medicinal for the treatment of acute and chronic phlegm conditions. Its acridity transforms phlegm, but it is the herb's bitter and cool nature that clears

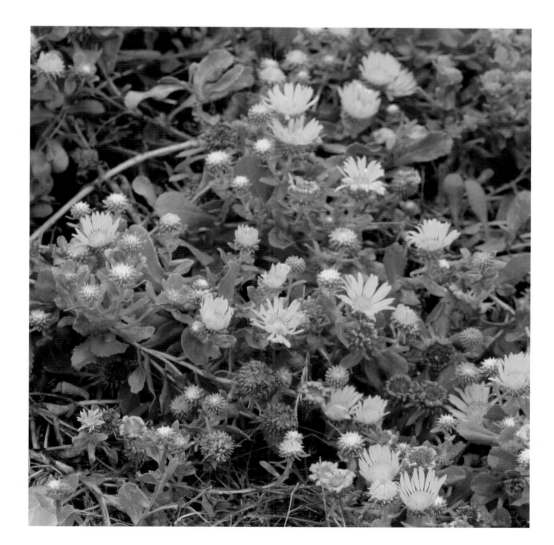

Grindelia (*Grindelia* sp.)

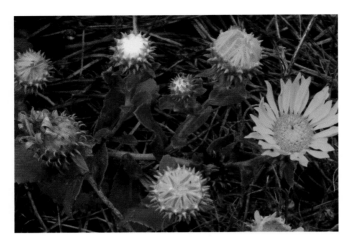

Close-up of grindelia flowers (*Grindelia* sp.)

heat and constraint. Thus, grindelia is excellent for constrained phlegm conditions.

- **Clears heat in the lower burner.** Grindelia is employed to treat heat patterns affecting the bladder. Grindelia is bitter and cool and thus drains and clears heat. It has a long history of medicinal use for biomedically defined kidney and bladder inflammation. The fresh plant tincture is best for this purpose.

- **Used externally for wind-heat-toxin.** Another use for grindelia is the treatment of wind-heat-toxin caused by poison oak *(Toxicodendron diversilobum)* and other sources of contact dermatitis. With acridity, grindelia scatters wind; with bitter coolness, it clears heat and resolves toxins. Grindelia is classically combined with yerba santa for poison oak.

CAUTIONS

Grindelia should not be used for extended periods of time, as it has a tendency to uptake selenium from the soil. That and the plant's high resin content may aggravate the kidneys.

Dosage and Preparation

Use 3–9 g in decoction; 2–4 ml tincture.

Both decoction and tincture are acceptable dosage forms for grindelia, taken either internally or externally. The fresh plant tincture is my favorite. For those who have problems with alcohol, the decoction works nicely, although tincture is still superior.

Gather the budding tops in spring and early summer. Because the plant is quite sticky, take care when drying it. Be sure to spread it out evenly; best results will be achieved in moderately warm and very well-ventilated conditions. Good-quality dried herb is green-to-light green with at least 50 percent flower content and less than 5 percent open flowers. It is perferrable to have no open flowers, seeds, or large stems.

Note that *G. squarrosa* in particular has been found to concentrate selenium and is considered toxic. Based on this, is probably best to avoid this species.

Major Combinations

- Combine with California spikenard and yerba santa for cough or panting with copious clear or white sputum. This combination is especially useful for chronic cases in which the *yáng qì* is weak.

- Combine with marsh mallow and pleurisy root for cough with thick, yellow, difficult-to-expectorate sputum.

- Combine with bluecurls for panting with difficult breathing (e.g., asthma).

- Combine with yerba santa, yarrow, arnebia, and plantain for wind-heat-toxin caused by poison oak. This preparation is primarily for external application, but can also be used internally.

Commentary

Grindelia is an extremely valuable U.S. native medicinal. While definite in its action, it is safe enough to use in full doses with children. It is an excellent addition to many formulas for cough associated with heat patterns. Grindelia is especially helpful for chronic conditions in which lung *yīn* has been damaged. Although it does not directly nourish lung *yīn,* it does clear heat without drying or further damaging lung *yīn.* This is an exceptional attribute for a medicinal with such strength in transforming phlegm.

Native peoples of the Americas employed this genus extensively, often having multiple uses for the species growing near them. As an example, the Flathead Indians of Idaho and western Montana used *G. squarrosa* extensively as a cold remedy, cough medicine, pulmonary aid (for whooping cough and pneumonia), respiratory aid (for bronchitis and asthma), tuberculosis treatment, and veterinary medicine.[4]

The genus name *Grindelia* comes from that of the German physician, plant pharmacist, and botanist D. H. von Grindel. Dr. C. A. Canfield of Monterey, California, first wrote about grindelia in *Pacific Medicine and Surgery* about 1863, but the herb wasn't regularly employed in American medicine until around 1875, when James G. Steele of San Francisco presented a paper to the American Pharmaceutical Association.

Grindelia was an official drug in *The United States Pharmacopoeia* from 1882–1926 and was official in *The National Formulary (U.S.)* from 1926–1960.

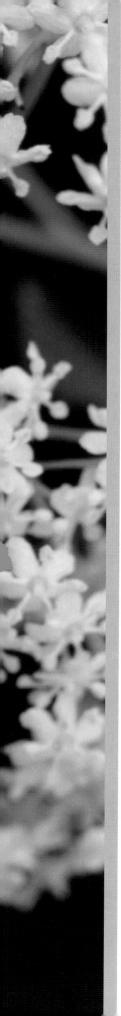

HERBS THAT AROMATICALLY TRANSFORM DAMPNESS

This special category of medicinals in Chinese medicine is similar to that known as "carminatives" in Western herbal medicine. These medicinals have a strong aroma and are rich in essential oils and often in resins as well. The main function of this category of medicinals is to arouse the spleen when it has been encumbered by turbid dampness, obstructing its ability to transform fluids. The transformation of dampness is accomplished by the aromatic nature of the medicinals, which penetrates the turbidity and moves *qi*, specifically the spleen *qi*. These medicinals tend to be warm, which gives them a stronger action, because warm dries dampness. Signs and symptoms of dampness include low appetite, fullness after eating, a pale, often wet tongue, and a soggy pulse.

This text includes only one Western medicinal representative of this category, but it is an important one. Western sweet cicely *(Osmorhiza occidentalis)* is acrid, bitter, sweet, warm, and aromatic. This combination of flavors and nature gives the medicinal the ability to move *qi* with acridity, drain with bitterness, act on the spleen and stomach with sweetness, dry with warmth, and transform with aroma. Thus it provides an entire suite of attributes that make it an outstanding member of this category.

Western Sweet Cicely

Osmorhiza occidentalis

Apiaceae

Osmorhizae Occidentalis radix et rhizoma

Also called sweet root, osmorrhiza

Flavor and *Qi:* acrid, bitter, sweet, warm, aromatic
Channels Entered: spleen, stomach, large intestine
Actions: antibacterial, antifungal, carminative

Functions and Indications

- *Aromatically transforms dampness and downbears qì.* Western sweet cicely is effective in the treatment of dampness obstructing the middle burner, with symptoms such as regurgitation, abdominal pain, nausea, bloating, gas, lack of appetite, and fullness and oppression in the chest. Western sweet cicely is acrid, bitter, and aromatic. Its acridity and aroma stimulate the movement of *qi* and aromatically transform dampness, while its bitterness downbears the *qi*. This combination of flavors converges with the medicinal's aroma and warm *qi* to restore the stomach's downbearing function, revive the spleen, and allow the small intestine to take charge of humor, separating the clear from the turbid.

- *Fortifies the spleen and harmonizes the stomach.* By drying the spleen, transforming damp, and downbearing *qi,* Western sweet cicely fortifies the spleen, assisting it when it is encumbered by dampness in upbearing the clear. In this way, it harmonizes the

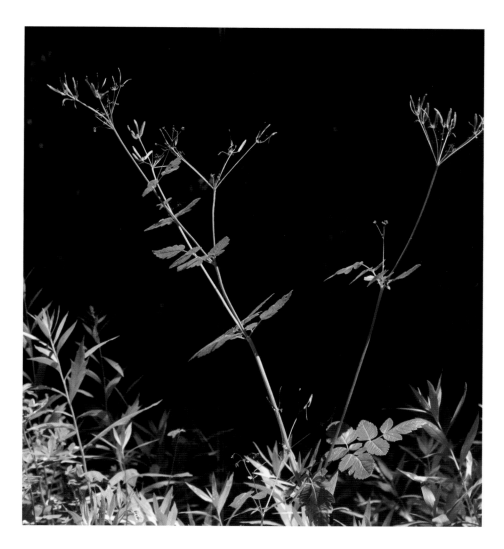

Western sweet cicely *(Osmorhiza occidentalis)*

stomach, assisting the downbearing action of the stomach *qi* on the turbid. These functions allow this medicinal to treat glomus, fullness, distention, and oppression in the stomach duct; belching; and vomiting of sour fluid.

- **Dries dampness and assists the dài mài.** Western sweet cicely is used to treat dampness pouring downward with vaginal discharge and a bloated, cold, and painful feeling in the lower burner. Although Western sweet cicely is warm, it can be used in damp-heat conditions when combined with the appropriate herbs.

CAUTIONS

Use Western sweet cicely with caution for those with *yīn* vacuity heat signs, especially stomach *yīn* vacuity.

Dosage and Preparation

Use 3–9 g in light decoction or strong infusion; 2–4 ml tincture.

Gather roots and rhizomes in autumn or early spring. They should be washed thoroughly and either cut and prepared as a fresh plant tincture or sliced and dried for storage. Good-quality dried root is strongly aromatic, with a sweet licorice or anise scent. The root has a lightly striated middle portion (a salt-and-pepper look) and a thin black or dark-brown skin.

Major Combinations

- Combine with atractylodes and white atractylodes to strengthen that combination's ability to revive and supplement the spleen while transforming damp.

- Combine with goldenseal for dampness and heat obstructing the middle burner, with symptoms such as regurgitation, nausea, and vomiting. If heat has begun to overcome the damp, add marsh mallow root.

Commentary

The genus name *Osmorhiza* comes from the Greek and means "sweet root." This is a small genus of ten or so species, with most species (eight) found in North America. The others come from Asia. Western sweet cicely is relatively unknown in commerce; in fact, it may be difficult to procure. I have been harvesting it since the early 1990s in the Sierra Nevada range of California and Nevada and in the Klamath-Siskiyou and Cascade ranges of Oregon. The plant has a rather large range and is abundant in many of the regions where it is native. I have not had any success with cultivation, but I have not tried to grow it in a mountainous area, which is its natural habitat. The herb has a sweet anise or licorice flavor with a distinctive, spicy bite.

The Paiute of the Great Basin and surrounding areas used this medicinal extensively. They administered a decoction for stomachaches, gas pains, indigestion, and as a "physic." They also employed the plant to treat colds and pulmonary afflictions with chills and fever. They applied it externally to relieve pain of toothache, swellings, and bruises, and chewed the root for sore throat.[1] The Shoshoni of the same region has similar applications for the plant, but also used it to regulate the menstrual cycle and took it as a tonic to prevent illness. They also combined Western sweet cicely with balsam root *(Balsamorhiza sagittata)* for what they called "heavy cough."[2] Both Western sweet cicely and balsam root are aromatic and dry dampness. Although Western sweet cicely aromatically dries damp and resolves phlegm to some extent, it is not a particularly strong phlegm-resolving medicinal. Balsam root, however, is a strong phlegm-resolving herb. This Shoshoni combination of the two might be likened to the classic Chinese formula Two Matured Ingredients Decoction *(èr chén tāng)*.

The Blackfoot people of Montana, Alberta, and Saskatchewan had another interesting gynecological use for Western sweet cicely, which I have not tried, that involves applying an infusion of the root to swollen breasts.[3] I do not know if this remedy was administered for premenstrual difficulties, but this seems likely, as the plant has *qi* regulating properties. These, I think, are primarily related to the essential oils in the root, some of which would be absorbed through the skin, thus regulating *qi* and relieving pain.

The well-known American herbalist Michael Moore suggests applying a diluted tincture of Western sweet cicely (which he calls "sweet root") externally for *Tinea* and other fungal infections. He also says, ". . . the tincture or root tea is definitely helpful for upper-intestinal candidiasis or lingering sulphurous burps from bad food or a low-level stomach infection." He recommends a douche or enema for yeast and candidiasis, respectively, further stating, "This seems especially effective when the infections have followed antibiotic or immunosuppressant anti-inflammatory therapy; it is less helpful in chronic immunodepression or when the infection is well established and regularly aggravated by sugar binging."[4]

A related species that is sometimes called sweet cicely *(O. chilensis)* is found throughout North America and in southern South America. The Cheyenne of Montana and Oklahoma included this medicinal as an ingredient in all medicines, and the Karok of Northern California considered it a panacea for all illnesses. The Karok also used an infusion of sweet cicely root as a bath for a grieving person. Furthermore, the Blackfeet served sweet cicely root to their mares in the winter to prepare them for foaling in the spring.[5]

Based on my ethnobotanical research and limited clinical experience with it, I think *O. chilensis* has great potential as a *qi*-supplementing medicinal. Because of its small size and unavailability in commerce, however, I have had little clinical experience with it to date.

Translation of Source Material

Chinese medicine uses one species of *Osmorhiza*. *Xiāng gēn qín (O. aristata)* is acrid and warm. It dissipates cold and effuses the exterior, stops pain, and is used to treat wind-cold common cold, headache at the vertex, and generalized body pain.

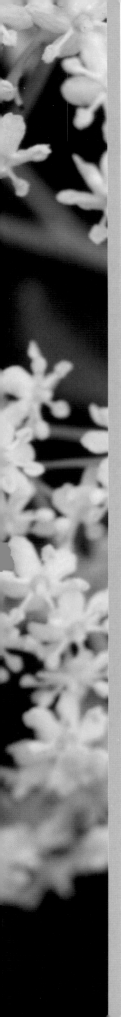

HERBS
THAT RECTIFY *QÌ*

To rectify the *qì* is to correct it. Correcting *qì* involves either moving it when it stagnates or changing the course of counterflow *qì*, for example, when counterflow downbearing *qì* manifests as cough or vomiting. The concept of *qì* includes an insubstantial yet dynamic quality. Thus an aberration of *qì* often requires the light and dynamic qualities of aromatic medicinals. Although this aromatic quality is frequently present it is not necessary. Some medicinals are quite serviceable at *qì* rectifying without the aromatic qualities. Medicinals with aroma are also found in the category of transforming dampness.

The two medicinals found in this category in this text are both extremely important additions from the Western materia medica. Vitex *(Vitex agnus-castus)* is closely related to several species used in Chinese herbal medicine; the one best known to Western practitioners is *màn jīng zǐ,* from the category of cool herbs that resolve the exterior. Although these two herbs from the genus *Vitex* are closely related botanically, they are employed medicinally in very different ways. *V. agnus-castus* is acrid and bitter and has a strong moving action, but it is also neutral and thus does not unnecessarily dry and damage humors.

Black cohosh *(Actaea racemosa)* is closely related to Chinese black cohosh *(shēng má),* but works in a slightly different manner. Again, Western practitioners of Chinese medicine will recognize that the Chinese relative comes from the category of cool herbs that resolve the exterior, but I believe this is a mere coincidence. Black cohosh was a difficult medicinal to categorize in this text, and I expect some may argue about its placement in this category. However, I have found that its main function is to move *qì*—and blood—while also lifting *yáng qì*. This last function is not traditionally considered within the category of rectifying *qì*, but I would argue that lifting the sunken does in fact rectify.

Vitex

Vitex agnus-castus

Verbenaceae

Vitex Agni-Casti fructus

Common names include chasteberry, monk's pepper

Flavor and *Qi:* acrid, bitter, neutral
Channels Entered: liver, heart
Actions: regulates hormonal balance

Functions and Indications

- ***Courses the liver and rectifies* qì.** Vitex is effective for binding depression of liver *qì* affecting the *rèn mài* and *chōng mài,* with symptoms of menstrual pain, menstrual block, premenstrual swelling of the breast, menstrual irregularities, ovulatory pain, and other premenstrual problems. Vitex is acrid and bitter. Its acridity courses the liver, dispersing binding depression of liver *qì.* Although it is not cooling, its bitterness gives it a downbearing action. When there is binding depression of liver *qì,* there is heat, and thus *qì* tends to rise. This herb's downbearing action helps to free the flow of *qì* and treat many manifestations of this pattern. Vitex is also helpful for other patterns associated with binding depression of the liver in which stagnation has affected other organ systems, either by impediment of *qì* or by the transference of heat from the liver due to long-term liver depression. An example of a pattern and condition treated in this way is heat in the stomach and lung that causes acne.

- ***Moves* qì, *frees depression, and opens the network vessels.*** Vitex is helpful for treating stoppage of or decrease in lactation due to liver depression *qì* stagnation, with distention and fullness of the breasts, anger,

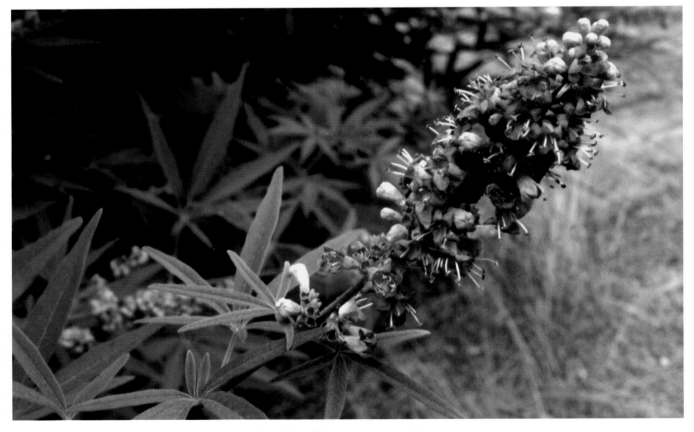

Vitex *(Vitex agnus-castus)*

resentment, irritability, thin tongue fur, and a string-like pulse. The herb is acrid and bitter in flavor and strongly resolves depression, yet its neutral *qì* makes it especially appropriate in cases like this, since this type of depression can often lead to heat, causing mastitis. This medicinal can also be used for simple, uncomplicated conditions even when they skim from vacuity. Because vacuity leads to stagnation, it is very appropriate to include vitex in a formula to treat stoppage or decrease of lactation in vacuity patterns.

CAUTIONS

Vitex should not be used by post-menopausal women. Two of its names, chasteberry and monk's pepper, come from its former application to decrease sexual cravings in men.

Dosage and Preparation

Use 3–9 g in decoction; 2–4 ml tincture; 1–3 ml fluid-extract; 0.5–2 g powdered extract.

Gather vitex fruits in late summer and early autumn, when they have ripened. They can either be ground and tinctured fresh or dried and stored for the future. Good-quality dried berries are whole, gray-black in color, and aromatic.

Major Combinations

• Substitute for bupleurum in Warm the Menses and Contain the Blood Decoction *(wēn jīng shè xuè tāng,* from *Fù Qīng-zhǔ's Gynecology)* for heavy menstruation that is behind schedule. In my clinical experience, this substitution results in a more effective formula.

• Substitute for bupleurum or add to Menses-Stabilizing Decoction *(dìng jīng tāng)* for menstruation that occurs at irregular intervals in association with a pattern of liver depression *qì* stagnation.

• Combine with black cohosh and cramp bark for painful menstruation caused by *qì* stagnation and/or blood stasis.

• Combine with *dāng guī* for milk stoppage due to *qì* stagnation. Add milk thistle to this combination for liver and spleen blood vacuity.

Commentary

Vitex is one of the most important allies for the menstrual cycle. Vitex "enhances corpus luteal development (thereby correcting a relative progesterone deficiency) via a dopaminergic activity on the anterior pituitary (which inhibits prolactin); normalizes the menstrual cycle, encourages ovulation. Indicated for any kind of premenstrual aggravation."[1]

Midwives often recommend vitex for women who are still nursing and have not yet resumed menses, but want to get pregnant again. For such cases, use tincture in 2.5 ml doses two to three times a day.[2] This treatment is also very reliable for women with a history of miscarriages who are trying to conceive.

In cases of irregular menstruation *(jīng shuǐ xiān hòu wú dìng qī),* *Fù Qīng-zhǔ* suggests that depression and binding of liver *qì* are the major pathogenic mechanisms. For this pattern, vitex is invaluable, and when used as a simple, often will regulate the menses on its own, without formulation. Of course, a complex of patterns is nearly always present, and therefore the most appropriate way to treat this condition involves the use of a formula, but I would not formulate for this disease or pattern without including this herb. Vitex is also invaluable for other patterns affecting the menstrual cycle, such as menstruation behind schedule *(jīng shuǐ hòu qī).* Its neutral nature and ability to resolve liver *qì* make it a welcome part of any formula intended to treat this disease pattern.

The origin of the genus name *Vitex* is unclear and appears to predate Linnaeus. However, the species name *agnus-castus* has origins in both the Greek and Latin languages, both of which refer to chastity. This plant was historically used to keep men's libido low and was incorporated by many ancient peoples in rituals for chastity. There is some speculation that this may be a dubious assertion, but I am not aware of any specific evidence to suggest vitex cannot be used for this purpose.

Black Cohosh

Actaea racemosa (formerly *Cimicifuga racemosa*)

Ranunculaceae

Actaea Racemosae rhizoma et radix

Other common names include black snakeroot, bugbane

Flavor and *Qi:* bitter, acrid, sweet, cool
Channels Entered: liver, spleen, lung, heart, large intestine
Actions: anti-inflammatory, antispasmodic, antitussive, diuretic, emmenagogue, hypotensive, sedative

Functions and Indications

- ***Moves* qì, *quickens the blood, and transforms stasis*.** Black cohosh is used to treat *qì* stagnation with blood stasis causing amenorrhea, dysmenorrhea, menopausal syndrome, abdominal pain, flank pain, mastitis, and chest impediment. Black cohosh is acrid and moving, quickening the blood and moving the *qì*. The activation helps resolve many issues related to the stagnation and stasis that are so prevalent in modern culture due to the sedentary lifestyle many people lead. It is frequently used to treat "female issues" tied to the monthly movement of blood and associated liver *qì*. Though black cohosh primarily stimulates the movement of both *qì* and blood, its sweet nature ameliorates the harshness that can be associated with medicinals that have this action. Furthermore, black cohosh's recent application for the treatment of menopausal symptoms suggests a possible use to nourish liver blood; I have found it beneficial as such in clinical practice. Thus, while black cohosh primarily moves blood, it also has nourishing properties.

- ***Lifts* yáng qì.** Black cohosh is used for the treatment of insufficient *yáng qì* causing aching, dull, or pulling pain in the lumbosacral area, muscles, or chest. This herb is also used for false labor (slippery fetus) in which a vacuity of *yáng qì* is unable to hold the fetus. Like its close relative *shēng má*, black cohosh has an upbearing action on the *qì* and is very effective for illnesses associated with spleen *qì* failing to upbear. Black cohosh has a long history of use for pulling pain in the lumbosacral area, which highlights its inherent ability to upbear *yáng qì*. Futhermore, its sweet flavor and gentle blood-nourishing action indirectly nourishes the *qì*, thus assisting the spleen and stomach. This makes black cohosh an important addition to formulas that supplement the middle. *Shēng má* holds an important place in Chinese medicine for the same purpose and is used in formulas like Supplement the Center and Boost the Qì Decoction *(bǔ zhōng yì qì tāng)*. This is a primary reason I believe the American species *(A. racemosa)* can be used as an analogue and may in fact be superior to the Chinese species *(A. foetida* and others).

- ***Dispels wind and dampness to treat wind-damp impediment*.** Black cohosh is effective in wind-damp impediment with symptoms such as muscle aches, lumbar pain, and joint pain. Black cohosh is also helpful for acute wind patterns, especially when complicated by dampness, with symptoms such as chilliness, heat effusion, stiff neck, headache, and body aches. Black cohosh's acrid and bitter nature effectively dispels wind and dampness and relieves pain. Combined with the appropriate medicinals, it is useful for impediment caused by either wind-damp-heat or wind-damp-cold. Because of its sweet flavor and nourishing action, it is effective in treating wind-damp conditions without damaging righteous *qì*. Black cohosh's ability to dispel external pathogens without plundering righteous *qì* make it a very important addition to the materia medica.

CAUTIONS

Use black cohosh with caution during pregnancy, especially during the first trimester. Note that an overdose of this herb may cause a dull frontal headache.

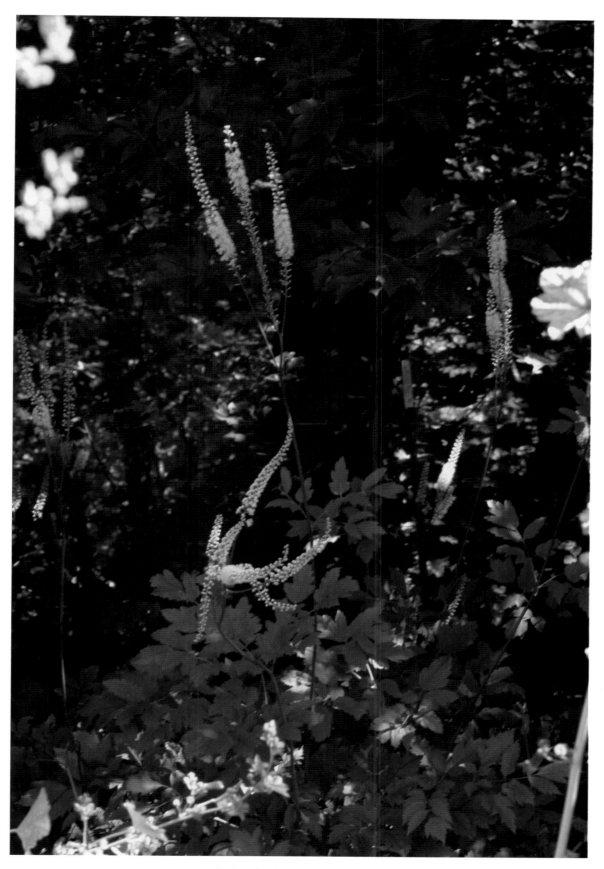

Black cohosh *(Actaea racemosa)*

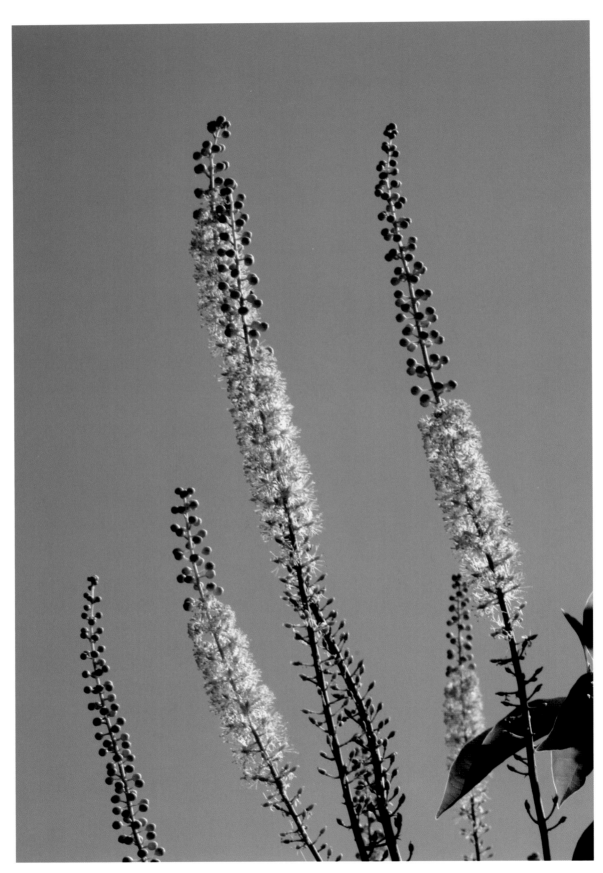

Black cohosh flowers *(A. racemosa)*

Dosage and Preparation

Use 3–9 g in decoction; 2–4 ml tincture.

Good fresh black cohosh root is quite sweet, as is fresh plant tincture, which is the preferred liquid medicine. Good-quality dried root has a black exterior and is grayish on the inside, with a sweetish smell. The taste should be bitter, slightly acrid, and slightly sweet. There should be very few extremely small rootlets, although small roots are acceptable to about 15 percent of the total weight. The rhizome should be hard and somewhat brittle, not pithy.

Major Combinations

- Combine with blue cohosh for a variety of menstrual disorders, including amenorrhea and dysmenorrhea, as well as for difficult labor and as preparation for labor.

- Combine with motherwort and bugleweed for chest impediment to treat blood stasis. This combination can be added to a larger formula to treat chest pain due either to vacuity or repletion. However, it is important to remember that nearly all chest pain has an underlying vacuity pattern.

- Combine with Chinese quince for cramping pain in the lower back or extremities.

- Combine with vitex, cyperus, and rose buds for dull, achy menstrual pain, flank pain, and breast tenderness.

- Combine with angelica duhuo and dipsacus for chronic low-back pain or other impediment syndromes with pain and cold-damp *yáng qì* vacuity patterns.

- Combine with red sage root and notoginseng for chest impediment with heart irregularities, palpitations, and pain.

Commentary

Black cohosh is indicated for dull, achy, crampy, or dragging pain anywhere in the body. It is used for rheumatism, headaches (including headaches due to eyestrain that have a sensation of a "bruised" feeling), amenorrhea, dysmenorrhea, and muscular pain. It is also an excellent antispasmodic for muscle spasm, false labor, whooping cough, and asthma. It is historically combined with blue cohosh and partridge berry herb and taken daily for the six weeks leading up to childbirth to help facilitate labor. Recently there has been some concern about the use of blue cohosh *(Caulophyllum thalictroides)*, an unrelated plant, during pregnancy. However, the single incident cited does not lead the author or the majority of the profession to believe blue cohosh is problematic, especially considering its long history of use in this manner. I have given this combination with additions to dozens of pregnant women and have never received an adverse report. To the contrary, reports are overwhelmingly positive from both moms and midwives—hundreds of midwives use this formula or some variation thereof every year without adverse effects.

Black cohosh is very closely related to *shēng má* and in many ways can be employed as an analogue for the Chinese herb. However, it is interesting to note that the American plant is much more widely used, and used for a broader variety of ailments, than the Chinese species. For instance, *A. racemosa* is indicated for a number of gynecological maladies, and in fact many consider it an extremely important medicinal in gynecology. According to traditional gynecology, black cohosh is helpful for amenorrhea, dysmenorrhea, menorrhagia, ovarian pain, mastitis, leukorrhea, labor pains, and after-pains. Recent research has secured black cohosh a very popular role in treating menopausal symptomatology and ovarian insufficiency; it may also be useful for conditions requiring a reduction in luteinizing hormone (LH) levels.[3]

Aside from gynecology, black cohosh is used for many spasmodic conditions. In Chinese medicine the word "spasm" *(jìng luán)* is not traditional, but rather is a Western medical term that has been adopted into Chinese medicine. However, this term can cover a lot of ground, as suggested in Wiseman and Feng's monumental *A Practical Dictionary of Chinese Medicine*. According to this text, spasm can mean any of the following in Chinese medicine:

- *Hypertonicity* usually attributed to wind, specifically wind-cold, but possibly a manifestation of blood or liquid vacuity depriving the sinew vessels of nourishment[4]

- *Cramp* due to insufficiency of *qi* and blood, fatigue, dampness, or cold[5]

- *Clenched jaw* due to wind-cold[6]

- *Arched-back rigidity* related to wind-cold-damp; or fire stagnating in the channels; or insufficiency of blood, fluid, and *qi* that allows vacuity wind to stir internally[7]

- *Tugging and slackening* caused by exuberant heat damaging *yīn,* with wind and fire exacerbating one another and leading to congestion of phlegm-fire; in febrile or summerheat disease, this is a sign of damage to the *qi,* and in epilepsy and lockjaw, is usually attributed to wind-phlegm or phlegm-heat, spleen-stomach vacuity, liver-cold, or blood loss[8]

As can be deduced from this list, three main factors in Chinese medicine appear to cause or contribute to much of what gets lumped under the Western term spasm: wind (generally with cold and/or damp), vacuity, and heat. *A. racemosa* is highly effective in resolving most of these issues. It dispels wind and damp, raises *yáng qi,* and treats vacuity. Although it does not strongly clear heat, it is cool, so does not resist attempts to clear heat in a formula. Furthermore, I believe this medicinal nourishes the blood, but because I am not certain of this function, I did not emphasize it in the text.

Black cohosh is also hypotensive and can be used to treat high blood pressure, especially when it's associated with anxiety and stress. The herb slows but strengthens the heartbeat in a manner similar to digitalis, but safely, with little chance that overdose will cause more than a dull headache.

The Cherokee of the western Carolinas and northern Georgia, where black cohosh is most abundant in the wild, had a plethora of applications for this plant. They used it to stimulate menstruation; to treat pain, colds, coughs, constipation, and fatigue; to help babies sleep; as a diuretic; and as a tincture for rheumatism. The Delaware of the East Coast of the United States combined black cohosh with elecampane and stone root as a tonic. The Iroquois of upstate New York and southern Ontario bathed in a decoction of black cohosh root to treat rheumatic pains. They also employed it as a blood purifier and to promote the flow of milk in women; they made a poultice of crushed leaves for babies with sore backs. Both the Micmac and the Penobscot took the root internally for kidney troubles.[9]

The former genus name *Cimicifuga* is a compound term consisting of *cimex,* meaning "bug," and *fuga,* meaning "repellent," a reference to the plant's apparent resistance to insect infestation. The species name *racemosa* is Latin for "cluster of grapes," based on the plant's appearance during fruiting.

Black cohosh is or has been official in the following texts: the *British Herbal Pharmacopoeia* (1996), *British Pharmaceutical Codex* 1934–73, *Pharmacopoeia of Brazil* (1926), Commission E Monographs (1989), *Martindale: The Extra Pharmacopoeia* (31st ed.), *Pharmacopoeia of Japan* (11th ed.), *The National Formulary (U.S.)* from 1955–1975, and *The United States Pharmacopoeia* from 1820–1936.

Translation of Source Material

Chinese medicine uses a number of species of *Cimicifuga.** *Sān miàn dāo (C. acerina)* is sweet, bitter, cold, and slightly toxic. It clears heat, quickens the blood, and resolves toxin. It is used to treat dry sore throat, knocks and falls, taxation damage, wind-damp pain in the lumbus and legs, and swollen boils.

Yě shēng má (C. simplex), which apparently has chemistry similar to that of *A. racemosa* (discussed in the main monograph above), is sweet, acrid, slightly bitter, and slightly cold. The medicinal dissipates wind, resolves toxin, upbears *yáng,* and outthrusts papules. It is employed to treat seasonal epidemic pestilence, *yángmíng* headache, sore throat, maculopapular eruption, wind-heat sore, enduring diarrhea with prolapsed anus, flooding and vaginal discharge, and childhood measles.

---

*Note: The name of this genus was changed recently from *Cimicifuga* to *Actaea;* however, much of the medical literature has not caught up with the botanical literature.

HERBS THAT REGULATE BLOOD

Regulating the blood refers to a general category of medicinals that return blood to its normal, regular activity. There are two main subcategories within this large category: stanching bleeding and quickening blood. Medicinals that quicken the blood make up an extremely important category in Chinese medicine, and a thorough understanding of their actions and functions will yield excellent clinical results in many chronic cases seen in the Western clinic. I have not included any medicinals specifically from the stanching bleeding subcategory in this text. However, there are several medicinals in the text that do staunch bleeding as a secondary action. Cayenne, which is listed in the Warm the Interior and Expel Cold category, and which is excellent for stopping bleeding externally, is an example.

Because of the importance of this category, it may be prudent to take a moment to explore the meaning behind the Chinese word *huó,* which I've treated here as "quicken" rather than "move or invigorate," as is done in many texts in the West. This is not my designation, but rather part of the work of Nigel Wiseman and Feng Ye as presented in their book, *A Practical Dictionary of Chinese Medicine.* In Chinese, *huó* means "alive" or "to be alive, active, or moving"; the underlying connotation is the active process of living. Thus, ascribing the meaning "alive *and* moving" to the word *huó* makes more sense than simply "to move or invigorate." From the perspective of Chinese medicine, aliveness is a critical aspect of the character of blood, and thus the category of regulating blood is a vital part of the practice of Chinese herbal medicine. (Don't confuse this concept with nourishing the blood, which is a more material aspect of the treatment of blood.)

Herbs that Quicken the Blood and Transform Stasis

The idea of blood stasis is central to the concept of regulating blood. Blood stasis indicates impairment or cessation of the normal flow of blood. The list of possible signs and symptoms related to this phenomenon is dizzying. However, some common manifestations include pain, masses and swellings, bleeding, a dark purple tongue with stasis speckles, and a fine and rough pulse.

There is a hierarchy of actions useful for dispelling stasis, of which quickening is the most common but the mildest. Three of the four medicinals discussed in this category have a primary action of quickening: cramp bark, motherwort, and red root. Next in strength in the hierarchy is transforming stasis. All of the medicinals discussed here transform stasis, but arnica has the strongest action. The third and final level in the hierarchy encompasses medicinals that break the blood, which are often insects in Chinese medicine. No medicinals in this text fall under that heading.

Arnica

Arnica montana, A. cordifolia,
A. latifolia, **and others**

Asteraceae

Arnicae herba cum radice (Arnicae flos)

Also known as wolf's bane

Flavor and *Qi:* acrid, very warm, slightly toxic
Channels Entered: heart, pericardium, liver
Actions: anti-inflammatory, stimulant

Functions and Indications

- ***Transforms blood stasis and relieves pain.*** Arnica effectively treats pain due to knocks and falls, with symptoms of swelling and bruising. Arnica may also help with other patterns of blood stasis causing pain. While primarily used externally, it may be applied internally or externally for any condition associated with static blood. Arnica has a strong transforming and dispersing action due to its acrid and very warm energy. Because of its very warm and slightly toxic nature, it can injure the stomach and cause a burning sensation. However, small doses can be used to good effect even in elderly patients, to help transform blood stasis associated with the normal aging process.

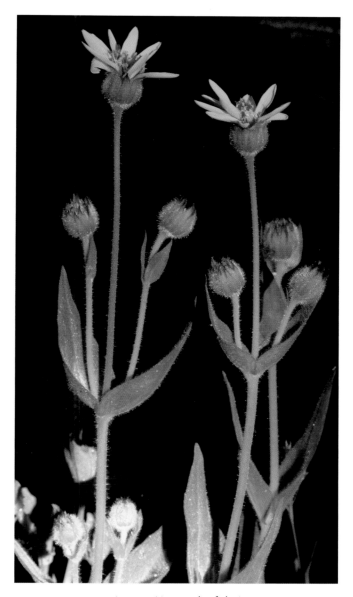

Arnica *(Arnica latifolia)*

CAUTIONS

Do not apply to open wounds. Arnica is not for extended use, either internal or external. Overdose can cause a burning sensation in the stomach. Other possible symptoms of overdose are dizziness, tremor, tachycardia, arrhythmia, and collapse.[1]

Dosage and Preparation

External: Apply oil and diluted tincture liberally for trauma and chronic pain. Internal: 5–20 drops of tincture.

Gather arnica flowers in summer at their peak. The entire plant can be harvested at the same time. If only the root is required, gather it in the autumn. The flower and herb are best processed fresh, though they can be dried carefully for future use. Good-quality dried arnica flower is slightly aromatic, bright yellow, and should not have gone to seed. Dried herb should be green and slightly aromatic. The root and rhizome should be clean and slightly aromatic when broken.

Major Combinations

- Combine with St. John's wort and cayenne for external application to treat swollen, painful joints and muscular pain due to strain. Prepare this formula as an oil or alcohol-based liniment.

- Combine with red sage root, *dāng guī,* safflower, peach kernel, or any other appropriate blood-quickening medicinal for patterns of blood stasis with pain.

- Combine with red sage root and safflower for chest impediment. For this purpose, combine tinctures in a 1:10:5 ratio and administer in 4 ml doses every 30 minutes until the pain is relieved.

Commentary

Arnica is primarily employed externally. Although it has important internal applications, exercise caution when using it in this manner.

Arnica is one of the most useful first-aid medications in the Western materia medica and should be in every first-aid kit. It is perhaps the most valuable herb for external treatment of bumps, bruises, and other trauma in which the skin is not broken. Arnica infused oil is most commonly used for this purpose, and dramatic results may be seen when the preparation is applied liberally to the affected area. Applying arnica oil quickens the blood and thus eases the pain. This action also stops or reduces bruising before it occurs and lessens any bruising that may have occurred already. Arnica tincture can be used externally for the same purpose in the form of a liniment, either alone or combined with other tinctures or essential oils.

The Catawba of the Catawba River region in the Carolinas used the roots of *A. acaulis* in an infusion for back pain.[2] The Thompson of Southwestern British Columbia mashed *A. cordifolia* and applied it for swellings and bruises and took an infusion of the plant internally for tuberculosis.[3] The famous philosopher, poet, and scientist Goethe is reported to have asked for arnica tea when he suffered from angina toward the end of his life.[4]

The genus name *Arnica* does not have ancient roots, and its specific origins are unknown. Some speculate the word comes from the Arabic language, while others guess it is either Latin or Greek. Apparently the name does not appear in any texts until the fourteenth century. The species name of the European species, *montana,* is Latin for "mountain." The name *cordifolia* comes from the Latin *cord,* meaning "heart," and *folia,* meaning "leaf," owing to the heart-shaped leaf of this species. The name *latifolia* comes from a Latin word meaning "broad" or "wide," a reference to the sometimes broad leaves of *A. latifolia.* Many other species are found throughout the western United States. I have used a number of them, and they all seem to have a similar action.

A. montana (whole plant) was official in *The United States Pharmacopoeia* from 1820–1851, but only the flowers were official from 1851–1925. The same plant was official in *The National Formulary (U.S.)* from 1926–1960. Arnica root was official in *The United States Pharmacopoeia* from 1882–1905. *A. montana, A. fulgens, A. sororia,* and *A. cordifolia* were all official in *The National Formulary (U.S.)* from 1947–1960. The listing of the three U.S. native species *(A. fulgens, A. sororia,* and *A. cordifolia)* reflected a need to find and use native medicinals after World War II ripped through Europe. Arnica flower is listed as official in the pharmacopoeias of Austria (including root), Belgium, France, Germany, Poland, Portugal, Romania, Spain, and Switzerland.

Cramp Bark

Viburnum opulus

Caprifoliaceae

Viburni Opuli cortex

Other common names include highbush cranberry, red elder, snowball tree, guelder rose

Flavor and *Qi:* bitter, acrid, slightly sweet, slightly cool, astringent

Channels Entered: liver, heart

Actions: antispasmodic, astringent, nervine, sedative

Functions and Indications

- ***Quickens and supplements the blood, relaxes the sinews, and opens the channels.*** Cramp bark is employed to treat pain and cramping associated with

blood stasis due to or in concert with blood vacuity. Cramp bark is especially useful for gynecological conditions, as well as cramping and tension in the sinews due to liver-blood vacuity causing pain in the limbs, torso, and internal organs, such as the intestines and bladder. With bitterness and acridity, cramp bark quickens the blood and opens the channels. With sweetness it nourishes the blood and relaxes the sinews. This combination of flavors works in an unusual manner to move, relax, and nourish, resulting in an action that is extremely useful in clinical practice. Furthermore, when used in tincture form at appropriate dosages, cramp bark can act swiftly, making it useful in acute conditions. I will often make a small "drink" consisting entirely or primarily of cramp bark for a patient who comes to the clinic compaining of menstrual pain, a treatment that can bring the patient significant relief within 30 to 120 seconds.

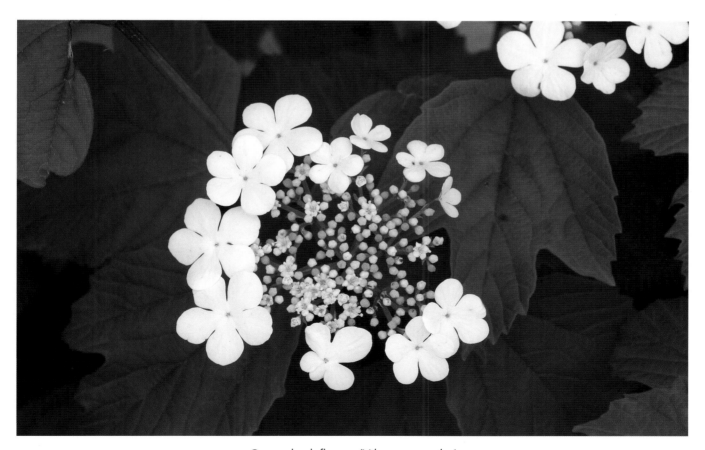

Cramp bark flower *(Viburnum opulus)*

- *Transforms stasis and stops bleeding.* Cramp bark is helpful for excessive menstrual bleeding and bleeding during pregnancy due to blood stasis. With acridity, cramp bark transforms stasis; with bitterness and coolness, it gently clears heat from blood depression. With its astringency, it stops bleeding when menstruation is excessive or when bleeding is inappropriate, such as during pregnancy. Its sweetness gives it a gently nourishing action that supports the right while treating the pathology, making it safe and effective during pregnancy. Many herbalists and midwives use a related species, black haw *(V. prunifolium),* for this function. Some herbalists consider black haw stronger medicine.

- *Nourishes the heart, quiets the spirit, and clears heat.* Cramp bark is used to treat heart-blood and/or *yīn* vacuity with symptoms of palpitations, insomnia, agitation, and anxiety. With sweetness and bitterness, cramp bark nourishes the heart and quiets the spirit, while also gently nourishing the heart blood. Its astringency helps to restrain *yīn,* thus preserving the right. Furthermore, the herb's bitterness supports its action both by directing the action to the heart and by gently draining heat from the heart; heat due to *yīn* vacuity and depression is often associated with this syndrome.

CAUTIONS

None noted.

Dosage and Preparation

Use 3–9 g in decoction; 3–10 ml tincture.

Gather cramp bark in the spring when the leaves are budding. It can be harvested at other times, but this is when the plant yields the best medicine, and it is easiest to peel the bark from the branch in the spring. Good-quality dried cramp bark is ash gray on the outside, with small black warts, and light brown inside. The taste is astringent and bitter.

Major Combinations

- Combine with motherwort, cyperus, and *dāng guī* for painful menstruation due to blood vacuity and stasis.

- Combine with black cohosh for muscle spasms and cramping due to stasis or vacuity. For more serious cases of spasms with wind involvement, add lobelia.

- Combine with albizia flowers, motherwort, and spiny zizyphus for anxiety, insomnia, and agitation due to heart-blood vacuity. Add cyperus to this combination for any accompanying liver-depression symptoms.

Commentary

Cramp bark's excellent ability to calm the spirit for those with pain caused by blood vacuity and stasis gives it a very useful clinical niche. Patients with pain due to vacuity are often agitated and irritable because of the discomfort as well as a lack of blood to nourish the heart and give the *shén* a proper house.

Cramp bark is a common plant in the central and eastern parts of the United States and adjacent Canada. It is also common in northern regions of Europe and Asia. Interestingly, cramp bark was used very little in Europe before the eighteenth century. Native Americans did employ it, none more than the Iroquois of upstate New York and southern Quebec. They found the plant helpful for a number of conditions, including hemorrhage after childbirth. They included it in a compound decoction to "regulate the heart." They also considered it an important blood medicine, and administered it in a compound decoction to improve prenatal strength.[5] However, it was likely the Chippewa people of the Great Lakes Region, who took cramp bark for stomach pain, who taught white settlers about cramp bark's effectiveness against pain. The Meskwakis of Iowa also used a decoction of cramp bark for pain over the entire body.[6]

Cramp bark has been cultivated for many decades and numerous varieties of *Viburnum* are available at nurseries. It is an attractive landscape plant, but only the named species should be used as medicine. Cramp bark was official in *The United States Pharmacopoeia* from 1894–1916, and in *The National Formulary (U.S.)* from 1916–1960.

Translation of Source Material

Chinese medicine has used many species of *Viburnum*. In the name of brevity I have included only a couple here. *Shān wǔ wèi zǐ (Viburnum foetidum* var. *ceanothoides)* is sweet and neutral. It clears heat, resolves the exterior, stops coughing, and treats headache and generalized body pain.

Xīn yè jiá mí gēn (V. cordifolium) is astringent and warm, and enters the liver channel. It is used to treat wind-damp numbness, sinew and bone pain, knocks and falls with congealed and static blood, and lumbus and rib-side *qì* distention.

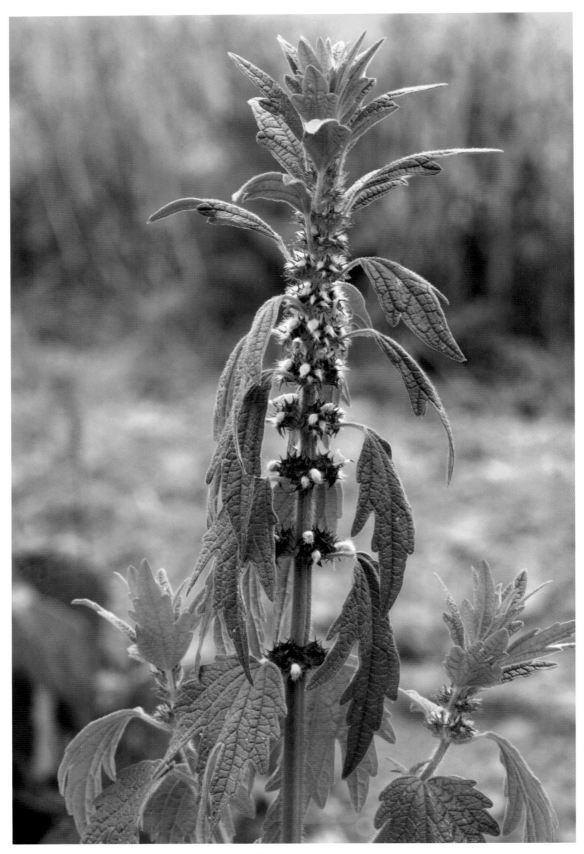

Motherwort flowers *(Leonurus cardiaca)*

Motherwort

Leonurus cardiaca

Lamiaceae

Leonuri Cardiacae herba

Flavor and *Qi:* bitter, acrid, slightly cold
Channels Entered: heart, liver, bladder, small intestine
Actions: antispasmodic, cardiac tonic, diuretic, emmenagogue, sedative

Functions and Indications

• ***Quickens the blood, transforms stasis, and stops pain.*** Motherwort is used in the treatment of blood stagnation with symptoms of pain in the uterus or chest or other pain syndromes related to blood stagnation. Motherwort is applied for almost any menstrual disorder, as it not only invigorates the blood but also regulates menses. The herb is bitter and acrid and directly enters the blood. It quickens blood with acridity, but does not harm it. It nourishes the blood without causing stagnation. If these functions appear to be much the same as for Chinese motherwort *(yì mǔ cǎo),* that is because they are! The main reason for using the Western species of motherwort is that high-quality organic herb is readily available.

• ***Nourishes heart blood and calms the spirit.*** Motherwort is helpful for palpitations, anxiety, insomnia, hysteria, and restlessness due to heart *yīn* and blood vacuity. Motherwort is a very important medicinal for treating heart vacuity with *shén* disturbances. This pattern of vacuity in the heart creates a lack of residence for the spirit, resulting in a restless or agitated *shén*. The bitter nature of the herb directs its action to the heart. As mentioned earlier, motherwort nourishes the blood, and its slightly cold nature clears heat due to vacuity. This medicinal enters the blood, and, because the heart governs blood, the heart. It acts on the heart to support the production of blood while directly nourishing the heart and calming the spirit.

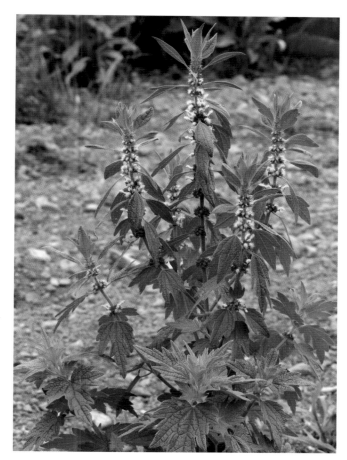

Motherwort *(L. cardiaca)*

• ***Promotes urination and clears heat.*** Motherwort is employed to treat heat in the heart and small intestine channels, with irritability; scanty, painful urination; and edema. Motherwort's cold and bitter nature drains heat and promotes urination. Although a secondary action, this is an important function that makes the herb useful both for *yīn* vacuity heat and replete heat in the heart and small intestine. Although it is slightly cold in nature, motherwort will not injure the spleen or right *qì*. It may also be used for early nerve pain due to herpes, before eruptions.

CAUTIONS

Use motherwort with caution during pregnancy. The herb is commonly used during pregnancy, but generally only in the third trimester and not during the first trimester.

Dosage and Preparation

Use 9–30 g in decoction; 2–6 ml tincture; 2–4 g powdered extract.

Gather motherwort in midsummer, when the flowering spikes have flowered about halfway up. Bundle the stems and hang them to dry, or strip the leaves and flowers to make fresh preparations. Once dried, the larger stems should be removed. Good-quality dried herb is a healthy green color and should be relatively whole and free from large stems. There should be no seeds, but small amounts of flowers are acceptable.

Major Combinations

- Combine with black cohosh for painful menstruation due to *qì* stagnation with blood vacuity. Add cramp bark to the above combination for dysmenorrhea with anxiety, irritability, and nervousness. To strengthen the ability of this combination to calm the spirit, add passionflower. Alternatively, combine with cyperus and *dāng guī* for painful menstruation due to *qì* stagnation.

- Combine with spiny zizyphus for anxiety and irritability due to heart *yīn* and blood vacuity.

- Combine with hawthorn and red sage root for palpitations and fearful throbbing in the chest, as well as dizziness, poor memory, and insomnia due to heart blood vacuity. If there is lassitude of spirit, shortness of breath, and spontaneous sweating due to heart *qì* vacuity, add codonopsis or red ginseng.

Commentary

Motherwort is commonly used to help facilitate birth for women who have either a history of difficult births or who are past their due date. The herb is very similar in function to the Chinese species *(Leonurus heterophyllus),* but because it has a broader range of use and is so widely known as a tonic in the West, I think of it as the superior species. I find it does all that Chinese motherwort does and then some, so I use it as a substitute for the Chinese species.

The Greek genus name *Leonurus* means lion's tail. The species name, *cardiaca,* also has Greek origins meaning "having life" or "heart disease." Motherwort is an herb of long repute and has been used in medicine since antiquity. Culpeper states, "There is no better herb to take melancholy vapours from the heart, to strengthen it, and make a merry, cheerful, blithe soul, than this herb."[7] Macer, a German writer from the twelfth and thirteenth centuries, is reported to have stated that it treats evil spirits in the heart.[8] In his tome from 1869, William Cook wrote, "As a tonic for nervousness, pains and palpitation of the heart, the sufferings peculiar to women, and habitual restlessness, it is an agent deserving of the first consideration."[9]

As one can see from these historical sources, motherwort has long been considered an extremely important plant. Today, in an age of high stress, early heart attacks, and exceedingly common menstrual problems, motherwort continues to find its way into numerous prescriptions, whether for gynecological problems, heart troubles, or nervous system disorders.

Motherwort is approved as medicine by the German Commission E.

Red Root

Ceanothus spp.

Rhamnaceae

Ceanothi cortex seu radicis

Also known as New Jersey tea, California lilac, buckbrush, Oregon tea tree

Flavor and *Qi:* bitter, slightly acrid, warm
Channels Entered: liver, spleen, gallbladder
Actions: antispasmodic, astringent, expectorant

Functions and Indications

- ***Quickens the blood, transforms blood stasis, resolves* qì *stagnation, and softens hardness.*** Red root is employed in the treatment of concretions and conglomerations; slow-healing ulcers; headache; painful, bleeding hemorrhoids; varicose veins; pain in the lower burner (e.g., prostate or cervical pain); breast cysts; and ovarian cysts. This is an important medicinal for the treatment of blood and *qi* depression. Red root enters the *qi* of the blood, quickening it and transforming stasis with bitterness and acridity. Its warm and acrid nature resolves *qi* stagnation. This combination of flavors and *qi* works to soften hardness and effectively treat concretions and conglomerations, as well as localized depression of blood and *qi* that causes conditions such as slow-healing ulcers, varicose veins, hemorrhoids, and various painful conditions of the lower burner.

- ***Quickens the blood and stops bleeding.*** Red root is used to treat bleeding patterns due to blood stasis with or without heat in the blood, with symptoms such as nosebleed, vomiting of blood, coughing blood, and excessive menstrual bleeding. When using red root to treat bleeding due to heat with stasis, remember that it does not have a cooling nature, and therefore must be used in combination with heat-clearing medicinals. However, this medicinal moves the blood in a fashion that lends itself to the treatment of bleeding due to stasis. Red root is also used as a gargle for sore throats.

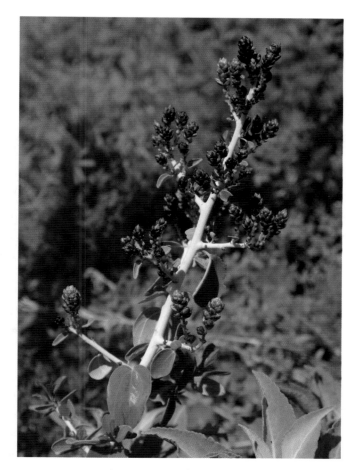

Red root *(Ceanothus oliganthus)*

CAUTIONS

None noted.

Dosage and Preparation

Use 3–9 g in decoction; 2–4 ml tincture.

Gather the root bark, and occasionally, stem bark, in early spring, before the plant has flowered. The bark can be chopped to make fresh plant tincture or allowed to dry for future use. Good-quality dried root bark of red root is brown, black, or gray outside, bright red to brownish red inside, and astringent in the mouth.

Major Combinations

- Combine with cleavers and figwort to treat swellings in the neck and throat.

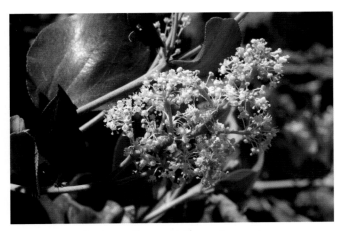

Red root flowers (*Ceanothus* sp.)

- Combine with ocotillo for hemorroids due to reple-tion. For stubborn or chronic cases, add moutan peony, peach kernel, or ligusticum to treat blood-heat, dryness, and wind associated with the condition.

- Combine with curcuma (*yù jīn*) and sparganium for concretions and conglomerations.

- Combine with cyperus and curcuma (*yù jīn*) for accumulations.

- Combine with echinacea and thyme as a gargle for painful sore throat due to wind heat. To make a pleas-ant and effective formula for this purpose, combine one part each red root, echinacea, thyme, osha, and black sage, and squeeze a little lemon juice into the mix.

Commentary

Red root is one of the most unique medicinals in North America, and consquently, this was one of the most dif-ficult herb entries to write. While extremely helpful, red root does not produce extremely obvious responses and is nearly always used in combination with other medicinals, even in the Western model. This makes it difficult to ascertain its exact actions from the perspec-tive of Chinese medicine. In his *Medicinal Plants of the Pacific West,* herbalist Michael Moore states, "Red root is one of the best examples of and recommenda-tions for using herbs in the subclinical grey area that precedes overt disease." This is not meant to imply that red root is not useful in overt disease—it is. Later in his monograph, Moore says, "It won't *cure* you—just make you better able to cure yourself." This implies the herb assists or encourages the body to make adjustments so it can heal. It acts on blood proteins and, according to Moore,

> It helps increase the quality of blood charge, thereby increasing the repelling charge of the capillary cells. With improved charges, there is improved transport of blood fluid out into the interstitial colloids and more efficient uptake of lymph, as well as return of fluid back into the blood exiting capillaries into the veins.[10]

This suggests an action on the blood and lymph, leading me to the conclusion that red root works on the blood as it is understood in Chinese medicine. When added to formulas composed according to the Chinese medical paradigm, red root is especially useful when there is obvious lymph involvement. However, I have learned that red root is an important part of most formulas designed to treat any accumulation of blood from *qi* stagnation, damp stagnation, or heat.

The Okanagon of Washington state and the Cana-dian border area, and the Thompson people of south-western British Columbia, administered *Ceanothus velutinus* both internally and externally for pain.[11] The Thompson also used this species to treat rheumatic complaints internally and externally.[12] The Alabama prepared a decoction of *C. americanus* root as a bath for injured legs and feet.[13] The Cherokee of the Carolinas used the same species as an infusion held in the mouth for toothache.[14] The Iroquois of upstate New York and southern Quebec took a decoction for delayed menses due to catching a cold, as well as to abort a fetus injured in the first two to three months of pregnancy.[15]

The genus name *Ceanothus* comes from a Greek word meaning thorny plant. The common name New Jersey tea refers to the historical use of the leaves of the East Coast red root species as a substitute for tea (*Camellia sinensis*) during the American Revolution.

HERBS THAT WARM THE INTERIOR AND EXPEL COLD

Warming the interior describes a category of medicinals used to dissipate cold that has penetrated the interior and caused debilitation of *yáng qì*. Disease patterns indicated here are mainly caused by external cold evil that has worked its way to the interior unchecked by either the body's inherent ability to right itself (e.g., with *yáng qì*) or by appropriate treatment. Otherwise, cold is due to a vacuity of *yáng qì*, which allows *yīn* to become exuberant. Some signs and symptoms of cold include a feeling of being cold, aversion to cold, little or no thirst except possibly for warm liquids, long voiding of clear urine, a slow or tight pulse, and a bluish tongue.

Invasion of cold *yīn* pathogen is marked by a tight pulse and symptoms affecting the digestion. Vacuity of *yáng qì*, which is more commonly seen in the clinic, is marked by more systemic cold symptoms, such as curling up in the fetal position, counterflow cold of the limbs, free draining of clear fluids through the anus and urinary system, and slow pulse.

The one medicinal in this category discussed here—cayenne pepper *(Capsicum annum)*—is native to the Americas, but is now found around the world. Cayenne is acrid, sour, and hot. It is excellent for treating cold, but due to its acrid and thus scattering nature, it must be used with care in vacuity patterns.

Cayenne

Capsicum annuum, C. minimum, C. frutescens

Capsici fructus

Solanaceae

Also called African bird pepper, hot pepper, chili pepper

Flavor and *Qi*: acrid, sour, hot
Channels Entered: kidney, heart, spleen, stomach
Actions: antiseptic, carminative, counterirritant, diaphoretic, rubefacient, stimulant

Functions and Indications

- **Warms the interior, expels cold, and rescues collapsed *yáng*.** Cayenne is used to treat sweating, cold skin, reversal cold of the limbs, apathy, and either no desire to drink or a desire for warm liquids. Cayenne scatters cold with acridity while warming and assisting *yáng* with its hot *qì*.

- **Disperses cold, warms the channels, and relieves pain.** Cayenne is helpful for wind-damp-cold obstructing the channels with pain and a feeling of cold. For this condition, cayenne is commonly applied externally in the form of an ointment. Cayenne disperses cold from the channels and penetrates them to relieve pain with its hot acrid nature.

- **Stops bleeding.** Applied topically, cayenne is very effective for stopping bleeding due to trauma. Its sour nature constrains blood to stop bleeding. It also stops bleeding by resolving stasis with its acrid and hot nature.

CAUTIONS

Do not use cayenne when there are heat signs related to vacuity.

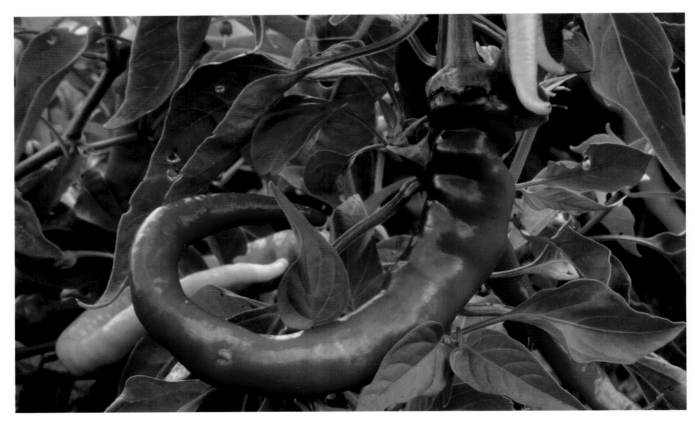

Cayenne pepper *(Capsicum frutescens)*

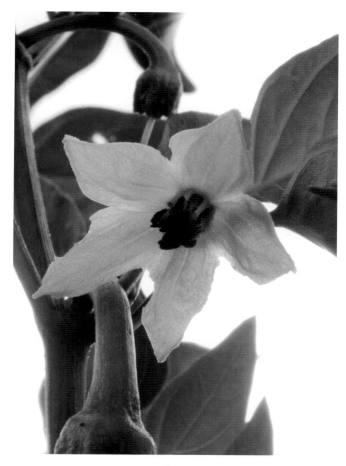

Cayenne pepper flower (C. frutescens)

Dosage and Preparation

Use 0.3–1.5 g in decoction or infusion; 0.25–1 ml tincture.

Major Combinations

- Combine with cinnamon bark to warm the middle and rescue *yáng*.

- Combine with turmeric and cinnamon twig to warm the channels and relieve pain caused by cold in the channels.

- Combine with hawthorn and red sage root for chest impediment due to blood stasis caused by cold.

- Combine with arnica, St. John's wort, and oil of wintergreen for pain due to knocks and falls. This is prepared as an external application in the form of an oil or cream.

Commentary

Cayenne is a common kitchen spice used around the world as both food and medicine. Although cayenne is a native plant of the Americas, it was quickly adopted as an important food by cultures around the world. In fact, all of the related peppers are also from the Americas, but if you go to Thailand or southern China you will find them in an extraordinary number of dishes. (Don't confuse these peppers with the true peppers of the genus *Piper*, such as black pepper and long pepper.)

Cayenne is an important medicinal for both internal and external use. However, when using it internally, be careful not to overdo it. Although it is not toxic, it is very hot in nature and can cause burning stomach and "hot" diarrhea, as well as acid reflux and other signs of heat in the middle that disrupt the *qì* dynamic.

Cayenne has become a very popular external medication for pain relief based on the oleoresin it contains; it is sold as "capsicum" or under various other names. It is extraordinarily good for this application and generally well tolerated. For this purpose, I use cayenne as a liniment, cream, or oil. I recommend applying a small amount of the product to a small patch of the patient's skin to be sure he or she will not react adversely.

Cayenne pepper is official in the pharmacopoeias of Austria, Belgium, Egypt, Europe, Germany, Hungary, Italy, Japan, Poland, Portugal, Spain, Switzerland, and the United Kingdom. It is listed in *The United States Pharmacopoeia* (26th ed.), the *British Herbal Pharmacopoeia, The National Formulary (U.S.)* (21st ed.), *Martindale: The Extra Pharmacopoeia* (33rd ed.), and *PDR for Herbal Medicines,* and is approved by the German Commission E.

Translation of Source Material

In Chinese medicine, *Capsicum frutescens (là jiāo)* is considered acrid, bitter, and hot. The medicinal warms the middle and downbears *qì*, dissipates cold and eliminates dampness, opens the stomach, disperses food, resolves phlegm depresson, and is used to treat cold stagnating in the abdomen, vomiting, diarrhea, frostbite, scab, and lichen *(jiè xiǎn)*.

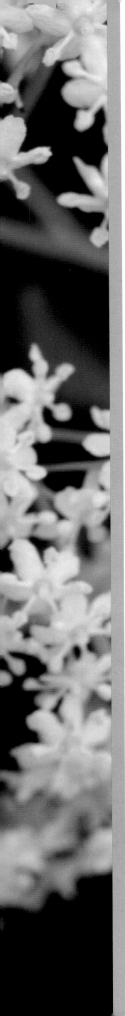

HERBS
THAT SUPPLEMENT

Supplementation is a method of treatment—one of the eight methods—used to treat vacuity. There are four subcategories within this main category, including supplementing *qì,* supplementing blood, supplementing *yīn,* and supplementing *yáng.* Although most Chinese materia medicas separate these actions into distinct groups, I have chosen not to, because there are only six medicinals in the entire group in this text. However, upon reading each herb entry, it should become apparent, at least in a general sense, which subcategory best describes each of these six medicinals.

Supplementation is a concept somewhat unique to Chinese medicine, and the number of supplementing medicinals found and commonly used in everyday Chinese herbal practice is significant. Students often learn early that one should not supplement when a pathogen is present. Unfortunately, this basic concept tends to stick firmly in people's minds to the point of making it absolute, which is not necessarily appropriate. Supplementation is an effective way of supporting the right *qì.* Thus, if a patient is too weak to overcome a pathogen, merely expelling the pathogen will not lead to true healing. In cases like this, effective treatment must take into account the principle that states, "By supporting the right, evils are dispelled."

The supplementing medicinals discussed here include elecampane *(Inula helenium),* a warm, acrid, and bitter medicinal that supplements the spleen *qì* and transforms damp; hawthorn *(Crataegus* spp.), a slightly warm herb that supplements the *qi* and blood, specifically of the heart; milk thistle *(Silybum marianum),* a bitter, sweet, neutral herb that supplements *yīn,* clears heat, and resolves toxins; marsh mallow *(Althaea officinalis),* a sweet, slightly bitter, and cold medicinal that works primarily to supplement the *yīn* of the lungs and stomach while also clearing heat; oat (*Avena* spp.), a sweet and neutral medicinal that nourishes both *yīn* and *qi* while also nourishing the heart; and finally damiana *(Turnera diffusa),* an acrid, sweet, and warm herb that primarily supplements the kidney and heart *yáng.*

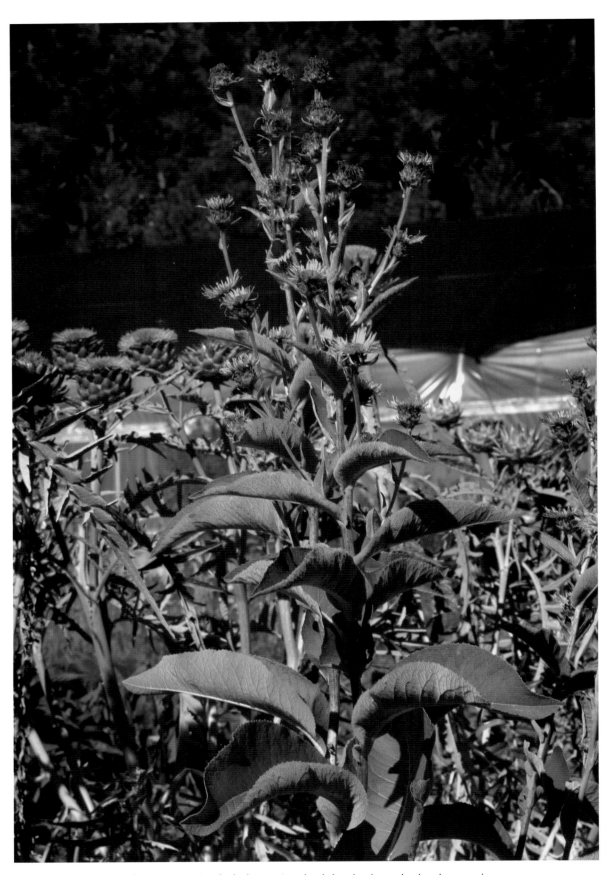

Elecampane *(Inula helenium)* with globe thistle in the background

Elecampane

Inula helenium

Asteraceae

Inulae Heleni radix

Other names include *tu mu xiang*

Flavor and *Qi*: bitter, acrid, warm
Channels Entered: spleen, stomach, lung
Actions: anthelmintic, diuretic, diaphoretic, expectorant

Functions and Indications

- ***Supplements* qì *and resolves dampness.*** Elecampane is helpful in the treatment of spleen *qi* vacuity causing indigestion, bloating, and diarrhea. For supplementing the spleen, elecampane should be honey mix-fried. When prepared in this way, it is sweet, bitter, slightly acrid, and warm. This combination of flavors and *qi* supplements without causing stagnation, while resolving damp accumulation due to spleen vacuity.

- ***Transforms phlegm.*** Elecampane is used to treat phlegm in the lungs and stomach in acute or chronic phlegm-damp, especially associated with cold. Elecampane opens with acridity and downbears with bitterness to effectively transform phlegm-damp. It is used for a variety of conditions where phlegm-damp obstructs the lungs and stomach, with symptoms such as cough with clear or white abundant sputum; wheezing; asthma; nausea and vomiting; and oppression in the chest with difficult breathing.

- ***Aromatically transforms dampness.*** Elecampane is effective for damp accumulation in the middle burner. With aroma, bitterness, and acridity, elecampane transforms dampness and revives the spleen. Furthermore, its nature causes stomach *qi* to descend, thus harmonizing the middle burner. This action is very similar to that of atractylodes *(cāng zhú),* and elecampane can be used as a replacement for that herb.

CAUTIONS

Elecampane's bitter, acrid, and warm nature can injure *yīn* and disperse *qì*. Therefore it should be used with caution for patients with *yīn* vacuity.

Dosage and Preparation

Use 3–9 g in decoction; 2–4 ml tincture. For use as a tonic, elecampane should be honey mix-fried to increase its supplementing action.

Gather elecampane root and rhizome in spring or autumn, after the plant has died back for the winter. The harvested material can either be sliced for drying or chopped for preparation of fresh plant tincture. Good-quality dried material is firm, light brown on the outside, and off-white on the inside with curved striations. The root should be strongly aromatic.

Major Combinations

- Use the honey mix-fried version of elecampane combined with white atractylodes and astragalus for spleen *qi* vacuity with bloating and diarrhea.

- Combine with pinellia and citrus peel for cough with copious amounts of white or clear sputum. For this purpose, use either the raw or honey mix-fried herb. The decision should be based on the amount of spleen *qi* vacuity present. If there is little vacuity, use the raw herb, which dries phlegm more strongly. However, in the presence of spleen *qi* vacuity, treating the spleen vacuity will resolve the problem more quickly and completely.

- Combine with trichosanthus root, red root, and Chinese skullcap for diarrhea with phlegm and blood in the stool due to heat and blood stasis in the intestines.

Commentary

Elecampane is closely related to *xuán fù huā (Inula britannica),* an herb used in Chinese medicine to descend *qi* and stop cough. Neither species is native to China, but *I. helenium* is now cultivated there, along with

I. britannica. The root of *I. helenium* is the plant part used in the West, primarily to treat phlegm in the lungs. However, when one looks closely at the way Western herbalists employ this herb through the lens of the Chinese medical paradigm, it appears that it functions as a supplementing herb. In my never-ending search for supplementing medicinals in the Western materia medica, it was natural for me to try it as a *qi* supplement. The results were somewhat but not totally satisfying, and applying *páo zhì* to enhance an action inherent in the herb seemed appropriate. Honey mix-frying the herb turned out to be an excellent choice, resulting in a product that was something like a white atractylodes–pinellia synthesis.

According to one source, this is one of the oldest medicinal plants known in Europe. All major writers of the past have discussed it as a significant medicinal. The Greek physician Dioscorides recommended it for cough, cramps, flatulence, sciatica, gastric weakness, and making loose teeth secure. He also calls it a "precious medicine" for stomach colds, asthma, chest congestion, cough, and digestive problems. William Cook states, "To the lungs it is warming and strengthening," and "while it answers an excellent purpose in subacute and chronic cases where the lung structure is relaxed and expectoration viscid or too profuse (as in humid asthma), it is not suitable for cases of any class where the lungs are irritated or dry—as it then increases the dryness, and gives a feeling of constriction."[1]

Elecampane is classified as endangered in Turkey. It is found in the *British Herbal Pharmacopoeia* (1996), the *British Herbal Compendium* (1992), the French Pharmacopoeia (1988), *Martindale: The Extra Pharmacopoeia* (33rd ed.), The Netherlands Pharmacopoeia V (1926), and *PDR for Herbal Medicine* (2nd ed.), and is approved by the German Commission E.

Translation of Source Material

Chinese medicine uses many species of *Inula*. Here I have only included the species discussed in the monograph above. *Tŭ mù xiāng (Inula helenium)* is acrid, bitter, warm, and enters the lung, liver, and spleen channels. It fortifies the spleen and harmonizes the stomach, moves *qi*, and stops pain. It is used to treat distention, fullness and pain in the chest and abdomen, vomiting and diarrhea, dysentery, and malaria.

Hawthorn

Crataegus laevigata, C. oxyacantha,
C. monogyna, C. douglasii

Rosaceae

Crataegi fructus seu flos et folium

Flavor and *Qi*: sweet, slightly bitter, bland,
slightly warm
Channels Entered: heart, pericardium
Actions: antisclerotic, cardiac tonic, hypotensive

Functions and Indications

- ***Supplements heart* qì.** Hawthorn supplements the
heart *qì* when there is a feeling of congestion and
oppression in the chest with tachycardia or bradycardia and shortness of breath on exertion. Hawthorn
is sweet, slightly bitter, and slightly warm. An ideal
supplementing medicinal, hawthorn supplements
the heart *qì* without causing stagnation. It is some-

what gentle but definite in its action, and it can be
used long term without causing problems. The herb's
blandness disinhibits dampness, which may accumulate due to heart *qì* vacuity. According to classic
patho-mechanisms, dampness accumulation associated with heart *qì* vacuity is due to kidney *yáng*
vacuity. However, I believe there are cases in which
there is accumulated dampness even in the absence
of kidney *yáng* vacuity. The heart and lung *qì* are
intimately connected, and a vacuity of heart *qì* often
is accompanied by a vacuity of lung *qì*. This can be
considered a dual vacuity of heart and lung in which
lung vacuity causes an accumulation of dampness due
to its function of regulating the waterways.

- ***Supplements and quickens the blood and calms the***
spirit. Hawthorn is employed in the treatment of
blood and *qì* vacuity leading to stagnation of blood
in the chest with angina, palpitations, and a choppy
pulse in the *cun* position. When the heart blood is
vacuous, the heart *qì* becomes vacuous. When the

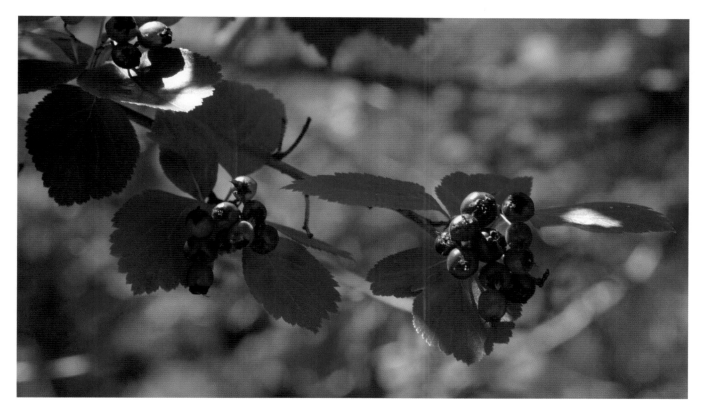

Hawthorn (*Crataegus* sp.)

heart *qì* becomes vacuous, the heart blood becomes vacuous. If this cycle occurs, the blood becomes static. Although not a particularly strong blood-quickening medicinal, hawthorn is an important treatment for heart-blood stasis.

CAUTIONS

Patients who are already taking digitalis must be monitored, as hawthorn may potentiate the effects of digitalis.

Dosage and Preparation

Use 3–9 g in decoction; 2–4 ml tincture; 1–3 ml fluid-extract; 2–3 g powdered extract.

Gather hawthorn fruits in late summer and early autumn when they are fully mature. They may be dried or processed fresh. Hawthorn leaves and flowers should be gathered in late spring and early summer when the flowers are mature. Leaves and flowers either can be processed fresh or carefully dried out of light and high heat. Good-quality fruits are fully dried, whole, and dark red. Leaves and flowers should be as whole as possible. Leaves should be green to dark green without stems. The flowers should be white to pink, not brown.

Major Combinations

- Combine with the classical formula Celestial Emperor Heart-Supplementing Elixir *(tiān wáng bǔ xīn dān)* to strengthen the formula.

- Combine with motherwort and red sage root for chest pain or impediment with pain, anxiety, and a choppy pulse. For chest impediment, add immature bitter orange *(zhǐ shí)* and trichosanthus peel *(guā lóu pí)*.

- Combine with raw rehmannia, *dāng guī,* and spiny zizyphus for anxiety, panic attacks, and insomnia due to heart-blood vacuity. Add motherwort and red sage root if palpitations are present.

Commentary

Although hawthorn is slightly warm, it is well tolerated by those with heat, especially when it is combined with other cooling herbs. Western species of hawthorn are significantly different from the primary species used in Chinese medicine, *Crataegus pinnatifida (shān zhā)*. First, Western hawthorn is more supplementing than Chinese hawthorn. Another difference between the Western and Chinese species of hawthorn is that Western hawthorn does not seem to have a history of use as a digestive remedy.

Western hawthorn is a true supplement in the sense that it takes time for its benefits to become apparent. The herb may be taken for extended periods of time with no known ill effects. One modern reference states, "In Western herbal medicine hawthorn is now considered to be the most significant herb for ischaemic heart disease and there is considerable objective evidence to support its status." The authors go on to list the following effects: "Increases force of myocardial contraction, increases coronary blood flow, reduces myocardial oxygen demand, protects against myocardial damage, hypotensive, improves heart rate variability, antiarrhythmic." [2]

In my experience using Western hawthorn as a supplementing medicinal, the flowers and leaves are the strongest for supplementing *qì* and moving the blood (flowers being the stronger of the two). The fruits, while also effective for supplementing *qì,* are best for supplementing and moving the blood.

Hawthorn has a long history of use, but did not become widely known in Western medicine until the nineteenth century, when an Irish doctor first described the effects of hawthorn in cardiac troubles.[3] Since that time, hawthorn has become a premier herbal remedy for heart trouble. The fruits, sometimes called haws, are made into jams and jellies as well as various alcoholic beverages. In England, hawthorn is a well-known hedgerow plant that forms thick, thorny fences within five to seven years. The specific origin of the genus name *Crataegus* is not known but probably comes from a Greek word meaning "hard" or "strong," in reference to its wood or its thorns.

Various species of hawthorn are listed as official in the pharmacopoeias of Belgium, Brazil, China, the Czech Republic, France, Germany, Poland, Portugal, Russia, Spain, and Switzerland. Hawthorn leaf and flower are approved as medicines by the German Commission E. In most cases, leaf, flower, and fruit are all listed; however, some pharmacopoeias, such as the *Pharmacopoeia of the People's Republic of China,* list only the fruit.

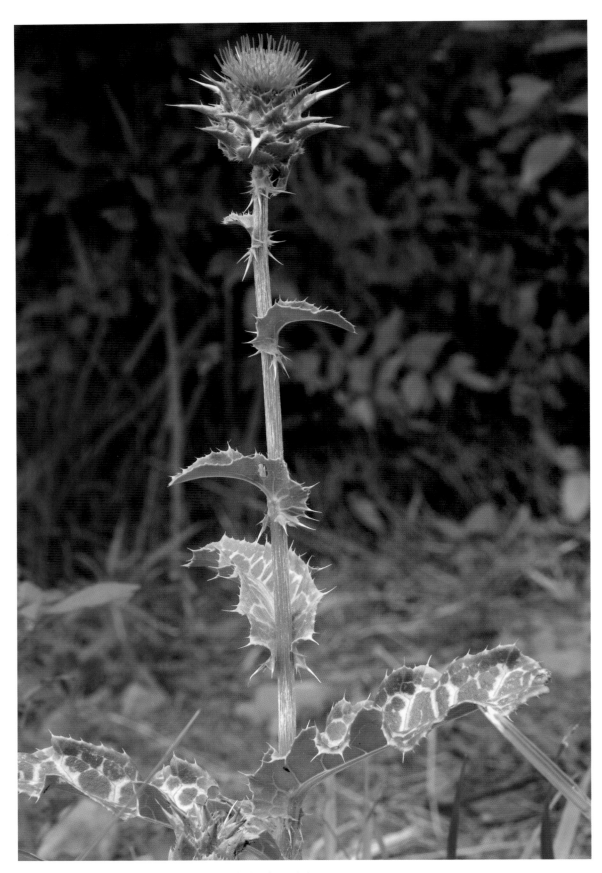

Milk thistle *(Silybum marianum)*

Milk Thistle

Silybum marianum

Asteraceae

Silybi Mariani semen

Flavor and *Qì:* bitter, sweet, neutral
Channels Entered: liver, spleen, stomach
Actions: cholagogue, galactogogue, hepatoprotective

Functions and Indications

- ***Supplements the liver-spleen blood and*** yīn, ***abates vacuity heat, and benefits spleen*** qì. Milk thistle is used in the treatment of symptoms associated with liver and spleen vacuity, such as malaise, lassitude, anorexia, dyspepsia, headache, low-grade fever, joint and tendon pain, tendon contracture, urticaria, and transient skin rashes. Milk thistle's bitter flavor abates vacuity heat, while the combination of its bitter and sweet flavors supplements the liver and spleen. Being neutral in nature, milk thistle is safe to use as a supplementing medicinal even in replete heat conditions. Milk thistle also helps improve the flow of scant breast milk associated with this pattern.

- ***Clears heat and resolves toxins.*** Milk thistle is employed to treat various toxic conditions, including poisoning by mushrooms, drugs, or other toxins that affect the liver. Although milk thistle is neutral in nature, its bitter flavor assists heat clearing and toxin resolving when combined with the appropriate medicinals. For this therapeutic effect, use a standardized extract or tincture. Alcohol and solid extracts are both available. The solid extracts are best for alcoholics and patients with serious liver impairment. Milk thistle is also commonly employed to treat a variety of other serious liver conditions, such as hepatitis C, for which it is invaluable.

CAUTIONS

None noted in the literature. However, I have heard reports of patients taking medications who seem to have metabolized those medications more quickly when taking milk thistle, so it may be important to watch such patients closely, especially if they are taking medications that are very dose sensitive.

Dosage and Preparation

Use 6–15 g in decoction (as a galactogogue); 3–6 ml tincture; 400–450 mg silymarin in standardized extract.

Gather milk thistle fruits (seeds) in midsummer when they are mature (shiny and slightly purple). Once the flowers have died, the seed heads must be gathered quickly, before the flowers reopen and disperse the seeds. Good-quality milk thistle seed is dark, whole, and shiny; dull-looking seeds are acceptable but of lesser quality. Good-quality tincture is yellow in color.

Major Combinations

- Combine with white peony, *dāng guī,* and cramp bark for tendon contracture due to blood vacuity.

- Combine with Chinese skullcap and yellow dock for urticaria and transient skin rashes.

- Combine with skullcap and Chinese skullcap for liver heat and toxin accumulation due to alcoholism.

- Combine with picrorhiza for hepatitis C.

Commentary

Milk thistle is commonly employed to detoxify poisons in the liver. The plant is so effective for this purpose that it is given intravenously in Europe for poisonings by *Amanita* mushrooms, which can be deadly. It is very beneficial for people with a history of alcoholism or drug abuse, as well as those who have been on medications that have damaged their liver. However, patients taking dose-sensitive medications should use milk thistle with

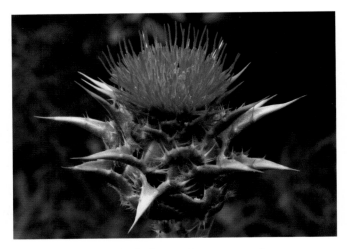

Milk thistle flower *(S. marianum)*

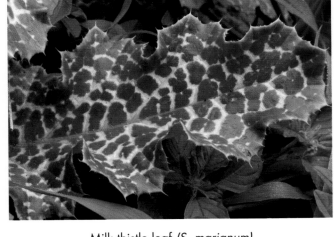

Milk thistle leaf *(S. marianum)*

caution, as it may encourage the liver to metabolize the drugs faster than usual, thus lowering serum levels of the drugs to a potentially dangerous level. I personally have never seen this happen, but have heard reports of it.

Research results suggest that silymarin (a complex of flavonoid compounds contained in milk thistle seed) has hepatoprotective, anti-inflammatory, and antiarthitic effects, as well as liver-regenerative properties that may produce beneficial effects in some types of hepatitis.[4]

Dioscorides, the famous Greek herbalist of the first century CE, said that milk thistle seeds are good for infants whose sinews had "drawn together." Ancient herbalists also employed milk thistle root, but I have no experience with it. Gerard said this about the root: "My opinion is that this is the best remedy that grows against all melancholy diseases." I find this statement very interesting, as did Mrs. M. Grieve, who speculated

that this ". . . was another way of saying that it had good action in the liver."[5]

The genus name *Silybum* comes from the Latin or Greek and refers to the fact that the plant is a thistle. The species name *marianum* is derived from a legend that tells how the Virgin Mary's milk dropped onto the leaf of a milk thistle plant, giving the leaf its milky veins. One has to wonder whether this also suggests that Mary used the plant in some way, either for herself or Jesus.

Tender young milk thistle leaves make an excellent spring green. The only problem is that they are well armed with spines, which you will need to cut off before cooking. Milk thistle became official in *The United States Pharmacopoeia* and in *The National Formulary (U.S.)* in 1999. Although it is used in a variety of proprietary products throughout Europe, only the German Commission E Monographs list it as official.

Marsh mallow

Althaea officinalis

Malvaceae

Althaeae Officinali radix

Flavor and *Qi:* sweet, slightly bitter, cold
Channels Entered: lung, stomach, kidney, bladder
Actions: demulcent, emollient, expectorant

Functions and Indications

- ***Supplements the lung and stomach* yīn *and clears heat.*** Marsh mallow is effective in the treatment of *yīn* vacuity of the lung and/or stomach, with symptoms such as dry cough; thirst; dry, sore throat; and burning sensation in the epigastrum. A premier *yīn* supplementing medicinal from the Western materia medica, marsh mallow root is one of the most popular medicinals with Western herbalists for treating symptoms of lung and stomach *yīn* vacuity with vacuity heat. Marsh mallow supplements *yīn* with sweetness and clears heat with bitterness and cold. This is a very important action for both stomach and lung *yīn* vacuity. It can also help with stomach heat, which will burn fluids to cause dryness and, eventually, *yīn* vacuity.

- ***Causes* yīn *vacuity heat to recede.*** Marsh mallow is used to treat *yīn* vacuity heat, with symptoms such as chronic urinary tract infections, thirst, and night sweating. Marsh mallow is bitter and cold and causes vacuity heat to recede. With its sweetness, it supplements the kidney *yīn* and moistens the bladder. Thus it is an effective treatment for the problematic chronic urinary tract infections that can occur when kidney *yīn* vacuity transfers vacuity heat to the bladder.

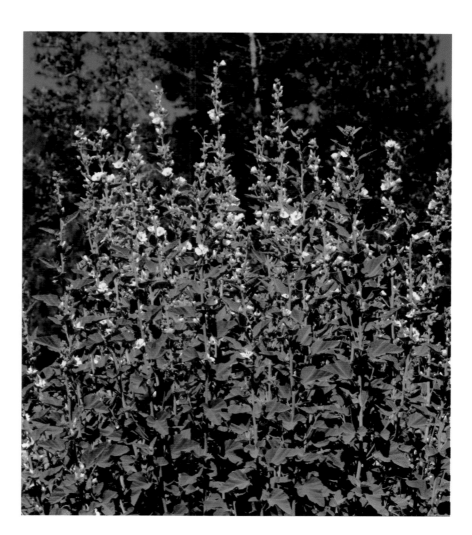

Marsh mallow *(Althaea officinalis)*

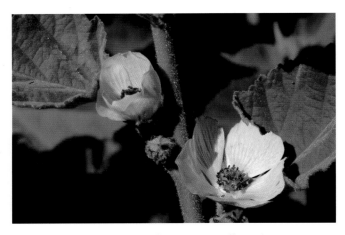

Marsh mallow flowers (A. officinalis)

CAUTIONS

Marsh mallow root is contraindicated in patients with spleen vacuity-damp conditions. Due to its bitter, cold, sweet nature, it should be used with caution in those with dampness, especially in the middle burner.

Dosage and Preparation

Use 2–6 g in decoction or infusion (up to 12 g); 2–5 ml tincture.

Gather marsh mallow root in fall after the plant has died back for the winter. Slice and dry the roots for tea or tincture them fresh. Good-quality dried marsh mallow root is whitish or dirty white, firm but lightweight.

Major Combinations

• Combine with ophiopogon and California figwort root for sore throat due to *yīn* vacuity.

• Combine with aucklandia and coptis for stomach *yīn* vacuity causing retching, burping, and vomiting.

• Combine with ophiopogon and mulberry leaf for dry cough due either to wind-dryness or lung *yīn* vacuity.

Commentary

Damp-heat patterns represent a combination of dampness and heat. With either acute or chronic conditions, the heat portion of the affliction can cause significant damage to tissue and *yīn*. Marsh mallow root is moistening and cold and is commonly used in damp-heat patterns such as strangury. Marsh mallow clears heat and nourishes *yīn,* thus protecting tissue against damage by heat.

In Western herbalism, marsh mallow is very popular for treating many types of heat syndromes. It is beneficial in most cases, but especially when either repletion-heat or vacuity-heat patterns have damaged *yīn*. Due to its high content of mucilage (10 to 20 percent), this herb cannot be decocted in large quantities because the mucilage will congeal, making the tea thick and slimy. Therefore, small doses are sufficient in most decoctions. To incorporate larger doses, add the medicinal at the end of the decoction or make a simple infusion.

The genus name *Althaea* comes from the Greek word *althae,* meaning "heal" or "cure." The species name *officinalis* was first recorded in the early nineteenth century and indicates that this is an official drug plant. This plant and its relatives have a long history of use in many cultures, including China. Many peoples have eaten the young tender leaves and shoots; in fact, the Bible mentions a mallow as a food source consumed during times of famine. Marsh mallow roots are made into syrups and candies, most of which are taken for sore throat and cough.

Many of the great herbalists of the past have written about marsh mallow, including Dioscorides and Pliny. According to Pliny, "Whosoever shall take a spoonful of the Mallows shall that day be free from all diseases that may come to him."[6]

Althaea was official as early as 1733 in the French pharmacopoeia, and remains official there today as well as in many other countries, including Austria, Belgium, Britian, Germany, Hungary, and Mexico. Althaea is listed in the *European Pharmacopoeia,* the *British Herbal Pharmacopoeia* (1996), the *British Herbal Compendium* (1992), *Martindale: The Extra Pharmacopoeia* (33rd ed.), and *PDR for Herbal Medicine.* Belgium and France also list the leaves and flowers as official; the German Commission E lists both the root and the leaf as approved medicines.

Oat

Avena sativa, A. fatua

Poaceae

Avenae semen immaturus

Flavor and *Qi:* sweet, neutral
Channels Entered: heart, kidney
Actions: antidepressant, cardiac tonic

Functions and Indications

- ***Supplements the kidney.*** Oat is used in *yīn* and *qì* vacuity with symptoms such as depression, poor sexual performance, lack of energy, and mental exhaustion. Oat, sometimes called wild oat, is sweet and neutral. Its sweetn   182

ess supplements *yīn* and *qì,* and because it is neutral, it does not aggravate *yīn* vacuity or disperse *qì*. Oat is extremely valuable for treating individuals exhausted by high-stress jobs, poor appetite, and lack of exercise.

- ***Nourishes the heart and calms the spirit.*** Oat is used in the treatment of disquieted heart *qì* for symptoms of anxiety, palpitations, forgetfulness, depression, listlessness, insomnia, and mental restlessness. The sweet flavor of oat can relax tension and stress caused by an undernourished heart that does not afford a safe place for the spirit to enter and reside. Oat's relaxing nature and its ability to nourish the heart and calm the spirit make it a premier medicinal for treating drug addiction. Furthermore, as already noted, oat nourishes the kidneys, an organ system that is often depleted in drug abusers.

CAUTIONS

None noted.

Dosage and Preparation

Use 9–30 g in decoction (up to 50 g); 1–4 ml tincture.

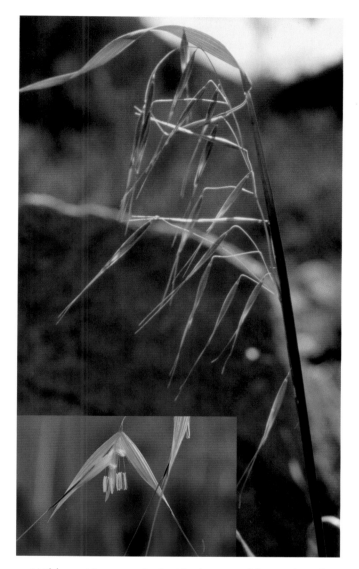

Wild oat *(Avena sativa)* with close-up of flower (inset)

Harvest oat spikelets (often called seeds or fruits) while they are in the milky stage—in other words, when squeezing the spikelet produces a white, milky juice. The seeds are immature at this stage, which lasts only five to eight days.

Major Combinations

- Combine with damiana and epimedium for male impotence and poor sexual performance.

- Combine with albizia flower, cyperus, and California poppy for liver *qì* depression with underlying kidney vacuity, with symptoms of insomnia and mental restlessness.

• Combine with skullcap for tobacco and other drug addictions. This is a very important combination for addiction treatment, and one that has proven effective for many patients, especially those addicted to tobacco (see below for more information).

Commentary

Oat is a gentle supplementing medicinal. Its action of supplementing both *yīn* and *qì* is somewhat unique and makes it appropriate for many patterns affecting an extraordinary number of patients in the West. Coupled with its quality to nourish the heart and calm the spirit, these supplementing properties make oat extremely important in modern practice. Oat can be very helpful for elderly people, especially those with sleeping problems. Taking the tincture throughout the day, with a double dose before retiring, helps patients sleep more deeply and wake less.

Oat has demonstrated significant benefits in many addictions, but most significantly in nicotine addiction. Although the herb can be employed in the form of a decoction for this purpose, I rarely use it as such, as I much prefer the fresh plant tincture. At least one study has shown the fresh plant tincture to be effective for treating nicotine addiction. In this study, a placebo-controlled clinical trial of four weeks duration, researchers observed a significant reduction in the number of cigarettes smoked by habitual tobacco users taking fresh wild oat alcoholic extract made from mature plants. The number of cigarettes smoked dropped from 19.5 to 5.7 cigarettes per day among those taking the wild oat tincture, compared with those in the placebo group, who went from 16.5 to 16.7 cigarettes per day.[7] I have used oat tincture in a variety of cases—in formulas as well as in combination with auricular acupuncture—and have seen very positive results.

While some authors suggest using oat straw (meaning the whole herb), the immature seeds are the most important medicinal part of the plant. The genus name *Avena* is Latin for "oats" and may come from the Sanskrit *avasa,* meaning "nourishment."

Translation of Source Material

Chinese medicine uses two species of *Avena,* including one from the monograph above. *Yàn mài căo (A. fatua)* is sweet, warm, and nontoxic. It can supplement vacuity detriment and is used to treat vomiting of blood, vacuity sweating, and menstrual flooding.

Qīng kē (A. nuda) is salty and cool. It downbears and rectifies *qì* while coursing depression, strengthens the sinews and benefits physical strength, eliminates damp sweating, and stops diarrhea.

Damiana

Turnera diffusa

Turneraceae

Turnerae Diffusae herba

Flavor and *Qi:* acrid, sweet, warm
Channels Entered: kidney, spleen, heart
Actions: antidepressant, aphrodisiac, stomachic

Functions and Indications

- ***Supplements kidney* yáng *and benefits the spleen.***
  Damiana is used to treat patterns of kidney *yáng*
  vacuity, with symptoms such as low sex drive; fatigue;
  poor appetite; spermatorrhea; and painful, cold
  lower back and knees. Damiana combines warm *qi*
  with sweet and acrid flavors to supplement *yáng* and
  lead water to its source. Although the herb primarily
  acts on the kidney, the warming and supplementing
  effects on the kidney also benefit the spleen. Futhermore, damiana's sweet and acrid nature leads it to the
  spleen, where it benefits *yáng* and assists the spleen in
  carrying out its function of transforming and trans-
  porting fluids.

- ***Benefits the kidney and strengthens heart* yáng.**
  Damiana is employed in the treatment of heart
  yáng vacuity with symptoms of depression and
  withdrawn behavior. Damiana has a sweet and acrid
  flavor and a warm *qi*. This combination of flavor
  and *qi* strengthens the heart *yáng* and warms the
  kidney, resolving depression associated with vacuity
  of *yáng*.

CAUTIONS

Use damiana with care when there are symptoms of heat
with dryness.

Dosage and Preparation

Use 3–6 g in decoction; 1–3 ml tincture.

Gather damiana leaf in spring before the flowers

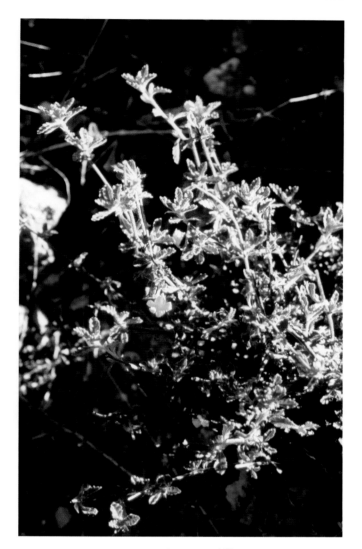

Damiana *(Turnera diffusa)*

emerge. Damiana can be either tinctured fresh or dried
for future use. Good-quality dried herb is grayish-
green, tomentose (covered with hair), aromatic, and
should not contain any large stems.

Major Combinations

- Combine with St. John's wort for heart *yáng* vacuity
  with depression.

- Combine with epimedium for kidney *yáng* vacuity
  with symptoms of low sex drive; withdrawal; and
  cold, painful lower back. This combination is also
  valuable for erectile dysfunction in men and infertility in women. For this use, morinda can be an important addition.

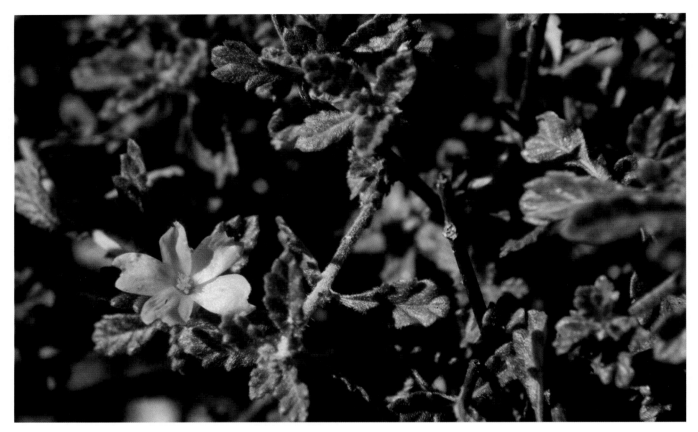

Damiana flower *(T. diffusa)*

• Combine with cuscuta *(tù sī zǐ)* and Licorice, Wheat, and Jujube Decoction *(gān mài dà zǎo tāng)* for non-interaction of the heart and kidney, with symptoms of heart vexation, insomnia, anxiousness, dream-disturbed sleep, and palpitations. This combination warms heart *yáng*, benefits the heart and kidney, secures the essence, and effectively treats depression and withdrawn behavior.

Commentary

Damiana's ability to help with a variety of reproductive dysfunctions has given it a unique and important place in the Western materia medica. Its historical applications by native peoples of Mexico suggest that it is a classic *yáng*-supplementing herb (from the Chinese perspective). It is useful not only for those with reproductive dysfunction, but also for the many patients who suffer from both kidney vacuity and emotional depression. The herb's ability to invigorate and warm *yáng* is key for all of the above indications.

The genus name *Turnera* comes from the name of the famous English botanist and naturalist of the mid-sixteenth century, William Turner. The medicinal properties of damiana were first reported by "a priest of known honesty and much experience," who said "that drinking a decoction of damiana made women fertile whom he had seen previously to be sterile and infecund."[8] The Mayans are thought to have long known about damiana's aphrodisiac effects, and native peoples of Mexico use the herb to "promote conception" and to "fortify the uterus," as well as for impotence, frigidity, sterility, sexual exhaustion, and "frio en la matriz" ("cold" uterus, infertility). Other applications include the treatment of diabetes, coughs and colds, scorpion stings, and inflammation.[9]

Damiana is official in the *British Herbal Compendium* (1992), the *British Herbal Pharmacopoeia* (1996), *Martindale: The Extra Pharmacopoeia* (33rd ed.), and *PDR for Herbal Medicine* (2nd ed.).

HERBS THAT
STABILIZE AND BIND

Many of the herbs in this category are known as astringents in Western herbal medicine. Their main application here, however, is to treat efflux desertion patterns. Because efflux desertion is considered a loss of some vital substance (either material or immaterial), the pattern is often associated with an inability to restrain. Treatment involves securing and astringing with medicinals that have astringent and supplementing properties. Some of the herbs in this category have both astringent and supplementing actions; others primarily have astringent qualities and are often combined with medicinals from the supplementing category.

In this text, I've included two medicinals from this category; one is a "pure" astringent, while the other is both astringent and supplementing. Bayberry *(Myrica cerifera),* a warm astringent, is also acrid. This makes it a clinically valued asset because it treats vacuity of *qi* and *yáng* with warmth and dampness and treats phlegm with warmth and acridity. Cranberry *(Vaccinium macrocarpon)* is sour, bitter, and only slightly warm. It is a strong astringent, but also supplements and has an action similar to cornus fruit in Chinese herbal medicine.

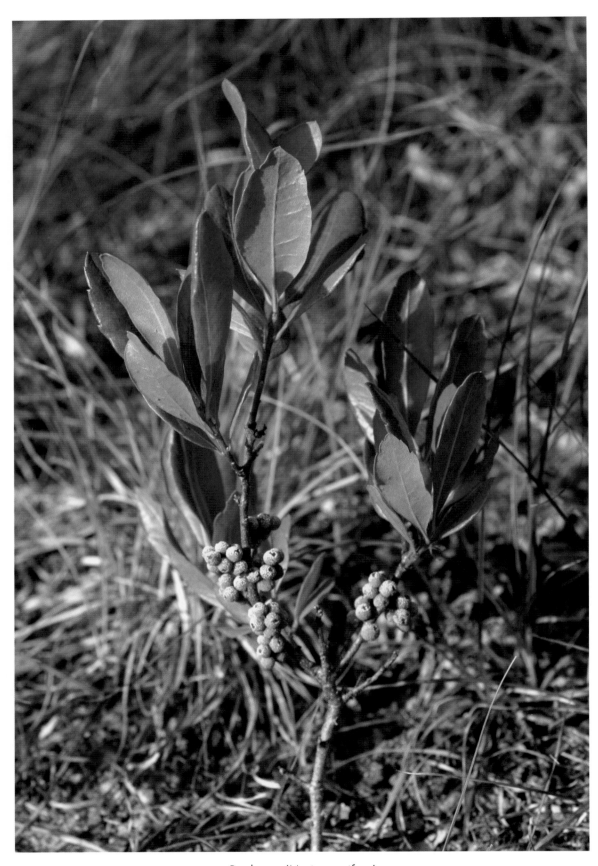

Bayberry *(Myrica cerifera)*

Bayberry

Myrica cerifera

Myricaceae

Myricae Ceriferae cortex seu radicis

Flavor and *Qi*: sour, acrid, astringent, warm
Channels Entered: large intestine, small intestine, liver, lung
Actions: astringent, diaphoretic (with large doses of tincture), stimulant

Functions and Indications

- ***Binds the intestines, warms the spleen, and stops diarrhea.*** Bayberry is effective against chronic cold-type diarrhea with mucus associated with spleen and kidney vacuity. Bayberry provides an interesting mix of flavors and *qi*. It is sour, acrid, astringent, and warm. With sourness and astringency, it binds and stops excessive flow. Yet it is also warm and acrid and thus dries and disperses dampness. This uncommon combination confers an action similar to that seen with the formula Four Spirits Pill *(sì shén wán),* without the supplementation aspect, and gives bayberry a unique niche in this materia medica.

- ***Transforms phlegm and restrains lung* qì.** Bayberry is used to treat chronic cough with either damp-phlegm or phlegm fluids congesting the lung, causing weakness of lung *qi* and disruption of the lungs' descending function. Bayberry transforms phlegm with warmth and acridity, while restraining the lung *qi* with sourness and astringency. By transforming phlegm in a case of chronic cough, the lung is freed to perform its downbearing functions; restraining the lung *qi* allows a preservation of right. This unusual mix of actions functions something like a combination of pinellia and schizandra.

- ***Stabilizes the kidneys and restrains essence.*** Bayberry treats leakage of fluids due to kidney vacuity, with symptoms such as leukorrhea, spermatorrhea, and nocturnal emissions. Bayberry stabilizes with sourness and astringency while warming the kidneys. We rely upon this function less today than in the past; however, adding this medicinal to kidney-supplementing formulas helps warm and restrain the kidney, an important function in cases of kidney *qi* and *yáng* vacuity.

- ***Assists in healing.*** Bayberry may be employed as a mouthwash or gargle for tender, spongy, bleeding gums and sore throat. It is also applied externally for ulcers that heal slowly. Bayberry is sour, acrid, astringent, and warm. With sour astringency, this medicinal contracts and astringes damaged tissue, stopping bleeding and reducing swelling. With warm acidity, it quickens the blood and disperses damp accumulation. These actions assist in the healing process for various slow-healing wounds, especially in the mouth and throat.

CAUTIONS

None noted.

Dosage and Preparation

Use 1–4 g in decoction; 2–4 ml tincture.

Gather bayberry bark in spring (this is ideal, although it can be gathered anytime) and either tincture it fresh or cut and dry it for future use. Good-quality dried material is firm, dark brown, astringent and pungent to the taste, and aromatic to the nose.

Major Combinations

- Combine with Calm the Stomach Powder *(píng wéi sǎn)* for cold-damp diarrhea.

- Combine with Six Gentlemen Decoction *(liù jūn zǐ tāng)* for cold-damp leukorrhea with concurrent spleen *qi* vacuity.

- Combine with Two Mature Ingredients Decoction *(èr chén tāng)* for phlegm fluids congesting the lung. Add astragalus for lung *qi* vacuity.

- Combine with Four Spirits Pill *(sì shén wán)* to strengthen the effects of the formula.

- Combine with True Man Viscus-Nourishing Decoction *(zhēn rén yǎng zàng tāng)* to replace *zhì yīng sùké* (prepared opium poppy husk). Bayberry can provide some of the binding action that was lost with the no-longer-available medicinal *zhì yīng sùké,* and will further assist with the transformation of phlegm.

Commentary

When I was a young boy on Cape Cod, bayberry bushes were a common sight. One fragrant bush bordered the southeastern portion of our yard. We gathered the berries in the late summer and fall and added them to melted wax to pour into sand molds to make sand candles. Adding bayberry wax made a sweet fragrant candle. To this day, when I go home for a visit, I like to pick some bayberry leaves and berries to place on the dashboard of the car. Unfortunately, this plant's habitat is in serious danger due to building and development.

Because of its warming and astringing action, bayberry is a valuable herb for vacuity leakage. Unlike many of the main astringing medicinals in the Chinese materia medica, bayberry provides an excellent drying action for excessive dampness due to its warm acridity, giving it important clinical applications. While many of the astringing medicinals in the Chinese materia medica are warming, their main job is to astringe, and practitioners rely on other herbs to drain or transform dampness or phlegm. Bayberry, on the other hand, is famous for both astringing and transforming dampness.

The etymology of the genus name *Myrica* is unknown; however, it may refer to the plant's resemblance to myrtle, or to a fragrant salve called *myron.* The species name *cerifera* comes from a Greek word meaning "wax-bearing."

Several Native American tribes, including the Delaware and the Mohegan of the northeastern United States, used bayberry for various kidney diseases.[1] Of its importance in the materia medica, William Cook wrote, "It combines stimulating and astringing powers in about equal proportions, is very decided and persistent in its action, and brings the whole frame under its influence."[2] After two-plus pages of discussion, Cook concluded, "This is somewhat extended praise to bestow on a single remedy, but this article fully deserves all here said of it."[3] Bayberry root bark was official in *The National Formulary (U.S.)* from 1916–1936 and is listed in the *British Herbal Pharmacopoeia* (1996), *Martindale: The Extra Pharmacopoeia* (33rd ed.), and *PDR for Herbal Medicine* (2nd ed.).

Translation of Source Material

Chinese medicine uses several species of *Myrica. Yáng méi (M. rubra)* is sweet, sour, and warm, and enters the lung and stomach channels. It engenders liquid and quenches thirst, harmonizes the stomach and disperses food, and is used to treat vexation and thirst, vomiting and diarrhea, dysentery, and abdominal pain.

Yáng méi shù (M. esculenta) is astringent and neutral. It disperses fire, promotes contraction, stops diarrhea, stops bleeding, stops pain, and is used in the treatment of dysentery, intestinal fire, flooding and spotting, and stomach pain.

Ai yáng méi (M. nana) is astringent and cool. (Note: both root bark and berry are used and called by the same name. I have included information only for root bark.) The medicinal disperses and transforms the impure; it is used in the treatment of dysentery, diarrhea, flooding and spotting, rectal bleeding, prolapsed anus, wind-damp impediment, and knocks and falls.

Cranberry

Vaccinium macrocarpon

Ericaceae

Vaccinii Macrocarpon fructus

Flavor and *Qi:* sour, bitter, slightly warm
Channels Entered: kidney, liver, bladder
Actions: astringent, tonic

Functions and Indications

- ***Supplements the kidneys and restrains essence.*** Cranberry is helpful in the treatment of incontinence, excessive urination, and excessive sweating. Cranberry is sour, bitter, and slightly warm. With sourness, it restrains essence. It benefits the essence and supplements kidney *qi*. Cranberry is similar in action to Chinese dogwood fruit and can be used as a substitute for that herb. Although I have successfully employed this substitution, I prefer to include both herbs in a formula, as I believe that Chinese dogwood fruit is likely a slightly better supplementing medicinal than cranberry.

- ***Strengthens the kidneys and liver.*** Cranberry is effective for *yīn* vacuity of the kidneys and liver with symptoms such as impotence, lower back pain, dizziness, and night sweats. Although cranberry is warm in nature, it is also bitter and sour. With bitterness it drains excess, and with sourness it restrains *yīn*. As a supplementing medicinal, it acts mainly on the kidney and to a somewhat lesser extent on the liver.

CAUTIONS

Although cranberry is commonly used to treat repletion, as mentioned above, it seems prudent to use caution when treating other types of repletion heat. I have never seen any side effects with this medicinal, but it is very acidic, and drinking the concentrated juice over a long period of time may cause stomach heat or stomach *yīn* vacuity.

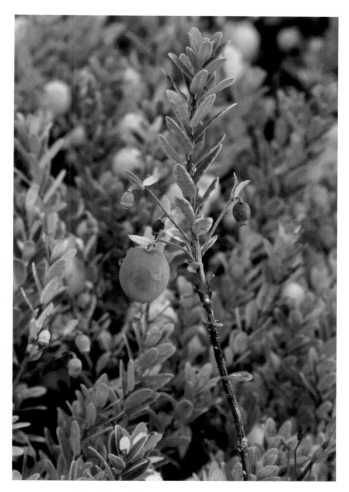

Cranberry *(Vaccinium macrocarpon)*

Dosage and Preparation

Use 2–9 g in decoction; 1–4 oz of pure (unsweetened) juice.

Gather cranberries in summer, when the fruit is completely ripe. The fruit resists drying unless the outside skin is cut; therefore, it is important to cut the skin of the fruits prior to drying. It is not necessary to cut it in any specific fashion, but it does need to be cut, broken, pierced, or otherwise breached. Good-quality dried berries are dark red, pliable, and very sour. It is best to avoid using the sweetened dry berries that are readily available in supermarkets.

Commentary

Another plant from my youth, cranberry is produced commercially in my native state of Massachusetts,

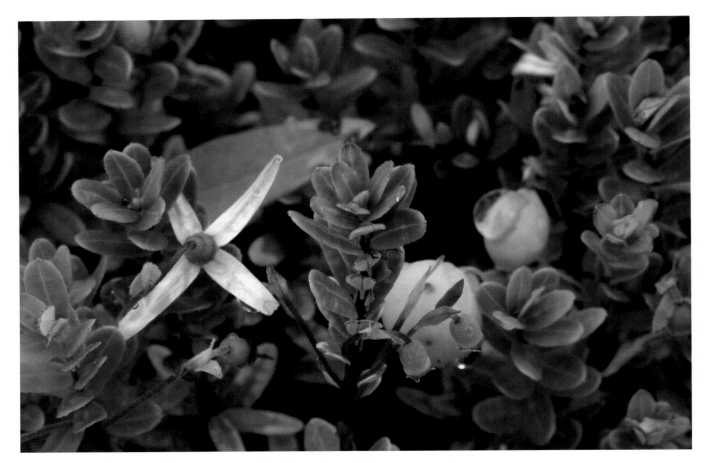

Cranberry flower *(V. macrocarpon)*

which is world-famous for cranberry production. When I was a boy, my family and I went to the cranberry festival and ate cranberries in every preparation possible, from pies to juice. There are still native cranberry bogs on Cape Cod and in surrounding areas, although most of them have been converted for commercial production. Cranberries were used extensively as a food by all the Native Americans in regions in which the plant is native (the northeastern United States and southeastern Canada). The berries were dried for use in the winter months, cooked into sauces, and eaten with corn preparations as a staple dish. It was likely one of the foods served to the Pilgrims at Plymouth, accounting for its continued popularity at Thanksgiving dinners throughout the United States.

Cranberry juice is commonly taken as a remedy for urinary tract infections. Recent research suggests that a compound in cranberry has the ability to ameliorate infection by preventing bacteria from clinging to the tissue of the urinary tract. (This principle has been employed in at least one commercial product marketed as a mouth-cleansing tincture.) This is an effective treatment and could be particularly helpful for chronic urinary tract irritation due to *yīn* vacuity.

Cranberry appears to be quite similar in function to the Chinese dogwood fruit as used in Chinese herbal medicine. Although I only have somewhat limited clinical experience with it, I believe this Western medicinal will prove very valuable for kidney and liver vacuity.

Cranberry is listed in *Martindale: The Extra Pharmacopoeia* (33rd ed.).

HERBS THAT
CALM THE SPIRIT

This category consists of medicinals that generally nourish the heart and quiet the spirit. The heart is the storage place for the spirit, if the heart is either replete or vacuous, the spirit may become disquieted. When the spirit is disquieted a patient may experience heart vexation, insomnia, palpitations, anxiety, susceptibility to fright, and even biomedically defined clinical depression.

The Western materia medica is replete with medicinals that fit into this category, perhaps because of our cultural predilection for stress, overwork, and undernourishment—physical, emotional, and spiritual. Seven medicinals are represented here. Each has its niche, but with the exception of passionflower, none of them are nourishing. California poppy *(Eschscholzia californica)* is bitter and draining, and thus is generally applied in conditions associated with heat, especially replete heat. Passionflower *(Passiflora incarnata)* is nourishing and can be used for all types of disquieted spirit. St. John's wort *(Hypericum perforatum),* kava *(Piper methysticum),* and valerian *(Valeriana officinalis)* are useful because of their *qi*-coursing actions. Although chamomile *(Matricaria recutita)* also courses the *qi,* this is a weaker action, and this plant will be more serviceable when digestive problems exist. Skullcap *(Scutellaria lateriflora)* is an exceptionally important medicinal native to the Americas. Skullcap is bitter, acrid, and cool. It quiets the spirit and resolves depression—both in the heart and liver. It is also helpful in the treatment of liver-wind conditions.

California Poppy

Eschscholzia californica

Papaveraceae

Eschscholziae Californicae planta

Flavor and *Qi:* acrid, bitter, cold
Channels Entered: liver, gallbladder, heart
Actions: anodyne, antispasmodic, anxiolytic, sedative

Functions and Indications

- ***Clears heat from the heart and quiets the spirit.*** California poppy is helpful in the treatment of anxiety, agitation, insomnia, vexation, agitation, irascibility, red tongue, and rapid pulse due either to repletion or vacuity. California poppy is acrid, bitter, and cold. It effectively clears heat, drains fire, and quiets *shén*. Although cold in nature, California poppy may be employed for both repletion and vacuity patterns due to the nature of heat in the heart. Whenever there is heat in the heart (whether due to repletion or vacuity) there will be an excess of fire, which is the five-phase orientation of the heart. Thus, either repletion or vacuity pathologies can lead to extremes of heat or fire in this organ system.

- ***Clears heat and resolves liver-gallbladder depression.*** California poppy is employed to treat depressed liver-gallbladder heat with symptoms of anxiety, heart vexation, dry mouth with desire to drink, sighing, irascibility, dizziness, headache, distention and pain in the rib or sides, yellow urine, dry stool, a red tongue (especially on the sides) with a thin yellow or slimy yellow coat, and a rapid, wiry pulse. California poppy is acrid, bitter, and cold and effectively resolves depression, drains heat, and resolves liver-gallbladder depression. The herb is also very helpful for general signs and symptoms of liver-depression affect disorder.

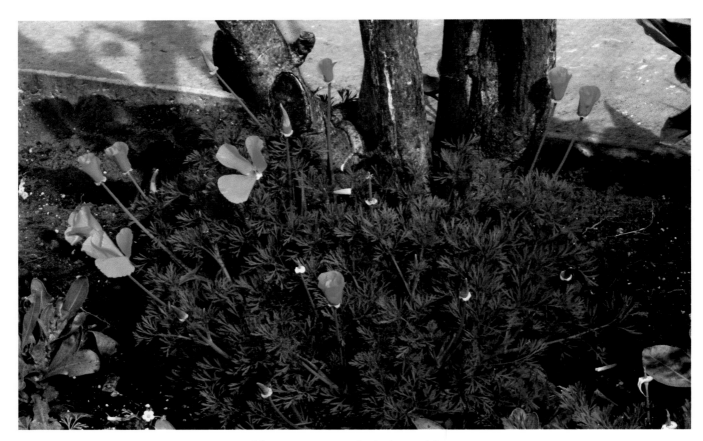

California poppy *(Eschscholzia californica)*

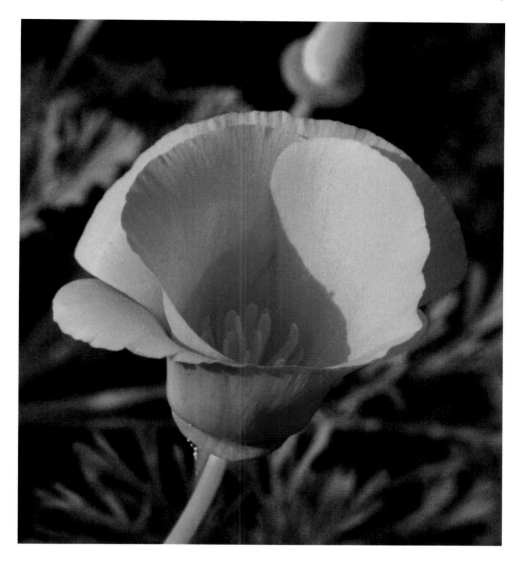

California poppy flower
(*E. californica*)

• **Relieves qì *stagnation and blood stasis, and reduces pain.*** California poppy is applied in a variety of painful conditions such as stomach pain, menstrual pain, toothache, colic, and other conditions related to stagnation of *qì* and blood stasis. California poppy disperses stagnation and stasis with acridity and bitterness, a common combination of dispersing, downbearing, and draining that moves *qì* and blood. The herb is cold in nature and therefore helps to cool the body, which commonly becomes overheated due to pain with anxiety and stress. For toothache, apply a slice of fresh California poppy root to the affected area and leave it there for 15 to 30 minutes. This is a temporary but very effective treatment to ease the pain until the patient can get to a dentist.

CAUTIONS

California poppy is cooling and most appropriate for conditions in which heat is present, either from vacuity or repletion.

Dosage and Preparation

Use 2–6 ml tincture; 4–12 g in decoction.

The fresh plant tincture is best; the tea, while acceptable, is not particularly palatable. Gather the entire plant when it is in full bloom (early to midsummer) and bears some seedpods, but before the pods mature. Good-quality dried material is light green with orange flower petals; the root (if present) should be orange to dark orange and free of dirt.

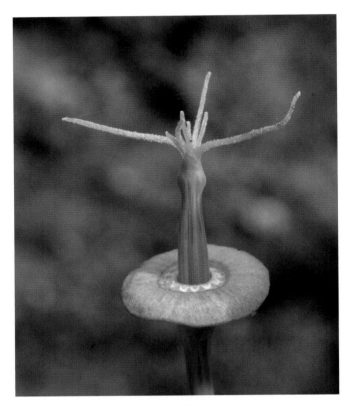

Close-up of immature California poppy seedpod
(E. californica)

Major Combinations

• Combine with chamomile and peppermint for hot, overexcited children. This combination is a simple and gentle calmative for rambunctious children and can be used either for overt pathology or when you're traveling and know it would be a nightmare otherwise.

• Combine with skullcap and kava for irritability, insomnia, and anxiety due to liver *qi* depression. This formula is especially useful when liver depression has affected the spleen and heart, causing digestive difficulties.

Commentary

California poppy is in the same family as opium poppy and has similar (but less potent) pain-relieving constituents, without the strength of chemicals like morphine and codeine. The chemical components of California poppy are non-narcotic, nonaddictive, and safe for long-term use without the worry of dependency. Popular in Europe, California poppy is one of the most prescribed herbs for anxiety in Germany.

California poppy is the state plant of California and is protected there; thus it cannot be legally harvested from the wild in that state. Fortunately the plant is very easy to cultivate and is readily available in the market as an organic herb. This is a very popular and useful plant for treating childhood insomnia and anxiety. The extract is safe and effective, although it can be difficult to administer because of its bitter taste. It is generally necessary to disguise the taste with sweet drinks, applesauce, or glycerin when giving it to children.

Native to California, the plant was employed by Native Americans throughout the state. In Southern California, the Cahuilla administered it to babies as a sedative, and in Northern California, the Mendocino Indians used it for similar sedative effects. They applied the root directly to a tooth and surrounding area for toothache. They treated stomachaches with the juice of the root, and applied that externally for suppurating sores and to dry up nursing women's milk.[1]

The genus name *Eschscholzia* commemorates the Russian naturalist J. F. Eschscholtz (1793–1831), and the species name obviously is derived from the plant's place of origin. California poppy is approved in the Commission E Monographs of Germany and is official in the *French Pharmacopoeia* (1988).

Passionflower

Passiflora incarnata and others

Passifloraceae

Passiflorae Incarnatae herba

Flavor and *Qi*: sweet, bitter, sour, cool
Channels Entered: heart, lung
Actions: antispasmodic, anodyne, hypnotic, hypotensive, sedative

Functions and Indications

- **Nourishes the heart and calms the spirit.** Passionflower is used to treat insomnia, palpitations, anxiety, agitation, mental restlessness, and a feeling of heat in the evening due to heart *yīn* vacuity. Passionflower is sweet and bitter, sour and cool in nature. With sweetness, passionflower nourishes the heart, while its cool bitterness clears heat due to *yīn* vacuity. The sour nature of the herb restrains *yīn* and acts to prevent further damage to heart *yīn*. This combination of flavors and *qì* nourish the heart and give the spirit a comfortable place to reside.

- **Nourishes *yīn*.** Passionflower is helpful in the treatment of persistent dry cough due to heat trapped in the lungs by chronic illness. Also used for hypertension and tachycardia when due to liver and heart *yīn* vacuity. Passionflower nourishes with sweetness, astringes with sourness, and drains vacuity heat with cool bitterness, a unique combination of flavors and *qì* that nourishes *yīn* while restraining it. By clearing vacuity heat, passionflower also treats the branch.

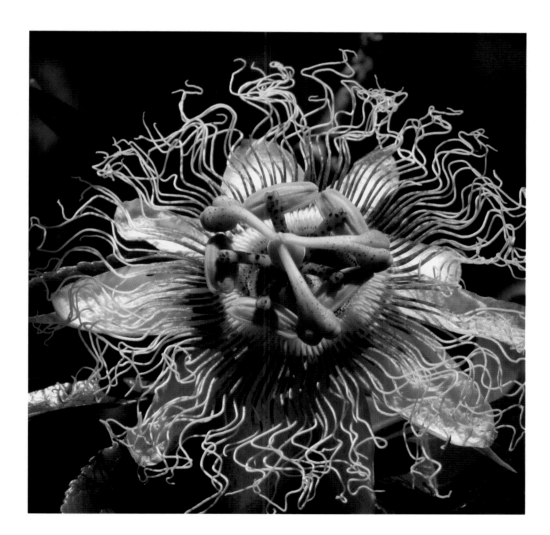

Passionflower (*Passiflora incarnata*)

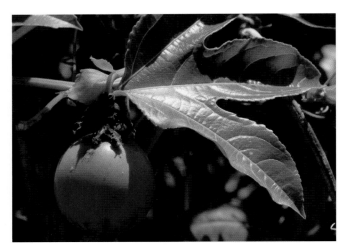

Fruit of the passionflower (*P. incarnata*)

CAUTIONS

None noted.

Dosage and Preparation

Use 2–4 ml tincture; 3–9 g in strong infusion.

Gather passionflower herb in early summer, before the flowers emerge. The herb can be prepared as a fresh plant tincture or dried carefully out of the sun and stored for future use. Good-quality dried herb is green to dark green and fresh looking. It should contain no large stems and few (if any) flowers.

Major Combinations

- Combine with Celestial Emperor Heart-Supplementing Elixir *(tiān wáng bǔ xīn dān)* for insufficient heart *yīn* and blood that does not afford the spirit a comfortable place to reside. The benefit of using a passionflower tincture in combination with *tiān wáng bǔ xīn dān* is that the passionflower can bring about an immediate response, helping to calm the patient down and thus allowing the nourishing actions of the other medicinals to take effect.

- Combine with Spiny Jujube Decoction *(suān zǎo rén tāng)* to strengthen its nourishing, calming, and heat-clearing actions and make it applicable for a wider range of patients.

Commentary

Passionflower holds an important place in the materia medica due to its ability to restrain *yīn* and nourish the heart. Its sour nature is key to its ability to restrain *yīn*, an action that has great value in *yīn* vacuity conditions.

Though passionflower is a native medicinal of the southeastern United States, little ethnobotanical information is available. The scant information that exists discusses applications for passionflower root only, yet we use only the herbaceous parts now. I have no experience using the root of this medicinal.

The Cherokee applied passionflower both internally and externally to treat boils and inflammations. They also administered an infusion into the ear for earaches and gave it to babies to help with the weaning process. The fruit of this and other species of passionflower, particularly *P. edulis,* were regarded as a great source of food and drinks. Passionflower juice is still popular today and can be found in specialty stores or combined with other juices in juice mixes. In Hawai'i, the fruits of several passionflower species are collectively called *liliko'i* and are eagerly gathered in the late summer for juice and fruit preserves.

The Eclectic phyisicians thought highly of passionflower. Some specific indications they listed include irritation of the brain and nervous system with atony; sleeplessness in the young and aged as well as that due to overwork, worry, or febrile excitement; neuralgic pains with debility; exhaustion from cerebral fullness or excitement; infantile nervous irritation; oppressed breathing; and cardiac palpitations due to excitement or shock.[2]

Passionflower is listed as official in the *British Herbal Compendium* (1992), the *British Herbal Pharmacopoeia* (1996), the *European Pharmacopoeia,* and the pharmacopoeias of Britain, Egypt, France, Spain, and Switzerland. Passionflower is included in *Martindale: The Extra Pharmacopoeia* (33rd ed.) and *PDR for Herbal Medicine* (2nd ed.), and is approved by the German Commission E. The pharmacopoeia of Brazil lists *P. alata* as its official species.

Skullcap
Scutellaria lateriflora

Lamiaceae

Scutellariae Lateriflorae herba

Other names include mad dog skullcap, blue skullcap

Flavor and *Qi:* bitter, acrid, cool
Channels Entered: liver, heart
Actions: anticonvulsant, antispasmodic, nervine, sedative

Functions and Indications

- ***Relieves heart depression and quiets the spirit.*** Skullcap is effective in nervousness, apprehension, and preoccupation, with choppy pulse due to disturbed heart *qi*. Skullcap is an excellent treatment for drug addiction in which the patient is full of apprehension, anxiety, worries, and preoccupations that injure the spirit. Skullcap enters the heart with bitterness and resolves depression with acridity. It combines bitter and cool properties to downbear and calm the spirit. Skullcap is well known for this function and is exceptionally effective in treating a host of

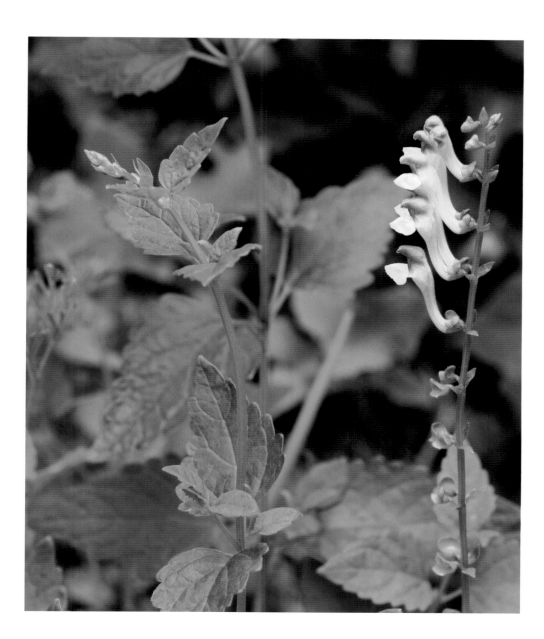

Skullcap *(Scutellaria lateriflora)*

ailments commonly seen in modern Western practice, many of which are related to emotional problems that lead to depression of the heart.

- **Clears heat in the heart and liver and resolves qì depression.** Skullcap is used to treat restlessness, insomnia, irritability, and emotional instability due to depressive heat in the heart and liver. Skullcap cools and clears with its bitter flavor and cool qì and resolves qì depression with its acridity. The primary focus here is on resolving depressive heat, but depressive heat leads to a disruption of the qì dynamic. Although this is a secondary action for skullcap, it is a welcome addition to formulas designed to treat such conditions. It may also be employed for patterns of liver depression qì stagnation and blood depression with symptoms such as menstrual pain (either premenstrual or during menstruation), flank pain, and chest pain.

- **Clears the liver, extinguishes wind, subdues liver yáng, and stops spasms.** Skullcap is an important herb for spasms, pain, and restlessness caused by internal movement of liver-wind associated with delirium tremens, withdrawal from drugs, epilepsy, palsy, shaking, Parkinson's disease, insomnia, and headache. Skullcap also helps relieve early nerve pain that occurs before herpes outbreaks.

CAUTIONS

Use skullcap with caution when there are signs of repletion heat with the "four bigs" of yáng-míng patterns.

Dosage and Preparation

Use 2–4 ml tincture; 2–9 g in decoction or strong infusion.

Gather skullcap from early summer through midsummer, from the time the plant is beginning to flower until it is in full bloom. The herb may be chopped and processed to make fresh plant tincture or bundled and dried for future use. Good-quality dried skullcap is vibrant green and includes some flowers, but is free (or nearly so) of seedpods.

Major Combinations

- Combine with Chinese red sage root and zizyphus for depressive heart patterns with anxiety, nervousness, preoccupations, and palpitations. This is also a good combination for the treatment of withdrawal from drugs. Consider adding passionflower and California poppy for cases in which heat is associated with this pattern. The combination of these five herbs with a bit of licorice makes an outstanding formula for treating drug withdrawal.

- Combine with bupleurum and white peony for depressive patterns of the liver with symptoms of dysmenorrhea, flank pain, and chest pain.

- Combine with kava, albizia, cyperus, and rose buds for heart and liver depressive patterns with depression, anxiety, vexation, sighing, and fullness and oppression in the chest and ribs or sides.

Commentary

Chapter 8 of *Líng Shū*, by Jing-Nua Wu, says, "Apprehension and anxiety, worries and preoccupations injure the spirit. . . . When the heart is prey to apprehension and anxiety, worried and preoccupied, then an injury to the spirit is produced."[2] These are primary feelings for a person undergoing drug withdrawal, all associated with fear. Skullcap's effectiveness in the treatment of drug addiction detoxification is related to its excellent ability to relieve heart depression, and therefore affect the greatest hurdles in the hell many people experience when trying to deal with a severe or long-term drug addiction. Furthermore, because of its profound effect on the liver, skullcap can help with many of the physical manifestations of withdrawal.

The Cherokee prepared skullcap as a decoction for "nerves and [for inclusion in a] compound for breast pain."[3] They also combined skullcap with three other herbs [unknown combination] to "promote menstruation."[4] One of the herb's old common names, mad dog

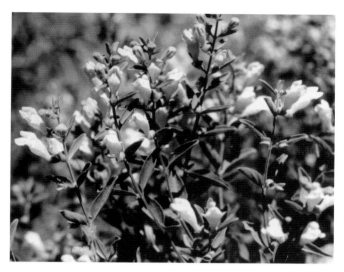

California skullcap (S. californica)

skullcap, comes from its application for hydrophobia (rabies) in the nineteenth century. It is doubtful that skullcap was a useful medicinal for this indication, and the claim has been refuted by many authors.

In addition to *Scutellaria lateriflora,* several other species of skullcap are native to the western United States. *S. californica* and, to a lesser extent, *S. antirrhi-* *noides* are two species I have used rather extensively. They are bitter and cold in nature and likely closely related in function to the Chinese species *S. barbata.* I have used these two Western natives similarly to the way the plant in this monograph is used but have not found it as effective in calming the spirit and relieving anxiety. However, they are better for clearing heat and thus relieving the depression associated with these patterns. They are quite effective when used in concert with other appropriate medicinals; however, I recommend using these species only when the pattern is associated with significant heat (i.e., a red, dry tongue and a rapid pulse). Other U.S. species used regionally include *S. galericulata* (marsh skullcap) and *S. nana,* and I am sure there are others.

Skullcap was official as a tonic, nervine, and antispasmodic in *The United States Pharmacopoeia* from 1863–1916, and in *The National Formulary (U.S.)* from 1916–1947. It is listed in the *British Herbal Pharmacopoeia* (1996), *Martindale: The Extra Pharmacopoeia* (33rd ed.), and *PDR for Herbal Medicine* (2nd ed.).

St. John's Wort

Hypericum perforatum

Hypericaceae

Hyperici Perforati herba seu flos

Flavor and *Qi*: bitter, sour, slightly acrid, cool
Channels Entered: heart, pericardium, liver, stomach
Actions: anti-inflammatory, anxiolytic, astringent, sedative

Functions and Indications

- ***Courses the liver, rectifies*** qì, ***and resolves depression.*** St. John's wort is used to treat binding depression of liver *qi* with symptoms such as anxiety, melancholy, indifferent expression, lack of interest in food, poor hygiene, and other signs of emotional depressive disorders. St. John's wort combines acridity and bitterness to course the liver and resolve depression. Combined with its cool nature, these actions help clear the heat associated with liver depression. St. John's wort has gained significant popularity in the last decade because of this function, a direct reflection of the amount of liver depression found in Western culture. St. John's wort is valuable in modern practice because of its ability to lift folks out of the doldrums, while other supportive therapies can assist in complete healing of this significant scourge.

- ***Clears heat, quickens the blood, and generates flesh.*** St. John's wort is helpful in a variety of conditions involving patterns of heat damage to the flesh and vessels, such as rashes, sunburn, ulcerations, acute trauma, and other inflammatory conditions. For this purpose, administer preparations of St. John's wort both internally and externally, in the form of tea, tincture, or infused oil.

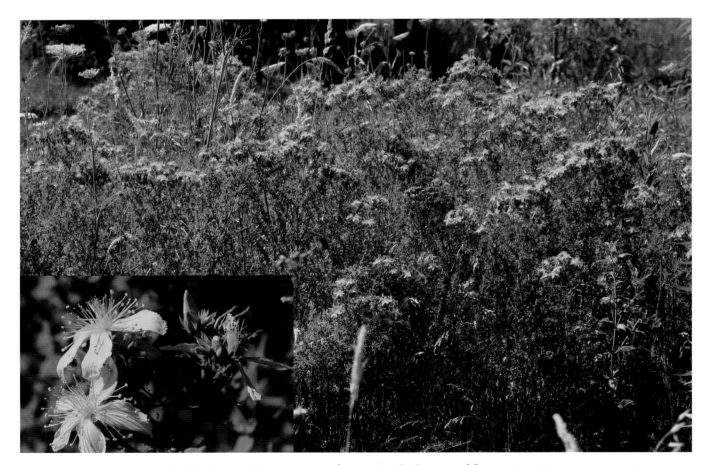

St. John's wort *(Hypericum perforatum)* with close-up of flowers (inset)

CAUTIONS

St. John's wort is not recommended for use during pregnancy. Those taking St. John's wort for extended periods of time or in large doses should avoid very strong or prolonged exposure to sunlight or similar light sources. Though phototoxicity is rare and generally overstated in many sources, there have been enough reports to warrant some caution. Those taking MAO inhibitors should not use this medicinal.

Dosage and Preparation

Use 2–4 ml tincture; 9–15 g in decoction; 2–4 g powdered extract; infused oil applied topically as needed. (Note: The infused oil can also be taken internally for problems in the GI tract.)

Gather St. John's wort in early summer through midsummer, when the flowers are just beginning to open. Harvest the top six to eight inches of the plant and either process it fresh or spread it to dry for future use. Good-quality dried herb has green leaves and yellow flowers. The product should be brightly colored and free of large stems.

Major Combinations

- Combine with Free Wanderer Powder *(xiāo yáo săn)* for depressive and withdrawn disorders concurrent with spleen vacuity.

- Combine with skullcap for liver depression and depression and anxiety disorders, especially those associated with drug abuse and withdrawal. This is an effective combination for treating such disorders, even in the absence of drug addiction issues.

- Combine with arnica and take either internally or externally for acute trauma with pain and inflammation.

- Combine with plantain and take either internally or externally for ulcerations, abrasions, or other conditions in which the integrity of the skin or digestive tract has been broken. This combination very effectively supports the healing process. For external conditions, add comfrey for swifter healing.

Commentary

St. John's wort has a long history of use, especially in Europe, where the plant is native. Though there are many references in the ethnobotanical literature to Native American uses of the plant, especially by the Cherokee people, Native Americans undoubtedly learned about the plant from white settlers. In Europe, St. John's wort has been used in medicine since antiquity. Dioscorides recommended taking it internally for sciatica and externally as a poultice for burns. Later, Paracelsus wrote that it was effective topical treatment for relieving the pain of wounds, contractures, and contusions. K. von Megenburg, a German writer of the Middle Ages, reported that St. John's wort strengthened the heart and liver, purified the kidneys, healed sores, and drew out poisons.[5] Culpeper wrote, "It is a singular wound herb; boiled in wine and drank, it healeth inward hurts or bruises; made into an ointment, it opens obstructions, dissolves swellings, and closes up the lips of wounds."[6] Other writers have recommended a St. John's wort tea for bedwetting.[7]

Modern writers describe similar uses for the plant, but there has been a trend toward administering St. John's wort to treat depressive states. American herbalist Michael Moore writes, "Hypericum is one of our best herbal therapies for depression and numbing frustration," and later states, ". . . I think of using *Hypericum* when someone whose circumstances have changed is unable to alter his ways of acting and responding." Moore further suggests, "The oil should be used topically when there is muscle or nerve pain that is distinct from joint or tissue inflammation, myalgia, and neuralgia."[8]

Positive results of modern clinical trials support the following indications for St. John's wort:[9]

- Mild-to-moderate depression

- Anxiety

- Adjunctive therapy administered along with pharmaceutical drug treatment for severe depression

- Adjunctive therapy given in combination with light therapy for seasonal affective disorder

- Psychological symptoms of menopause

- Aerobic endurance in athletes

Several other *Hypericum* species are used in various parts of the world, but *H. perforatum* has become or is becoming the species of choice, even in cultures in which that plant it is not native. Though its effects are relatively gentle, they are positive, and there is little or no ill effect, even when the herb is taken in large doses. Over the years, I have found myself using St. John's wort more and more frequently. It is an excellent anti-inflammatory and wound healer (vulnerary) and is part of many of the topical preparations I prescribe.

For internal anti-inflammatory and vulnerary effects, any preparation is suitable. However, for those who are able to tolerate taking oil orally, I have found *Hypericum*-infused oil to be very effective for gastric irritation and bowel complaints. In Chinese medicine, such complaints translate to stomach heat or fire, stomach *yīn* vacuity, intestinal wind bleeding, large intestine damp-heat, intestinal welling-abscess, and small intestine repletion heat.

The genus name *Hypericum* comes from the Greek *hypereikon,* which means something like "a taxon somewhat similar to heather."[10] The species name *perforatum* refers to the tiny perforations in the leaf, which allow light to shine through when the leaf is held up to the sun. St. John's wort is official in many pharmacopoeias, including the *British Herbal Pharmacopoeia* (1996), *The United States Pharmacopoeia* (26th ed.), *The National Formulary (U.S.)* (21st ed.), and the pharmacopoeias of the Czech Republic, France, Poland, Romania, Russia, and the United Kingdom. It is approved by the German Commission E and the European Cooperative on Phytotherapy (1997), and is also listed in the *European Pharmacopoeia, PDR for Herbal Medicines,* the *United States Herbal Pharmacopoeia,* and *Martindale: The Extra Pharmacopoeia* (31st ed.).

Translation of Source Material

Several species of *Hypericum* are used in Chinese medicine; I have included only the species discussed in the monograph above. *Guàn yè lián qiào (H. perforatum)* is considered acrid, slightly bitter, and neutral. It clears heat and resolves toxin, astringes and stops bleeding, disinhibits dampness, and is used to treat spitting of blood, vomiting of blood, intestinal wind with bleeding, bleeding due to external injury, wind-damp bone pain, mouth and nose sores, toxic swellings, and damage to the intestines due to fire.

Kava

Piper methysticum

Piperaceae

Piper Methystici radix et rhizome

Also called 'awa (Hawaiian)

Flavor and *Qi*: acrid, bitter, warm
Channels Entered: heart, liver, spleen
Actions: anxiolytic, muscle relaxant, sedative

Functions and Indications

- ***Rectifies qì and calms the spirit.*** Kava is helpful for patterns in which overthinking leads to *qi* stagnation, dampness, and phlegm. Dampness and phlegm impede the *qi* dynamic and adversely affect the spirit, leading to symptoms such as mental restlessness, nervous anxiety, and a feeling of being stressed all the time. Kava is acrid, bitter, and warm in nature. It rectifies the *qi* with acridity and bitterness. With acridity kava is upbearing and outthrusting, while at the same time downbearing with bitterness. Kava's warm nature assists the transformation of fluids, relieving stagnation and gently calming the spirit when the *qi* dynamic is impaired. Kava is very effective for this purpose and is an important addition to the materia medica.

- ***Dispels wind and dampness.*** Kava is used to treat wind-damp impediment with symptoms of aching muscular pain and tightness of the muscles and sinews. Kava is also helpful in the treatment of traumatic injury with soreness and muscle spasms. The herb is acrid, bitter, and warm. It outthrusts wind and damp with acridity and warmth, warming the collaterals and muscle layer. Like many medicinals of this nature, kava aggressively enters the channels to drive out the pathogenic factors.

- ***Rectifies qì, transforms damp, and relieves pain.*** Kava treats strangury patterns associated with *qi* stagnation and dampness, with symptoms of difficult, painful, or turbid urination. Kava is very helpful for damp stagnation with accumulation. With its combination of bitterness and acridity, kava rectifies *qi* and treats *qi* stagnation, relieving pain. It transforms damp with warmth and acridity and drains it away with bitterness, thus effectively treating strangury patterns.

- ***Relieves pain.*** Applied topically to gums and teeth, kava provides temporary relief of toothache. With

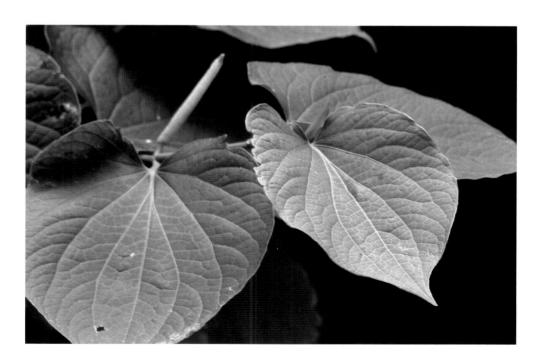

Kava *(Piper methysticum)*

acridity and warmth, the herb effectively treats minor to moderately severe pain due to *qi* stagnation and blood stasis. This provides temporary topical relief, but is not a curative action.

- **Transforms phlegm.** Kava is employed in the treatment of a variety of phlegmatic conditions, including phlegm in the lung and stomach and in the liver channel. Although kava is warm, it can be used for warm patterns when combined with the appropriate herbs. Acrid, bitter, and warm, kava warms the spleen and with acridity and bitterness transforms dampness and phlegm. For this function, the alcoholic extract seems to work best.

CAUTIONS

Kava is not recommended for use during pregnancy or nursing. Because of kava's warm, acrid nature, long-term use can damage *yīn* and blood, causing symptoms of dry, cracked skin and blurry vision. Avoid preparations that contain kava stems, leaves, or root peel, plant parts that may be associated with liver toxicity.

Dosage and Preparation

Use 2–4 ml tincture; 3–15 g in decoction; 2–4 g solid extract.

Though the traditional practice of chewing the root before consumption is rarely followed today, some details should be taken into account when making kava extracts. The best extracts employ a fat to emulsify active constituents; coconut milk or lecithin works well. Also, adding a small amount of peppermint tincture or essential oil to the preparation seems to intensify its effect, possibly by enhancing absorption. This mixture, unfortunately, is not particularly stable and therefore of little value, except for immediate administration in the clinic.

Because of its long history of cultivation, kava plants no longer produce seeds and therefore do not have a reproductive cycle. This allows harvesters to gather roots and rhizomes throughout the year.

Although kava root is acceptable for use, the rhizome (frequently called a "lateral root") traditionally is considered the most important plant part and generally provides the most potent medicine. It has a mild odor and is acrid and numbing to the mouth.

Good-quality dried material consists of peeled rhizome, which should be dark gray or black on the outside and whitish on the inside. The inside is pithy and striated.

Major Combinations

- Combine with California poppy for disquieted heart spirit with symptoms of vexation, insomnia, anxiety, and susceptibility to fright. This combination is balanced, as kava is warm and California poppy cool. Thus it is an effective and safe combination to add to myriad formulas.

- Combine with Licorice, Wheat, and Jujube Decoction *(gān mài dà zǎo tāng)* for restlessness and anxiety due to overthinking.

- Combine with wild oat and skullcap for anxiousness and depressive states related to withdrawal from tobacco or marijuana.

- Combine with black cohosh and St. John's wort for sore and tight muscles caused by overwork, strain, or trauma. For severe spasms, add lobelia.

- Combine with yerba mansa, sassafras, and black cohosh for wind-damp impediment with aching, sore muscles and joints. Add turmeric if there is more significant joint involvement. Add lobelia for spasms associated with this syndrome.

Commentary

Kava has gained a significant reputation for effectiveness in the treatment of anxiety in the West over the last decade or so, although some recent reports of liver toxicity have delivered a big blow to the sales of the herb. The herb has a long history of use in the South Pacific, but recent use in the West has led to the isolation of specific phytochemicals and the marketing of highly concentrated products. I am not aware of any problems associated with use of raw herb or simple extracts. However, it is important to note that the problem with liver toxicity has been directly linked to companies using the entire plant rather than only the rhizome. The leaves and stem peelings have significant amounts of an alkaloid called pipermethystine, which has been shown to be hepatotoxic but is undetectable in the rhizome or root. It has also been speculated that the use of solvents other than water, such as ethanol or acetone may increase the risk of toxicity. This is in part because the antioxidant glutathione, which appears to have a protective action on cells, is present in much higher levels in extracts produced using water.[11]

Kava is native to Melanesia and was later introduced into Polynesia (except New Zealand and Easter Island) as early voyagers migrated to the islands of the Pacific. It is said to relieve anger and frustration, stress, and bad mood, among other problems. In addition to its use as a medicine, kava also has special ritual significance through the Pacific islands. It was, and to a certain extent still is, used by the Hawaiians as a way of showing hospitality to visitors and is served during feasts. (This practice was historically essential but is much less followed today.)[12] In other parts of western Polynesia, the consumption of the drink carried implications of social rank. According to Handy and Handy, Hawaiians used the lateral roots medicinally to treat "congestion in the urinary tract" as well as rheumatism and asthma.[13] These authors also suggest that

although the *kāhuna* (learned men) drank kava during ceremony, those who did heavy physical labor drank it to help relieve sore muscles and relax. It was also a common beverage for chiefs to drink before meals.

In spite of its history of ritualistic use, kava is served at bars in some cultures, much the way alcohol is sold in other parts of the world. In fact, it is the national drink of Tonga and Fiji and is consumed much the same as coffee is consumed in Western cultures.[13] There is some evidence that recreational overuse of kava may lead to problems similar to those associated with alcohol abuse, along with a skin disorder called "kava dermopathy." Adverse effects of kava abuse are not as severe as those caused by alcohol abuse, and one must consume much more than normal therapeutic doses of kava for extended periods of time for these problems to arise. Although some consider kava an intoxicant, it does not seem to have the same toxic effects on the nervous system as other intoxicants.

The genus name *Piper* comes from the Sanskrit *pippali,* meaning "peppercorn," while the species name *methysticum* comes from a Greek root meaning "to intoxicate," "intoxicating drink," or simply "intoxicating."

Kava came into use as a medicine by physicians in the United States and Europe in the late nineteenth and early twentieth centuries. It is currently official in the *British Herbal Pharmacopoeia* (1996), *Martindale: The Extra Pharmacopoeia* (33rd ed.), *PDR for Herbal Medicines,* and *WHO Monographs on Selected Medicinal Plants,* and is approved by the German Commission E.

Valerian

Valeriana officinalis and others

Valerianaceae

Valerianae Officinali rhizoma et radix

Flavor and *Qi:* acrid, slightly bitter, warm
Channels Entered: heart, liver, spleen, stomach
Actions: hypnotic, hypotensive, nervine, sedative

Functions and Indications

- ***Quiets the spirit, courses the liver, and relieves depression of the heart and liver.*** Valerian is used to treat nervousness, poor memory, depression, insomnia, giddiness, restlessness, agitation, and nausea with stagnation of liver *qi* impinging on the heart. As valerian is warm and somewhat stimulating, it is especially useful when the *qi* is depressed and the *yáng* is vacuous, or if there is a concurrent cold pattern. Valerian is acrid, slightly bitter, and warm. It courses the liver and resolves depression with warm acridity; it also downbears with bitterness, thus quieting the spirit. Valerian is a warming and drying medicinal and therefore must be used carefully, as it can exacerbate problems in patients with vacuity heat, making the condition worse. However, it is very good for resolving depression. Thus, with proper formulation, it can be helpful for individuals with repletion-heat patterns.

- ***Courses the liver and harmonizes the liver and spleen-stomach.*** Valerian is helpful in the treatment of *qi* stagnation and disharmony between the wood and earth phases, with symptoms of glomus and fullness after eating, sloppy diarrhea, abdominal distention, smaller-abdominal distention, and oppression in the chest with rib-side pain. Valerian is especially useful when these symptoms are associated with nervous disorders. The herb is warm, acrid, bitter, and slightly drying in nature. This combination of flavor and *qi* helps to dry dampness associated with the pattern. When the liver *qi* invades the spleen, dampness accumulates, causing oppression and pain. Valerian treats the branch with its warm and slightly dry nature, and treats the root with acidity and bitterness.

- ***Relieves pain.*** Valerian is acrid and warm. It courses *qi* and calms the spirit. It can be administered to treat pain due to many different etiologies. For pain relief, larger doses of valerian may be employed. When using valerian for pain, I usually give patients a simple tincture and instructions to use the full dosage range as frequently as needed, starting with a lower dose and working up to a higher dose as needed. Larger doses can cause drowsiness and caution should be used when driving or performing other tasks that require keen awareness and full motor function.

CAUTIONS

Because of valerian's warm and stimulating qualities, it should be used with caution when there is heat from repletion or especially vacuity. Large doses can cause drowsiness.

Dosage and Preparation

Use 2–8 ml tincture; 6–15 g in strong infusion or decoction.

Gather valerian roots and rhizomes in the autumn after the aerial parts of the plant have died back for the winter. The roots and rhizomes can be chopped to make fresh plant tincture or sliced and dried for future use. Good-quality dried root is firm and has a peculiar odor (some say it smells like old socks). The material should be free of foreign matter, such as dirt.

Major Combinations

- Combine with skullcap and passionflower for nervousness, anxiety, agitation, and insomnia due to liver *qi* impinging on the heart.

- Combine with sweet flag and polygala for poor memory, giddiness, insomnia, and nausea associated with liver and heart depression.

- Combine with St. John's wort and arnica for pain associated with blunt trauma. Although both of

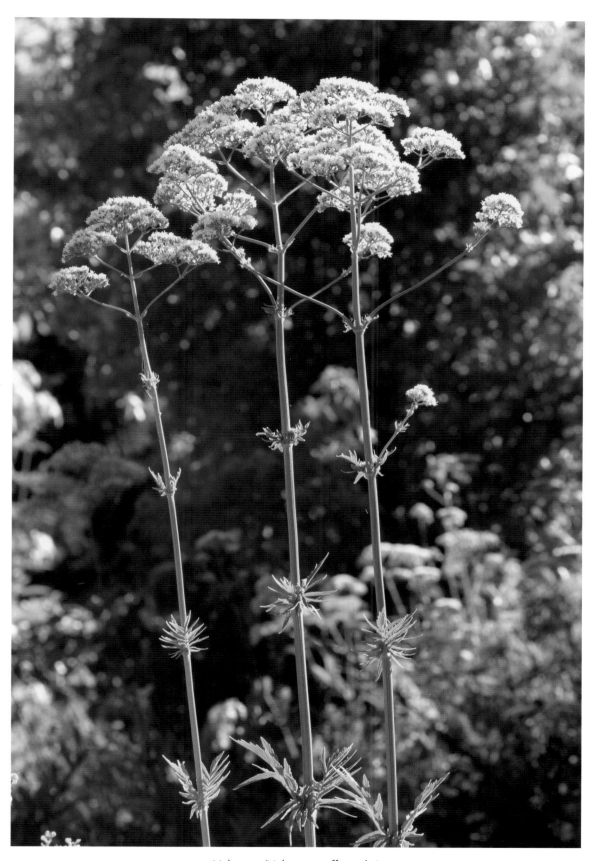

Valerian *(Valeriana officinalis)*

these herbs are often applied externally for this purpose, they are also very effective when combined with valerian and taken internally. (See page 155 for more information on using arnica internally.)

Commentary

Qi depression eventually leads to heat. Due to valerian's warm nature, it can sometimes cause excitation by worsening heat that is already present. But if you account for its heat when formulating, this medicinal can be used very safely in heat conditions. I have heard many stories from people who said valerian kept them up at night or made them feel agitated. The problem does not lie with the herb, but rather with the improper use of the herb. Valerian's warming nature makes it especially useful for situations in which the *yáng qi* is weak or there is repletion cold. If the *qi* mechanism is depressed with heat—the most commonly seen clinical picture—excellent results can be achieved by prescribing valerian along with other herbs that are cooling and perhaps nourishing to the heart. The real strength of the herb, however, is in treating colder, damp conditions.

As an herbalist in the northwestern United States, I have used a number of species of valerian for many years, but mainly *V. sitchensis*. This plant is very common throughout the mountains of northwestern California—north to Alaska and west to Montana and Colorado. The Okanagon of northern Washington and southern Canada prepared a decoction of valerian root for pain. The Thompson Indians of southwestern British Columbia also administered valerian for pain as well as for stomach troubles, diarrhea, and colds. Both tribes also applied the root externally to wounds, bruises, and inflamed areas.[15]

Dioscorides considered *V. officinalis* a warming stimulant to the menstrual cycle, as well as a diuretic for strangury and as a treatment for stitches in the side. Pliny said that the medicinal "helps all stoppings and stranglings in any part of the body, whether they proceed of pains in the chest or sides, and takes them away." Culpeper included valerian in a formula with licorice, raisins, and anise seed for "those that are short-winded, and for those that are troubled with the cough, and helps to open the passages, and to expectorate phlegm easily." He further stated, "It helps expel the wind in the belly." This, I believe, speaks to valerian's warming and drying nature.

Many authors throughout history have written about the application of valerian for cramps and spasms. Although the herb is an antispasmodic, this action is weak and the relief is related mainly to relaxing effects on the entire system.

Valerian is officially listed in many pharmacopoeias, including the *British Herbal Pharmacopoeia* and the pharmacopoeias of Belgium, Egypt, France, Norway, the Netherlands, Portugal, and Spain. Valerian is included in the German Commission E Monographs, *Martindale: The Extra Pharmacopoeia* (31st ed.), and the *WHO Monographs on Selected Medicinal Plants*.

Translation of Source Material

In Chinese medicine, *Valeriana officinalis, V. coreana, V. stubendorfi, V. amurensis,* and *V. hardwickii* are all used, although *V. officinalis (xié căo)* is listed as the main species in the *Grand Dictionary of Chinese Medicinals*. This medicinal is considered acrid, bitter, warm, and slightly toxic, and enters the heart and liver channels. It expels wind and resolves tetany, engenders flesh and stops bleeding, and is used to treat disquieted heart spirit, weak stomach, lumbar pain, menstrual irregularities and stopped menstruation, knocks and falls, and stomach and intestinal cramping.

Chamomile

Matricaria recutita

Asteraceae

Matricarii Recutitae flos

Flavor and *Qi:* bitter, acrid, cool
Channels Entered: liver, heart, stomach
Actions: anti-inflammatory, antispasmodic, nervine, sedative

Functions and Indications

- ***Quiets the spirit and clears depressive heat in the heart and liver.*** Chamomile is used to treat restlessness, insomnia, irritability, and peevishness due to repletion or vacuity heat. Chamomile downbears with bitterness while clearing heat with coolness. Its acridity assists the action of other medicinals in

treating depression, making chamomile an important medicinal for depressive disorders with heat.

- ***Courses the liver and harmonizes the stomach.*** Chamomile helps treat disharmony between the liver and stomach for symptoms such as flank pain, flatulence, lack of appetite, and epigastric pain. Chamomile courses the liver with cool acridity and harmonizes the stomach with bitterness and acridity. Its cool nature also helps to clear stomach heat associated with this pattern. Chamomile is very valuable for treating this pattern. Unfortunately, many people don't realize its power, probably due to the use of inadequate dosages or poor-quality material.

- ***Clears heat in the stomach and intestines.*** Chamomile can be employed for heat due to either vacuity or repletion. The herb clears and drains heat with cool bitterness and relieves pain with acridity. Mental

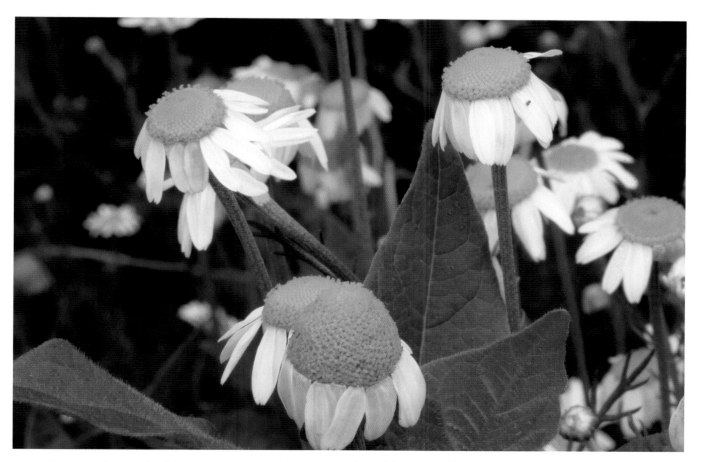

German chamomile (Matricaria recutita). Note that the broad leaves visible here are not those of chamomile. The finely cut leaves visible on the lower right are the chamomile leaves.

restlessness is a common symptom accompanying heat and pain in the stomach, small intestine, or large intestine. Repletion of *yáng-míng* is *yáng* in nature, and the upbearing *yáng qì* (heat) can cause mental restlessness. Thus, with chamomile we can cool both the *yáng-míng* and the mental restlessness. This action also makes chamomile effective in treating mental restlessness and abdominal pain due to repletion heat in the small intestine and for abdominal pain due to damp-heat in the large intestine.

• ***Disperses milk/food accumulation, abducts stagnation, and harmonizes the spleen and stomach.*** Chamomile is helpful in the treatment of feeding accumulation and is commonly used for colic and other digestive disorders, as well as for crying without any perceivable pathology. As already noted, when the *yáng-míng* is replete there will be mental restlessness, which in children translates to crying. Chamomile clears heat, harmonizes the middle burner, and calms the spirit, a function that is extremely helpful in pediatrics.

CAUTIONS

Use chamomile with care in conditions associated with cold.

Dosage and Preparation

Use 2–4 ml tincture; 3–9 g (up to 15 g) in strong infusion. The infusion can be used as a steam inhalation for cough with dry irritated lungs due to either dry evil or *yīn* vacuity. The glycerite tincture proves very useful in pediatric disorders because its sweetness helps mask the bitter flavor of the chamomile. Also, using a chamomile glycerite as the base for a formula makes it easy to add other herbs that may be otherwise challenging to give infants and young children.

Gather chamomile from late spring through summer, when the flowers are in full bloom. The flowers can either be processed fresh or carefully dried for future use. Good-quality dried herb smells sweet and fruity and is bright with clear, white ray flowers, not brown or musty smelling.

Major Combinations

• Combine with Chinese red sage root and motherwort for depressive heat in the heart and liver with restlessness, insomnia, and irritability. This combination is also good for dysmenorrhea due to *qì* stagnation and blood stasis associated with heat.

• Combine with coptis and licorice for stomach and intestinal heat patterns with lack of appetite, epigastric pain, and irritability.

• Combine with lemon balm for colic and other digestive disorders in children. This combination is also helpful for crying, including night crying.

• Combine with Harmony-Preserving Pill (*bǎo hé wán*) or Stomach-Calming Powder (*píng wèi sǎn*) for feeding accumulation with vomiting of sour milk, crying, and diarrhea or constipation.

Commentary

This monograph is specific to the German chamomile (*Matricaria recutita*), which should be distinguished from Roman chamomile (*Chamaemelum nobile*). The latter species is used in medicine and skin care products, but is generally considered to be inferior to the former species.

German chamomile is an old remedy in European herbalism. In fact, one source suggests chamomile was a medicine from the Teutonic tribes of the Baltic region of Denmark, southern Norway, and southwestern Sweden, having been used in prehistoric times.[16] Dioscorides recommended chamomile for menstrual pain, urinary difficulty and stones, jaundice, flatulence, liver ailments, thrush, bladder infections, and periodic fevers. Culpeper suggested a decoction to "take away pain and stitches in the side." He further stated,

It is profitable for all sorts of agues that come either from phlegm, or melancholy, or from an inflammation of the bowels, being applied when the humours causing them shall be concocted; and there is nothing more profitable to the sides and region of the liver and spleen than it.[17]

Chamomile is one of the gentlest yet effective medicinals in any materia medica. Though sweet smelling, it is somewhat bitter. It simultaneously clears and moves heat and *qi*, respectively, so is calming and soothing to both tissue and the mind. Weiss recommends using an infusion of chamomile flowers as an anti-inflammatory douche.[18] He also suggests gargling the hot tea for oral and throat inflammations.[19] He further includes chamomile flowers in a formula with mistletoe, hawthorn flowers, and valerian root for hypertension or angina.[20] A poultice of chamomile flowers is helpful for eye inflammation and other local heat due to various etiologies.

Chamomile is invaluable in pediatrics. Because it is so gentle, it does not disturb the underdeveloped digestive system of the infant, yet it applies enough medical action to gain the desired result. This is when dosage becomes extremely important. Children need a smaller dosage than adults, and although I have never seen difficulty with giving a child too much chamomile, it would behoove the practitioner to be aware of the cooling and *qi*-moving nature of this medicinal.

Chamomile is very important for all digestive complaints associated with heat. I find it helpful to prescribe large doses of the herb as an adjunctive tea for patients to drink ad lib for disorders such as irritable bowel syndrome and ulcerative colitis. When treating ulcerative colitis, I often add ½ part plantain to the combination. Chamomile is cooling, soothing, and natural in taste, so it is not difficult to take. I find that whatever other therapy I am utilizing to treat ulcerative colitis is greatly enhanced if the patient can consume about one quart of this combination per day.

The blue chamomile essential oil (see page 37 [yarrow herb entry] for additional information) is a very important anti-inflammatory additive for external preparations. Unfortunately, it is quite expensive. Chamomile is also included in many skin and hair care products.

German chamomile can be found in many pharmacopoeias, including the *British Herbal Pharmacopoeia* (1996) and the pharmacopoeias of Argentina, Brazil, Egypt, Germany, Hungary, the Netherlands, Portugal, Poland, Romania, and Yugoslavia. It is listed in the German Commission E Monographs, *Martindale: The Extra Pharmacopoeia* (29th ed.), and the *WHO Monographs on Selected Medicinal Plants*.

Translation of Source Material

In Chinese medicine, *Matricaria chamomilla** (*mǔ jú*) is considered sweet, neutral, and nontoxic. It is said to expel wind and resolve the exterior and is used to treat common cold and wind-damp pain.

---

*Matricaria chamomilla is a synonym for *Matricaria recutita*, the species discussed in the monograph above.

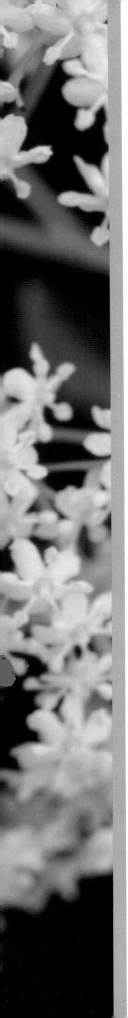

HERBS THAT EXTINGUISH WIND

Extinguishing wind in Chinese medicine refers to treating an internal stirring of liver-wind. Liver-wind arises when there is a severe imbalance of *yīn* and *yáng* or of blood and *qì,* particularly in the liver. In essence, it is the internal movement of *yáng qì* upward. Thus, it is a vacuity of *yīn* or blood that is often responsible for this pattern. However, fire may also be a factor due to its rising nature. Some signs and symptoms of stirring of internal wind are severe dizziness, headache with a pulling sensation, stiffness in the neck, tingling or numbness in the extremities, and twitching.

One medicinal from this category is included here. Lobelia *(Lobelia inflata)* is another native American medicinal that has a relative in Chinese medicine, *bàn biān lián,* but has little or no relationship in its clinical function. Lobelia is acrid, bitter, and cold. It is an exceptionally effective medicinal for treating most manifestations of internally stirring liver-wind. Its wind-coursing and *qì*-resolving actions are strong enough to use in many other important clinical situations, most notably afflictions of the lung.

Lobelia

Lobelia inflata

Campanulaceae

Lobeliae Inflatae herba seu semen

Flavor and *Qi:* acrid, bitter, cold
Channels Entered: liver, lung, triple burner, stomach
Actions: demulcent, diuretic, emollient, refrigerant

Functions and Indications

- ***Extinguishes wind and alleviates spasms and convulsions.*** Lobelia is used to treat liver-wind stirring internally, of any etiology. Lobelia causes wind with acridity and downbears with cold bitterness. This is a very important herb for all types of spasm, convulsions, tremors, and seizures. Lobelia is exceptional for the treatment of these conditions.

- ***Diffuses and disinhibits the lung*** qì, ***downbears phlegm, and suppresses cough and panting.*** Lobelia is helpful for spasmodic cough, tightness in the chest, shortness of breath, flaring nostrils, and difficulty breathing. Lobelia is acrid, bitter, and cold. Because it is very acrid, it strongly diffuses the lung *qì*. Because it is bitter and cold, it also strongly downbears the lung *qì*. Cough and panting occurs when the lung *qì* loses its depurative downbearing action and its ability to diffuse. Because lobelia treats this pattern so efficiently, it may be used for associated conditions of any etiology, including wind-cold fettering the exterior, wind-warmth invading the lung, and effulgent fire distressing the lung. Lobelia is also very helpful for treating whooping cough in children.

- ***Courses wind, resolves the exterior, and disperses wind-heat.*** Lobelia is employed in the treatment of exterior invasion of wind-heat, with symptoms such as heat effusion, slight aversion to cold, headache, slight sweating, cough, a red-tipped tongue with either a thin white or yellow coat, and a floating, rapid pulse. Lobelia strongly courses external wind and resolves the exterior with its cool acridity. Although gener-

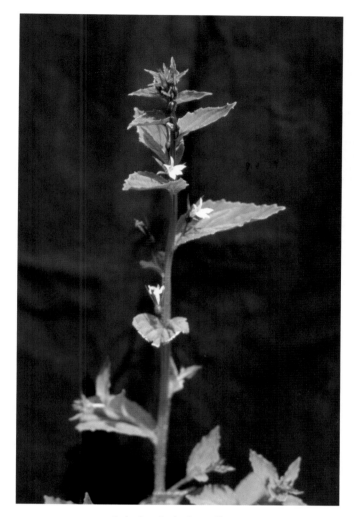

Lobelia *(Lobelia inflata)*

ally used for invasions of wind-warmth, lobelia can be effective against invasion of wind-cold when combined with the appropriate medicinals.

- ***Induces vomiting.*** Lobelia can be effectively applied as ejection therapy to treat either phlegm-drool obstructing the throat and hampering breathing or stagnation of food causing distention, fullness, and pain. When using lobelia for ejection therapy, administer it in small frequent doses until nausea occurs. Then it should be pushed with one-and-a-half to two times the dosage until ejection ensues. Be aware that the patient is likely to perspire profusely with the ingestion of this quantity of lobelia. The patient may also experience oppressive prostration and relaxation of the muscular system and have a vacuous pulse, but this state is short-lived and the ensuing relief significant. The infusion of this medicinal is generally considered the best preparation and apparently, some of the above side effects—such as profuse perspiration—may be avoided if one uses the infusion rather than the tincture. My only experience with this medicine for ejection therapy has been with tincture, in part because the taste of this medicinal is quite acrid. See Commentary for more information about using lobelia for ejection therapy.

- *Quickens blood, resolves* qì *stagnation and depression, and relieves pain.* Lobelia may be applied externally as a liniment for a variety of conditions, including pain with or without swelling or inflammation, sharp pain in the chest made worse with breathing, and dull, aching pain. A tincture of lobelia seed is most effective for external application.

CAUTIONS

Avoid use of lobelia in patients with severe heart *yáng* or *qì* vacuity. Exercise caution when using lobelia in patients who are very weak, the elderly, and the very young. When treating the elderly or very young, be sure to modify the dosage according to specifications of these populations. Also note that ejection therapy is not appropriate for these patients.

Dosage and Preparation

Use 0.5–2 ml tincture (up to 3.5 ml as a simple or 0.5 ml in formula); 0.5–2 g in infusion (up to 4–6 g to cause ejection).

Gather the herb in mid- to late summer, when the seedpods have ripened but before they open. Good-quality dried material is dark green to slightly brown (a natural color of the plant), but not "dead brown" looking. The herb should contain seeds, although this is not required. The seeds are very small and can go unnoticed, but herb that contains seeds is likely to have a stronger action. Some practitioners prefer the seeds to the herb, while some prefer the seeds for external preparations.

Major Combinations

- Combine with pleurisy root and ginger for heat effusion due to external invasion by either wind-heat or wind-cold.

- Combine with blue cohosh and cayenne for tugging and slackening.

- Combine with skullcap and passionflower for tobacco addiction. It is also appropriate to add a constitutional formula in the form of a patent medicine for any patient who is trying to move away from tobacco—for example, Ophiopogon Decoction *(mài mén dōng tāng)* or All-the-Way-Through Brew *(yī guàn jiān)*.

Commentary

Lobelia has generated controversy over the years. At one time, it was one of the most widely prescribed herbs in American and British herbalism. Partially because of its ability to cause nausea and vomiting, it has since fallen out of vogue to some extent. Nevertheless, lobelia remains one of the most useful herbs in the Western and certainly the American materia medica. Although some may consider it toxic, I have used it to treat cough in children, including my own, with great success and no adverse reactions. Dosage is critical, and, as with any medication, makes the difference between therapeutic value and toxicity. When the herb is prepared correctly, only a small amount of lobelia is needed to affect a significant change in a patient's condition. The change can be profound and lasting.

Lobelia came to the attention of white Americans in the early nineteenth century by way of Samuel Thomson. This man was quite revolutionary for his time and created an entire movement in medicine called the Thomsonian System. Estimates suggest that in the middle part of the nineteenth century, about one-fifth of the American population relied on Thomsonian herbalism as their main method for treating illness. Thomson used only a few herbs, and lobelia was his standby. While Thomson's branch of

American herbalism had declined significantly by the late 1860s, the use of lobelia was perpetuated through the Physio-medical and Eclectic schools of medicine.

Lobelia contains a chemical constituent, lobeline, that is very similar in structure to nicotine and is said to bind to the same receptor sites. For this reason, lobelia can prove very useful in treating tobacco addiction. For this purpose, it can be smoked or, preferably, taken as a tincture. I add lobelia to tincture formulas as a standard practice when assisting those with tobacco addiction and have found it to be quite helpful.

For antispasmodic effects, no better medicinal is available. Anytime there is spasm, anywhere in the body, lobelia is both effective and efficient. For muscle spasms, it is helpful administered either internally or externally, and will prove most efficacious when both methods are employed simultaneously. A lobelia seed tincture is best for external use as a liniment.

The Cherokee had many uses for lobelia. They applied a poultice of the root for body aches and rubbed lobelia leaves on aching body parts and stiff neck. They administered boiled plant material externally to bites and stings and took the herb internally as an emetic and to treat colic. Lobelia was smoked to "break tobacco habit," to treat asthma, and as a ceremonial medicine.[1]

Lobelia was official in *The United States Pharmacopoeia* from 1820–1920 and is still official in the *British Herbal Pharmacopoeia*. It is listed in *Martindale: The Extra Pharmacopoeia* (29th ed.) as well as the pharmacopoeias of Austria, Belgium, Brazil, Egypt, France, Portugal, Poland, and Spain.

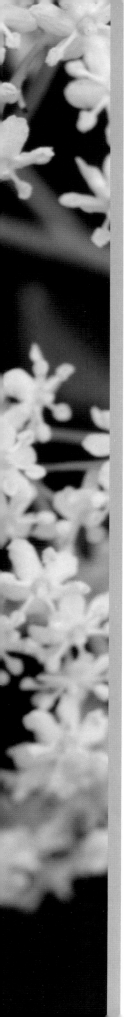

APPENDIX I

WESTERN ANALOGUES OF CHINESE HERBS

Including Chinese Herbs that Grow in the West

Here you will find a list of common Chinese medicinals found growing in the West, either wild or under cultivation, as well as some related Western species that may be used in similar ways or even as substitutes for their Chinese relatives. Some of the plants included here are discussed at length within the main body of the text, while others are mentioned only in this appendix. This list is not meant to be exhaustive. It is my hope that you will use the information to further the work I have begun in this text, and that it will help you see the value of some of the plants growing around you, even if you live in a city. I have harvested and used many of these plants, although there are a few that I have not had the opportunity, yet, to pick myself.

Note: When a specific species is listed with the Chinese name in the heading, this indicates that the same species found in the West is used in Chinese medicine.

Albizia julibrissin (hé huān huā/hé huān pí). Albizia is an extremely common cultivar throughout most of the United States. It is commonly seen on roadsides, parks, and as plantings in yards.

Arctium lappa (niú bàng zǐ). Native to Eurasia, burdock is naturalized in many parts of North America. See page 69 for more information.

Bupleurum americanum. This species of bupleurum is native to the northwestern United States and western Canada. I have not used this Western species, but according to Michael Moore in his *Medicinal Plants of the Pacific West,* "Chinese medicine uses a close relative . . . and the constituents of the two Bupleurums are virtually identical."[1]

Capsella bursa-pastoris (jì cài). Commonly known as shepherd's purse, this plant is a European native that is employed as medicine throughout Asia, Europe, North America, and Australia. It is considered a weed in most parts of North America. The fresh plant tincture is used primarily to stop internal bleeding, including excessive menstrual bleeding. In Chinese medicine, the herb is employed to stop bleeding due to heat in the blood, drain heat through the urine, and lower high blood pressure.

Clematis spp. *(wēi líng xiān).* At least three species of *Clematis* are used in Chinese medicine; others are used in Western herbalism. Although I have used three different species found in the West, I do not have enough information to be able to say whether or not they may be analogous.

Coix lacryma-jobi (yì yǐ rén). This is a common weed in the Hawaiian Islands, where the seeds are used to make seed *leis* that are draped around the necks of people to honor them.

Coptis spp. *(huáng lián).* The North American *Coptis* species are very similar to the Chinese species in action and indeed may be considered analogous. Unfortunately, these species are quite small and probably not worth cultivating; rather, *huáng lián* should be cultivated and used.

Cuscuta spp. *Cuscuta* is native throughout the world. Western herbal practitioners have used the herbaceous portions of the plant as an emetic. The seeds of our native species are so small that I have never attempted to gather enough to try as medicine, but due to restrictions on the importation of seeds, it may be worth a cultivation attempt. A species of *Cuscuta* native to Hawai'i is used there to make *leis po'o* (head lei).

Cyperus rotundus (xiāng fù). This is a common weed found throughout the world. It grows quite commonly in the southwestern United States and is considered a pest because of its growth around waterways.

Dioscorea bulbifera (huáng yào zǐ). This plant is a Polynesian introduction to Hawai'i. It was used in time of famine as a survival food after being washed with water. It grows on O'ahu, Maui, Kaua'i, and Moloka'i.

Dipsacus fullonum and D. sativus. These plants are both native to Europe but widely naturalized in North America, especially in the West. I have used these species as *xù duàn* for many years now and find them to be reasonably analogous, although I don't think they are quite as good for treating pain.

Eclipta prostrata (hàn lián cǎo). A common weed throughout the world, *Eclipta prostrata* is found most abundantly in the southwestern United States and on all the islands of Hawai'i.

Ephedra spp. Western use of *Ephedra* differs from Chinese use in that Western herbalists primarily employ the herbaceous material, rather than the whole plant (including the root) as in Chinese medicine. However, the root of several Western species appears to be nearly the same as that of the Chinese species in terms of astringency. See page 55 for more information.

Epilobium spp. This is a common plant in mountainous regions of the western United States and Europe. Various *Epilobium* species are used as a mild anti-inflammatory in Western herbal medicine. Several *Epilobium* species are used in Chinese medicine. One of the species used, *Epilobium cephalostigma (xiā fá cǎo),* is sweet and neutral, clears heat, courses wind, eliminates dampness, and disperses swelling. It is used to treat hoarseness or loss of voice due to wind damage, sore and swollen throat, excessive menstruation, and edema.

Eriogotrya japonica (pí pá yè). Also known as common loquat, this plant is cultivated throughout much of the southern United States and in California south of San Francisco as a landscape plant. The fruits are delicious and are made into syrups, jellies, and pies.

Equisetum spp. Widely known as horsetail, *Equisetum* is a common plant throughout the world. There are many species, most of which have been used by local people, although I know of no other group of people who use horsetail as a cool acrid herb to relieve the exterior in the way the Chinese use their species *(mù zéi)*. I no longer use this plant in medicine, for ecological reasons. I do not know if any other species could be used as the Chinese use theirs.

Glehnia littoralis (běi shā shēn). This Chinese medicinal is native to the northwestern United States coastal area from Northern California to Alaska, but I have never gathered or used it.

Houttuynia cordata (yú xīng cǎo). This is a common cultivated plant in the United States, grown as a ground cover. The one most frequently seen in landscapes has variegated leaves of red, yellow, and orange. I do not recommend using this cultivar, as it is unclear whether or not it has the same medicinal action as the standard species. However, the standard species is also common, so if you want to grow it, look for the non-variegated variety at your local nursery.

***Ligusticum* spp.** Occuring throughout North America, the most famous of the Western species is *L. porteri,* known as osha. See page 47 for more information.

Ligustrum lucidum (nǚ zhēn zǐ). Ligustrum is widely cultivated throughout most of the United States. Commonly known as privet, it is found along streets, used as a hedge in yards, and planted in fields.

Lonicera japonica (jīn yín huā). Honeysuckle is a twining, trailing, shrubby perennial that grows throughout much of the United States. It is most common from Maryland south to Florida and west to Texas. The flowers are picked when they are still in the bud stage and either dried for tea or tinctured fresh.

Lycopodium clavatum. Commonly known as clubmoss, this species is very similar and used in essentially the same way as several species used in Chinese medicine. The main Chinese species, *L. japonicum,* is known as *shēn jīn cǎo* and is in the category of medicinals that resolve wind-dampness.

Mentha arvensis (bò hé). This native mint is quite widespread throughout North America. I have seen it along creeks and rivers in Northern California, upstate New York, and Wisconsin.

Paeonia californica, P. brownii. These native Western peony species are very similar to *chì sháo* and *bái sháo.* They are used in bioregional herbalism in the western United States, where they grow from Southern California to Oregon.

***Pedicularis* spp.** A number of *Pedicularis* species are used as medicine in China. *Pedicularis daviddii (tài bái shēn)* is sweet, slightly bitter, and warm; it is used to supplement vacuity, fortify the spleen and stomach, disperse heat and stop pain, nourish kidney *yīn,* supplement the center, and boost *qi*. It is helpful for treating body weakness, lack of appetite, steaming bone disorder, and joint pain. *Pedicularis resupinata (mǎ xiān hāo)* dispels wind, overcomes dampness, disinhibits water, and treats wind-damp joint pain, inhibited urination, kidney stones, and leukorrhea. *Pedicularis rex (wǔ fēng zhǎo yáng cǎo)* clears heat, resolves external toxins, and is used to treat measles. This medicinal is neutral, bitter, and acrid.

I have used several U.S. native species of *Pedicularis,* all harvested in Oregon or California, including *P. attollens* (little elephant's head), *P. densiflora* (Indian warrior), *P. groenlandica* (elephant's head), *P. racemosa* (leafy lousewort), and *P. semibarbata.* Each species has its own applications, although many are used similarly. The primary use for the first three species I've listed here is as a muscle relaxant. For this, a tea or tincture may be employed. Alternately, the leaves or flower heads (preferred) can be smoked to achieve a state of relaxation. This method is also commonly employed for the fourth species listed, *P. racemosa.*

I have harvested P. semibarbata several times. I use the entire plant, root and all, similar to the way the Chinese use tài bái shēn. I had begun to work this out before gaining access to the Chinese literature. However, due to lack of clinical evidence, I cannot present a monograph at this time.

Phytolacca americana (chui xu shang lu). Known as poke root in the West, this plant is native to the eastern United States. It is applied both internally and externally to treat lymphatic conditions. Use caution with this medicinal, as it has some toxicity.

Phragmites communis (lú gēn). Phragmites is a common weed that occurs around the world. It can be found growing in many places in the western United States, although the rhizomes look different from those I am accustomed to seeing in Chinese pharmacies. Although I have dug this plant, I have not used it in clinical practice.

***Polygala* spp.** The famous Senega snakeroot *(P. senega)* was used by the people of the eastern United States long before

Europeans arrived. Various *Polygala* species grow throughout the United States, and several species are native to the western United States. I have used *P. cornuta* with success as a substitute for *yuǎn zhì*. The fresh rhizome and tincture have a decided wintergreen aroma, which lessens with time.

***Polygonatum* spp.** Known as Solomon's seal, this herb is common in eastern North America. I have used two species, *P. biflorum* and *P. pubescens*. Of the two, only *P. biflorum* is available commercially; I personally have wildcrafted and transplanted the other species into my garden. Both are very similar to *yù zhú*, although I believe *P. pubescens* to be closer. However, several species are listed in the Chinese materia medica, and it is likely that either of the American species could be used as *yù zhú*. I have not tried to process either of these in the way *huáng jīng* is processed, but I would suspect *P. biflorum* might be the best species to try. Another commonly cultivated species is *P. multiflorum*, which is native to Europe. I have no experience with this species, but it has a long tradition of use in Europe similar to *yù zhú*.

Polygonum cuspidatum (hǔ zhàng). *Polygonum* species are common weeds throughout North America. *P. cuspidatum* is in fact considered a noxious weed and has overgrown some native plants in sensitive areas. I have seen it in various places in California, Oregon, and the northeast United States, but have not gathered this plant from the wild.

Prunella vulgaris (xià kū cǎo). Commonly called self-heal or heal-all in the West, this plant is a common weed throughout the world. It is little used in modern Western herbalism.

Pueraria lobata, P. montana (gé gēn). Kudzu is considered a noxious, nonnative weed in the southeastern United States and is also present in the Hawaiian Islands. I have not gathered this plant from the wild.

***Pyrola* spp. (lù xián cǎo).** At least one of the species of *Pyrola* used in China grows in the West. *P. minor (duǎn zhù lù tí cǎo)* is used in Heilongjiang, Jilin, and Xinjiang.[2] Many other *Pyrola* species are listed in *Chinese Herbal Medicine: Materia Medica* (3rd edition), leading one to believe that other species are likely applicable for the same indications. In China, the plant is used to dispel wind-dampness, strengthen bones and sinews, and stop bleeding.[3]

Scrophularia californica. This U.S. native species of figwort mainly is found close to the coast of California and Oregon. Western herbalists use the entire herb; in contrast, the Chinese use only the root of their species. However, I believe the root and rhizome of *S. californica* to be analogous to *xuán shēn* and recommend the substitution. See page 66 for more information.

Sonchus arvensis. Native to Europe, sow thistle is a common weed found throughout North America and in Hawai'i. The plant is used in northern China as *bài jiàng cǎo*.[4]

***Tremella* spp.** These fungi grow throughout North America and elsewhere. I have gathered the species called witch's butter *(T. mesenterica)* and used it in the same manner as *T. fuciformis (bái mù ěr)*. The latter, the official species in Chinese medicine, grows throughout Asia and in warmer climates around the world, including the southern United States.[5]

Viscum album. European mistletoe is abundant in Europe and parts of California, where it has naturalized. This *Viscum* species, native to Eurasia, is closely related to the one used in China, *V. coloratum (hú jì shēng)*, which is often used interchangeably with *Taxillus chinensis (sāng jì shēng)*.[6] Mistletoe has a long tradition of use in Western herbal medicine for hypertension and as a cardiac tonic, sedative, and antispasmodic. Most recently, it has been applied in the treatment of cancer. The fresh plant tincture is an excellent simple for hangovers. The most common species of mistletoe in North America are from the *Phoradendron* genus; Native Americans used them in various ways similar to the Chinese use of *sāng jì shēng*. Although I have never used any of the native species, I suspect they could be used as a substitute.

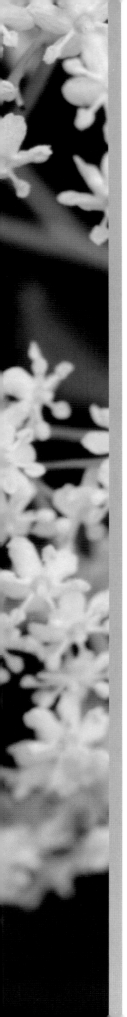

APPENDIX II

INDEX OF HERBS BY COMMON (ENGLISH) NAME

Common Name	Latin Name	Chinese Name
Aconite	*Aconitum carmichaeli*	*fù zǐ*
Agrimony	*Agrimonia eupatoria*	
Akebia fruit	*Akebia trifoliata*	*bā yuè zhá*
Albizia bark	*Albizia julibrissin*	*hé huān pí*
Albizia flower	*Albizia julibrissin*	*hé huān huā*
Ambrosia	*Ambrosia dumosa* and others	
Angelica	*Angelica arguta, A. breweri*	
Angelica, Chinese	*Angelica dahurica*	*bái zhǐ*
Angelica duhuo	*Angelica pubescentis*	*dú huó*
Apricot kernel	*Prunus armeniaca*	*xìng rén*
Arnebia	*Arnebia euchroma, A. guttata*	*zǐ cǎo gēn*
Arnica	*Arnica montana, A. cordifolia,* and others	
Artichoke, globe	*Cynara scolymus*	
Astragalus	*Astragalus membranaceus*	*huáng qí*

Common Name	Latin Name	Chinese Name
Atractylodes	*Atractylodes lancea*	*cāng zhú*
Atractylodes, white	*Atractylodes macrocephala*	*bái zhú*
Aucklandia	*Aucklandia lappa*	*mù xiāng*
Balsam root	*Balsamorhiza sagittata*	
Bamboo shavings	*Bambusa tuldoides* and others	*zhú rú*
Bayberry	*Myrica cerifera*	
Bitter orange	*Citrus aurantium*	*zhǐ shí*
Black cohosh	*Actaea racemosa* (formerly *Cimicifuga*)	
Black cohosh, Chinese	*Actaea foetida, A. dahurica* (formerly *Cimicifuga*)	*shēng má*
Blue cohosh	*Caulophyllum thalictroides*	
Bluecurls	*Trichostema lanatum, T. lanceolatum*	
Boneset	*Eupatorium perfoliatum*	
Buckthorn	*Rhamnus californica*	
Bugleweed	*Lycopus virginicus*	
Bupleurum	*Bupleurum chinense*	*chái hú*
Burdock	*Arctium lappa*	*niú bang gēn*
California poppy	*Eschscholzia californica*	
California spikenard	*Aralia californica*	
Cayenne pepper	*Capsicum annuum, C. frutescens*	
Chamomile	*Matricaria recutita*	*mǔ jú*
Chinese black cohosh	*Actea foetida, A. dahurica* (formerly *Cimicifuga*)	*shēng má*
Chinese dandelion	*Taraxacum sinicum* and *T. mongolicum*	*pú gōng yīng*
Chinese dogwood	*Cornus officinalis*	*shān zhū yú*
Chinese figwort	*Scrophularia ningpoensis*	*xuán shēn*
Chinese hawthorn	*Crataegus pinnatifida*	*shān zhā*
Chinese mistletoe	*Taxillus chinensis*	*sāng jì shēng*
Chinese mistletoe	*Viscus coloratum*	*hú jì shēng*
Chinese quince	*Chaenomeles speciosa*	*mù guā*
Cinnamon bark	*Cinnamomom cassia*	*ròu guì*
Cinnamom twig	*Cinnamomom cassia*	*guì zhī*
Citrus peel	*Citrus reticulata*	*chén pí*
Cleavers	*Galium aparine*	*bā xiān cǎo*
Coix	*Coix lacryma-jobi*	*yì yǐ rén*

Common Name	Latin Name	Chinese Name
Coptis	*Coptis chinensis*	*huáng lián*
Corn silk	*Zea mays*	*yù mǐ xū*
Cramp bark	*Viburnum opulus*	
Cranberry	*Vaccinium macrocarpon*	
Curcuma	*Curcuma wenyujin, C. aromatica*	*yù jīn*
Curcuma rhizome	*Curcuma phaeocaulis, C. kwangsiensis*	*é zhú*
Cyperus	*Cyperus rotundus*	*xiāng fù*
Damiana	*Turnera diffusa*	
Dandelion	*Taraxacum officinale*	
Dandelion, Chinese	*Taraxacum sinicum, T. mongolicum*	*pú gōng yīng*
Dang gui	*Angelica sinensis*	*dāng guī*
Dipsacus	*Dipsacus asperoides, D. fullonum*	
Dogwood, Chinese	*Cornus officinalis*	*shān zhū yú*
Echinacea	*Echinacea purpurea*	*song gua gu*
Elder	*Sambucus mexicana, S. canadensis, S. nigra*	
Elecampane	*Inula helenium*	*tǔ mù xiāng*
Elecampane flower	*Inula britannica*	*xuàn fù huā*
Ephedra	*Ephedra californica, E. viridis*	
Ephedra, Chinese	*Ephedra sinensis*	*má huáng*
Epimedium	*Epimedium brevicornum* and others	*yín yáng huò*
Figwort	*Scrophularia nodosa*	
Figwort, California	*Scrophularia californica*	
Figwort, Chinese	*Scrophularia ningpoensis*	*xuán shēn*
Forsythia	*Forsythia suspense*	*lián qiào*
Fringetree bark	*Chionanthus virginicus*	
Fritillaria	*Fritillaria thunbergii*	*zhè bèi mǔ*
Fritillaria, Sichuan	*Fritillaria cirrhosa*	*chuān bèi mǔ*
Gardenia	*Gardenia jasminoides*	*shān zhī zǐ*
Gentian	*Gentiana lutea, G. calycosa*	
Gentian root, large	*Gentiana macrophylla*	*qín jiāo*
Ginger	*Zingiber officinale*	*shēng jiāng*
Ginseng	*Panax ginseng*	*hóng rén shēn*
Ginseng, American	*Panax quinquefolius*	*xī yáng shēn*

Common Name	Latin Name	Chinese Name
Goldenseal	*Hydrastis canadensis*	
Grindelia	*Grindelia squarrosa*	
Hawthorn	*Crataegus* spp.	
Hawthorn, Chinese	*Crataegus pinnatifida*	*shān zhā*
Hemp seed	*Cannabis sativa*	*huǒ má rén*
Honeysuckle	*Lonicera japonica*	*jīn yín huā*
Horse chestnut	*Aesculus hipppocastanum*	
Isatis	*Isatis indigotica*	*bǎn lán gēn*
Juniper	*Juniperus communis*	
Kava	*Piper methysticum*	
Lavender	*Lavandula angustifolia*	
Lemon balm	*Melissa officinalis*	
Leopard lily	*Belamcanda chinensis*	*shè gān*
Licorice	*Glycyrrhiza glabra, G. uralensis*	*gān cǎo*
Ligusticum	*Ligusticum chuanxiong, L. wallichii*	*chuān xiōng*
Lobelia	*Lobelia inflata*	
Magnolia buds	*Magnolia biondii, M. denudate*	*xīn yí*
Marsh mallow	*Althaea officinalis*	
Meadowsweet	*Filipendula ulmaria*	
Milk thistle	*Silybum marianum*	
Mint	*Mentha arvensis, M. x piperita*	*bò hé*
Mistletoe, Chinese	*Taxillus chinensis*	*sāng jì shēng*
Mistletoe, Chinese	*Viscum coloratum*	*hú jì shēng*
Mistletoe, European	*Viscum album*	
Morinda	*Morinda officinalis*	*bā jǐ tiān*
Mormon tea	*Ephedra californica, E. viridis*	
Motherwort	*Leonorus cardiaca*	
Motherwort, Chinese	*Leonurus heterophyllus*	*yì mǔ cǎo*
Mulberry leaves	*Morus alba*	*sāng yè*
Mulberry rootbark	*Morus alba*	*sāng bái pí*
Mullein	*Verbascum thapsus*	
Myrrh	*Commiphora mol mol, C. myrrha*	*mò yào*
Nettle	*Urtica dioica, U. urens*	

Common Name	Latin Name	Chinese Name
Notoginseng	*Panax notoginseng*	*sān qī*
Oat	*Avena sativa, A. fatua*	
Ocotillo	*Fouquieria splendens*	
Ophiopogon	*Ophiopogon japonicus*	*mài mén dōng*
Osha	*Ligusticum grayi, L. porteri*	
Oregon grape root	*Mahonia* spp. (formerly *Berberis*)	
Passionflower	*Passiflora incarnata*	
Partridge berry	*Mitchella repens*	
Peach kernel	*Prunus persica*	*táo rén*
Peony, California	*Paeonia californica, P. brownii*	
Peony, moutan	*Paeonia suffruticosa*	*mŭ dān pí*
Peony, white	*Paeonia lactiflora*	*bái sháo*
Peppermint	*Mentha* x *piperita*	
Phellodendron	*Phellodendron amurense, P. chinense*	*huáng băi*
Picrorhiza	*Picrorhiza scrophulariiflora*	*hú huáng lián*
Pinellia	*Pinellia ternata*	*zhì bàn xià*
Plantain	*Plantago lanceolata, P. major*	
Pleurisy root	*Asclepias tuberosa*	
Polygala	*Polygala tenuifolia* and others	*yuăn zhì*
Poria	*Poria cocus*	*fú líng*
Prickly ash	*Zanthoxylum americanum*	
Quince, Chinese	*Chaenomeles speciosa*	*mù guā*
Red clover	*Trifolium pratense*	*sān xiāo căo*
Red root	*Ceanothus* spp.	
Red sage root	*Salvia miltiorrhiza*	*dān shēn*
Rehmannia (raw)	*Rehmannia glutinosa*	*shēng dì huáng*
Rehmannia (steamed)	*Rehmannia glutinosa*	*shú dì huáng*
Rhubarb	*Rheum palmatum*	*dà huáng*
Rose	*Rosa rugosa*	*méi guī huā*
Safflower	*Carthamus tinctorius*	*hóng huā*
Sage	*Salvia officinalis*	
Sage, black	*Salvia mellifera*	
Sage, white	*Salvia apiana*	

Common Name	Latin Name	Chinese Name
Sarsaparilla	*Smilax* spp.	
Sassafras	*Sassafras albidum*	
Saw palmetto	*Serenoa repens*	
Scented Solomon's seal	*Polygonatum odoratum*	*yù zhú*
Schizandra	*Schisandra chinensis*	*wǔ wèi zǐ*
Skullcap	*Scutellaria lateriflora*	
Skullcap, Chinese	*Scutellaria baicalensis*	*huáng qín*
Skullcap, Chinese	*Scutellaria barbata*	*bàn zhī lián*
Shepherd's purse	*Capsella bursa-pastoris*	*jì cài*
Sparganium	*Sparganium stoloniferum*	*sān léng*
St. John's wort	*Hypericum perforatum*	*guàn yè lián qiào*
Sundew	*Drosera rotundifolia*	
Sweet cicely	*Osmorhiza chilensis*	
Sweet cicely, Western	*Osmorhiza occidentalis*	
Sweet flag	*Acorus calamus*	*chāng pú*
Thyme	*Thymus vulgaris*	*shè xiāng cǎo*
Trichosanthus fruit and root	*Trichosanthus kirilowii*	*guā lóu*
Turmeric	*Curcuma longa*	*jiāng huáng*
Usnea	*Usnea* spp.	*sōng luó*
Uva-ursi	*Arctostaphylos uva-ursi*	
Valerian	*Valeriana officinalis, V. sitchensis*	*xié cǎo*
Vervain	*Verbena lasiostachys* and others	
Vitex	*Vitex agnus-castus*	
Vitex, Chinese	*Vitex rotundifolia, V. trifolia*	*màn jīng zǐ*
Water plantain root	*Alisma orientalis*	*zé xiè*
White atractylodes	*Atractylodes macrocephala*	*bái zhú*
Wild ginger	*Asarum caudatum, A. canadensis*	
Wild ginger, Chinese	*Asarum heterotropoides, A. sieboldii*	*xì xīn*
Wild yam	*Dioscorea villosa*	
Willow bark	*Salix* spp.	
Wintergreen	*Gaultheria procumbens*	
Yarrow	*Achillea millefolium*	*yáng she cao*

Common Name	Latin Name	Chinese Name
Yellow dock	*Rumex crispus*	*niú ěr dà huáng*
Yerba mansa	*Anemopsis californica*	
Yerba santa	*Eriodictyon californicum*	
Yucca root	*Yucca* spp.	
Zizyphus, spiny	*Zizyphus spinosa*	*suān zǎo rén*

APPENDIX III

INDEX OF HERBS BY LATIN NAME

Latin Name	Common Name	Chinese Name
Achillea millefolium	yarrow	*yáng she cao*
Aconitum carmichaeli	aconite	*fù zǐ*
Acorus calamus	sweet flag	*chāng pú*
Actaea racemosa (formerly *Cimicifuga)*	black cohosh	
Aesculus hipppocastanum	horse chestnut	
Agrimonia eupatoria	agrimony	
Albizia julibrissin	albizia bark	*hé huān pí*
Albizia julibrissin	albizia flower	*hé huān huā*
Alisma orientalis	water plantain root	*zé xiè*
Althaea officinalis	marsh mallow	
Ambrosia dumosa and others	ambrosia	
Anemopsis californica	yerba mansa	
Angelica arguta	angelica	
Angelica breweri	angelica	
Angelica dahurica	Chinese angelica	*bái zhǐ*
Angelica pubescentis	angelica duhuo	*dú huó*

Latin Name	Common Name	Chinese Name
Angelica sinensis	dang gui	*dāng guī*
Aralia californica	California spikenard	
Arctostaphylos uva-ursi	uva-ursi, bearberry, kinnikinick	
Arctium lappa	burdock	*niú bang gēn (zǐ)*
Arnebia euchroma, A. guttata	arnebia	*zǐ cǎo gēn*
Arnica montana, A. cordifolia	arnica	
Asarum caudatum, A. canadensis	wild ginger	
Asarum spp.	Chinese wild ginger	*xì xīn*
Asclepias tuberosa	pleurisy root	
Astragalus membranaceus	astragalus	*huáng qí*
Atractylodes lancea	atractylodes	*cāng zhú*
Atractylodes macrocephala	white atractylodes	*bái zhú*
Aucklandia lappa	aucklandia	*mù xiāng*
Avena sativa, A. fatua	oat	
Balsamorhiza sagittata	balsam root	
Bambusa tuldoides and others	bamboo shavings	*zhú rú*
Belamcanda chinensis	leopard lily	*shè gān*
Bupleurum chinense	bupleurum	*chái hú*
Cannabis sativa	hemp seed	*huǒ má rén*
Capsella bursa-pastoris	shepherd's purse	*jì cài*
Capsicum annuum, C. frutescens	cayenne pepper	*là jiāo*
Caulophyllum thalictroides	blue cohosh	
Ceanothus spp.	red root	
Chaenomeles speciosa	Chinese quince	*mù guā*
Chionanthus virginicus	fringetree bark	
Cinnamomom cassia	cinnamon bark	*ròu guì*
Cinnamomom cassia	cinnamon twig	*guì zhī*
Citrus aurantium	bitter orange	*zhǐ shí*
Citrus reticulata	citrus peel	*chén pí*
Coix lacryma-jobi	coix	*yì yǐ rén*
Commiphora mol mol, C. myrrha	myrrh	*mò yào*
Coptis chinensis	coptis	*huáng lián*
Cornus officinalis	Chinese dogwood fruit	*shān zhū yú*

Latin Name	Common Name	Chinese Name
Crataegus spp.	hawthorn	
Crataegus pinnatifida	Chinese hawthorn	*shān zhā*
Curcuma longa	turmeric	*jiāng huáng*
Curcuma phaeocaulis, C. kwangsiensis	curcuma rhizome	*é zhú*
Curcuma wenyujin, C. aromatica	curcuma	*yù jīn*
Cynara scolymus	globe artichoke	
Cyperus rotundus	cyperus	*xiāng fù*
Dioscorea villosa	wild yam	
Dipsacus asperoides, D. fullonum	dipsacus	
Drosera rotundifolia	sundew	
Echinacea purpurea	echinacea	*sōng guǒ jú*
Ephedra californica, E. viridis	ephedra, Mormon tea	
Ephedra sinensis	Chinese ephedra	*má huáng*
Epimedium brevicornum and others	epimedium	*yín yáng huò*
Eriodictyon californicum	yerba santa	
Eschscholzia californica	California poppy	
Eupatorium perfoliatum	boneset	
Filipendula ulmaria	meadowsweet	
Forsythia suspense	forsythia	*lián qiào*
Fouquieria splendens	ocotillo	
Fritillaria cirrhosa	Sichuan fritillaria	*chuān bèi mǔ*
Fritillaria thunbergii	fritillaria	*zhè bèi mǔ*
Galium aparine	cleavers	*bā xiān cǎo*
Gardenia jasminoides	gardenia	*shān zhī zǐ*
Gaultheria procumbens	wintergreen	
Gentiana lutea, G. calycosa	gentian	
Gentiana macrophylla	large gentian root	*qín jiāo*
Glycyrrhiza glabra, G. uralensis	licorice	*gān cǎo*
Grindelia squarrosa	grindelia	
Hydrastis canadensis	goldenseal	
Hypericum perforatum	St. John's wort	*guàn yè lián qiào*
Inula helenium	elecampane	*tǔ mù xiāng*
Inula britannica	elecampane flower	*xuàn fù huā*

Latin Name	Common Name	Chinese Name
Isatis indigotica	isatis	*bǎn lán gēn*
Juniperus communis	juniper	
Lavandula angustifolia	lavender	
Leonurus cardiaca	motherwort	
Leonurus heterophyllus	Chinese motherwort	*yì mǔ cǎo*
Ligusticum chuanxiong, L. wallichii	ligusticum	*chuān xiōng*
Ligusticum grayi, L. porteri	osha	
Lobelia inflata	Lobelia	
Lonicera japonica	honeysuckle	*jīn yín huā*
Lycopus virginicus	bugleweed	
Magnolia biondii, M. denudate	magnolia buds	*xīn yí (huā)*
Mahonia spp.	Oregon grape root	
Matricaria recutita	chamomile	
Melissa officinalis	lemon balm	
Mentha arvensis, M. x *piperita*	mint	*bò hé*
Mentha x *piperita*	peppermint	
Mitchella repens	partridge berry	
Morinda officinalis	morinda	*bā jǐ tiān*
Morus alba	mulberry leaves	*sāng yè*
Morus alba	mulberry rootbark	*sāng bái pí*
Myrica cerifera	bayberry	
Ophiopogon japonicus	ophiopogon	*mài mén dōng*
Osmorhiza chilensis	sweet cicely	
Osmorhiza occidentalis	Western sweet cicely	
Paeonia californica, P. brownii	California peony	
Paeonia lactiflora	white peony	*bái sháo*
Paeonia suffruticosa	moutan peony	*mǔ dān pí*
Panax ginseng	ginseng	*hóng rén shēn*
Panax notoginseng	notoginseng	*sān qī*
Panax quinquefolius	American ginseng	*xī yáng shēn*
Passiflora incarnata	passionflower	
Phellodendron amurense, P. chinense	phellodendron	*huáng bǎi*
Picrorhiza scrophulariiflora	picrorhiza	*hú huáng lián*

Latin Name	Common Name	Chinese Name
Pinellia ternate	pinellia	*zhì bàn xià*
Piper methysticum	kava	
Plantago lanceolata, P. major	plantain	
Polygala tenuifolia and others	polygala	*yuǎn zhì*
Polygonatum odoratum	scented Solomon's seal	*yù zhú*
Poria cocus	poria	*fú líng*
Prunus persica	peach kernel	*táo rén*
Rehmannia glutinosa	rehmannia (raw)	*shēng dì huáng*
Rehmannia glutinosa	rehmannia (steamed)	*shú dì huáng*
Rhamnus californica and others	buckthorn	
Rheum palmatum	Chinese rhubarb	*dà huáng*
Rosa rugosa	rose	*méi guī huā*
Rumex crispus	yellow dock	*niú ěr dà huáng*
Salix spp.	willow bark	
Salvia apiana	white sage	
Salvia mellifera	black sage	
Salvia miltiorrhiza	red sage root	*dān shēn*
Salvia officinalis	sage	
Sambucus mexicana, S. canadensis, S. nigra	elder	
Schisandra chinensis	schizandra	*wǔ wèi zǐ*
Sassafras albidum	sassafras	
Scrophularia californica	California figwort	
Scrophularia nodosa	figwort	
Scrophularia ningpoensis,	Chinese figwort	*xuán shēn*
Scutellaria baicalensis	Chinese skullcap	*huáng qín*
Scutellaria barbata	Chinese skullcap	*bàn zhī lián*
Scutellaria lateriflora	skullcap	
Serenoa repens	saw palmetto	
Silybum marianum	milk thistle	
Smilax spp.	sarsaparilla	
Taraxacum officinale	dandelion	
Taraxacum sinicum, T. mongolicum	Chinese dandelion	*pú gōng yīng*

Latin Name	Common Name	Chinese Name
Taxillus chinensis	Chinese mistletoe	*sāng jì shēng*
Thymus vulgaris	thyme	
Trichosanthus kirilowii	trichosanthus fruit and root	*guā lóu*
Trichostema lanatum, T. lanceolatum	bluecurls	
Trifolium pratense	red clover	*sān xiāo cǎo*
Turnera diffusa	damiana	
Urtica dioica, U. urens	nettle	
Usnea spp.	usnea	
Vaccinium macrocarpon	cranberry	
Valeriana officinalis	valerian	*xié cǎo*
Valeriana sitchensis	valerian	
Verbascum thapsus	mullein	
Verbena lasiostachys and others	vervain	
Viburnum opulus	cramp bark	
Viscum album	mistletoe, European	
Viscum coloratum	Chinese mistletoe	*hú jì shēng*
Vitex agnus-castus	vitex	
Vitex rotundifolia, V. trifolia	vitex, Chinese	*màn jīng zǐ*
Yucca spp.	yucca root	
Zanthoxylum americanum	prickly ash	
Zea mays	corn silk	*yù mǐ xū*
Zingiber officinale	ginger	*shēng jiāng*
Zizyphus spinosa	spiny zizyphus	*suān zǎo rén*

GLOSSARY OF CHINESE MEDICAL TERMS

This glossary is intended to serve as a quick reference for those less familiar with the terminology presented in this book or with Chinese medicine in general. It is not meant to provide comprehensive coverage of all the terminology found in this book, nor are all of the defintions meant to be complete in scope.

It is through the graciousness of Nigel Wiseman and Feng Ye, authors of *A Practical Dictionary of Chinese Medicine,* as well as Bob Felt of Paradigm Publications, that I am honored to be able to offer the Chinese medical terms glossed herein. Out of respect for the authors and publisher, I have kept the list short. Hence, you will find definitions (for the most part) only for primary concepts, treatment methods, and patterns. For some of the more complex disease patterns for which I did not provide a specific definition, you will be able to extrapolate some information from the material provided. For example, there is no entry for heart *qi* vacuity, but the definitions provided for heart, *qi,* and vacuity should give one some idea about the disease pattern called heart *qi* vacuity.

However, I leave you with a strong word of caution: be careful about trying to define concepts on which you are unclear without referring to the primary reference to confirm your speculations. For entries that would require more space to cover fully, the reader is referred to *A Practical Dictionary of Chinese Medicine,* in which all of these definitions originate, for a more detailed discussion of complex topics, including key concepts, disease patterns, and treatment methods.

accumulation: Gathering, amassment; specifically: 1. a type of abdominal lump (see concretions, conglomerations, accumulations, and gatherings); 2. accumulation of food in the digestive tract.

acridity: One of the five flavors. Acridity enters the lung; it can dissipate and move. See five flavors.

affect: 1. Any natural movement of the heart, such as joy, anger, or grief. 2. The seven specific emotional and mental activities (joy, anger, anxiety, thought, sorrow, fear, and fright), which in excess can cause disease.

ascendant hyperactivity of liver *yáng*: An imbalance of the liver's *yīn* and *yáng* aspects that occurs when vacuity of liver-kidney *yīn* lets liver *yáng* get out of control and stir upward excessively. This pathomechanism may be exacerbated when depression, anger, and anxiety impair free coursing; when free coursing is impaired, depressed *qì* transforms into fire, fire damages *yīn*-blood, and *yīn* has no power to restrain *yáng*.

binding depression of liver *qì*: Stagnation in the liver and liver channel resulting from impairment of the liver's function of free coursing. It arises when affect-mind frustration leads to depression and anger that damage the liver and impair free coursing.

bitterness: The flavor of burnt things; the flavor associated with fire. Bitterness enters the heart; it can drain and dry. See five flavors.

bladder: One of the six bowels; the organ in the smaller abdomen that stores and discharges urine. The bladder stands in exterior-interior relationship with the kidney.

bladder damp-heat: A disease pattern that arises when damp-heat causes inhibited bladder *qì* transformation that manifests in frequent urination, painful urination, red or yellow murky urine, or bloody urine.

blandness: Mild flavor, or the absence of a predominating flavor; the flavor associated with damp-percolating and water-disinhibiting medicinals. See five flavors.

blood: The red fluid of the body that, according to traditional explanations, is derived from the essential *qì* from food by the stomach and spleen; it becomes red blood after being transformed by construction *qì* and the lung.

blood-aspect pattern: Any warm disease pattern that arises when an evil enters the blood aspect. Signs include a deep crimson tongue coloring and indications of frenetic movement of the blood, such as bleeding and purple maculopapular eruptions.

blood-heat: A condition characterized by heat and blood signs, mostly occurring in externally contracted heat (febrile) diseases, though not uncommon in miscellaneous diseases. When blood-heat scorches the vessels, it can cause extravasation of the blood, bloody stool or urine, nosebleed, or menstrual irregularities.

blood stasis: Impairment or cessation of the normal free flow of blood. Blood stasis may arise when knocks and falls, bleeding *qì* stagnation, *qì* vacuity, blood-cold, or blood-heat impair free flow, causing local blood stasis.

blood vacuity: The manifestation of insufficiency of the blood. Blood vacuity may develop from excessive loss of blood before replenishment is complete. It may also be caused by insufficiency of blood formation stemming from splenic movement and transformation failure. A further cause is failure to eliminate static blood and engender new blood. Blood vacuity is characterized by a pale white or withered yellow facial complexion, dizzy head, flowery vision, relatively pale tongue, and a fine pulse.

chest impediment: 1. A disease pattern characterized by fullness and oppression in the anterior chest, with pain reaching to the back in severe cases and panting that prevents the patient from lying down. It is caused by *yīn* evils, such as phlegm turbidity and static blood, that congeal and bind, preventing diffusion of chest *yáng*. 2. A pattern characterized by fullness and oppression in the anterior chest, pain on swallowing, and, in some cases, occasional vomiting.

clearing heat: A method of treatment used to address heat using cool and cold medicinals, in accordance with the principle stated in *Elementary Questions (sù wèn)* as "heat is treated with cold." Clearing heat is used in the treatment of interior heat patterns, such as *qì*-aspect heat, blood-aspect heat, damp-heat, and *yáng* sore patterns. Clearing heat is a generic term that corresponds to *clearing* in the Eight Methods. It includes clearing heat (in a more specific sense), draining fire, and resolving toxin.

cold damage: 1. Externally contracted heat (febrile) diseases. 2. A specific form of externally contracted heat (febrile) disease, such as cold damage, wind stroke, damp warmth, heat disease, and warm disease.

cold impediment: An impediment *(bì)* pattern attributed to wind-cold-damp, with a prevalence of cold, that invades the joints and channels; it is characterized by acute pain in the joints that is exacerbated by exposure to cold and relieved by warmth. There may also be hypertonicity of the extremities.

cold pattern: Any disease pattern characterized by cold signs, such as aversion to cold, a somber white or green-blue facial complexion, slow or tight pulse, no thirst or a desire for warm fluid, and long voidings of clear urine.

concretions, conglomerations, accumulations, and gatherings: Four kinds of abdominal masses associated with pain and distention. Concretions and accumulations are masses of definite form and fixed location, associated with pain of fixed location. They stem from disease in the viscera and blood aspect. Conglomerations and gatherings are masses of indefinite form that gather and dissipate at irregular intervals and are attended by pain of unfixed location. They are attributed to disease in the bowels and *qì* aspect. Accumulations and gatherings chiefly occur in the center burner. Concretions and conglomerations chiefly occur in the lower burner, and in many cases are the result of gynecological disease. In general, concretions and gatherings arise when emotional depression and dietary intemperance causes damage to the liver and spleen. The resultant organ disharmony leads to obstruction and stagnation of *qì,* which in turn causes static blood to collect gradually. Most often the root cause is insufficiency of right *qì.*

conglomerations: See concretions, conglomerations, accumulations, and gatherings.

course: To enhance flow (of *qì,* especially depressed liver *qì*); to free (the liver or digestive tract of *qì* stagnation and depression); to eliminate (evils, such as wind in the exterior); to free (the exterior or channels from evils such as wind).

coursing the exterior: A method of treatment used to free the exterior of evil without necessarily causing the patient to sweat.

coursing the liver and rectifying *qì:* To restore the normal free coursing of liver *qì* in the treatment of depression of liver *qì,* which is characterized by rib-side pain and distention, oppression in the chest, mental depression, pain and distention in the stomach duct, nausea and vomiting, poor appetite, menstrual irregularities, bitter taste in the mouth, stringlike pulse, and thin tongue coating.

damp depression: One of the six depressions. See six depressions for more information.

damp-heat: A combination of dampness and heat. Damp-heat may be of external or internal origin or a combination of both. It can cause a variety of different diseases and is characterized by signs of both dampness and heat.

damp impediment: 1. An impediment *(bì)* pattern arising when wind, cold, and predominantly dampness invade the channels and joints. Damp impediment is characterized by heaviness of the limbs, stubborn numbness of the skin, and pain in the joints in fixed locations that is triggered by *yīn*-type (dull, wet) weather. 2. Leg *qì* with pain and numbness in the legs.

dampness: 1. One of the six *qì* (i.e., dampness as an environmental phenomenon). 2. One of the six excesses (i.e., environmental *qì* as a cause of disease). 3. Dampness as an evil in the body. Dampness in the body is qualitatively analogous with and causally related to dampness in the natural environment. It is associated with damp weather or damp climates and with stagnant water in places where ground drainage is poor. Dampness has a number of characteristics: 1. It is clammy, viscous, and lingering. Dampness diseases are persistent and difficult to cure. 2. Dampness tends to stagnate. When dampness evil invades the exterior, the patient may complain of physical fatigue; heavy, cumbersome limbs; and heavy-headedness. If dampness invades the channels and joints, the patient may complain of aching joints and inhibited bending and stretching. 3. The spleen is particularly vulnerable to dampness evil. 4. There may be general or localized stagnation or accumulation of water-damp, such as water swelling, leg *qì,* vaginal discharge, or exuding sores, such as eczema. 5. Over time, dampness can gather to form phlegm.

depression: Stagnation; reduced activity. In physiology, depression refers either to depressed *qì* dynamic (frustrated physiological activity) or to flow stoppage due to congestion. The term also describes inhibition of normal emotional activity that expresses itself in the form of oppression, frustration, and irascibility. In practice, depression is usually *qì* stagnation due to affect damage, and is therefore more restricted in meaning than *qì* stagnation, which may be due to other causes.

disinhibit: To promote fluency, movement, or activity (i.e., to treat inhibited flow of *qì*, blood, fluids, or inhibited physical movement).

dispel: Eliminate (evils). See drain.

disperse: To break up, dispel. See dispersion; drain.

dispersion: One of the eight methods; the gradual breaking up of accumulations of substances in the body, using medicinals that abduct and disperse, soften hardness, and transform accumulations.

downbear: To descend or cause to descend.

drain: 1. To eliminate evils in the body that manifest in repletion patterns. 2. Specifically, to eliminate fire and lower burner damp-heat. 3. To cause the stool to flow.

dryness: 1. The opposite of moisture. 2. One of the six *qì*; dryness as an environmental phenomenon and a potential cause of disease, associated with autumn in China. 3. One of the six excesses; dryness as an environmental *qì* causing disease. 4. A state of the body resulting from contraction of dryness in the environment. 5. A state of the body arising from depletion of *yīn*-humor and presenting signs similar to those created by environmental *qì* dryness.

effuse (effusion): To move outward, as sweat through the interstices; to induce such movement. For example, "effuse the exterior" means to induce sweating so that evils located in the exterior can escape.

ejection: One of the eight methods; a method of treatment that involves induction of vomiting, either by the use of medicinals or by mechanical means (e.g., tickling the throat with a feather) in order to expel collected phlegm or lodged food. In clinical practice, ejection is used when phlegm-drool obstructs the throat and hampers breathing or when food stagnates in the stomach after voracious eating, causing distention, fullness, and pain.

essence: That which is responsible for growth, development, and reproduction and determines the strength of the constitution; it is manifested physically in the male in the form of semen. Essence is composed of earlier heaven essence (congenital essence), which is inherited from the parents and constantly supplemented by later heaven essence (acquired essence) produced from food by the stomach and spleen. Pathologies of essence include congenital insufficiency, late or improper maturation, premature senility, or sexual and reproductive dysfunctions.

evil: Any entity from outside or within that threatens health. Evils include the six excesses or six *qì* (wind, cold, fire, summerheat, dampness, and dryness) in terms of their capacity to cause disease. Evils also include the warm evils described by the warm heat school and the various kinds of toxin.

excess: Any of the six *qì* (wind, cold, fire, summerheat, dampness, and dryness) in excess.

exterior: The outer part of the body as opposed to the interior; it includes the fleshy exterior (i.e., the skin and exterior muscles of the head, limbs, and trunk) and bowels, which are the organs of the exterior through which the essences of grain and water (nutrients in food) are absorbed and waste is expelled.

fire: 1. One of the five phases; the phase associated with summer, south, red, the heart, and joy. 2. In physiology, a transmutation of *yáng qì* explained as a vital force (e.g., sovereign fire, ministerial fire, and lesser fire). 3. One of the six *qì*; hot weather. See heat. 4. One of the six excesses, which when invading the body, can cause the following signs: 1. Pronounced generalized or local signs of heat, such as high fever, aversion to heat, desire for coolness, flushed complexion, reddening of the eyes, reddish urine, red tongue, yellow coating, rapid pulse, or, in sore patterns, redness, heat, pain and swelling. 2. Thick, sticky excreta, such as thick snivel, thick yellow phlegm, sour watery vomitus, murky urine, blood and pus in the stool, acute diarrhea, or foul-smelling stools, often with a burning sensation on discharge. 3. Damage to the fluids characterized by a dry tongue with little liquid, thirst with desire for cold fluids, and dry hard stool. 4. Bleeding and maculopapular eruptions that occur when fire evil scorches the blood and causes frenetic blood movement. 5. Disturbances of the spirit and vision.

five flavors: Acridity, sourness, sweetness, bitterness, and saltiness. Medicinals and foodstuffs with different flavors have different actions. Acridity can dissipate and move;

sourness can contract and astringe; sweetness can supplement and relax (i.e., relieve pain and tension); bitterness can drain and dry; saltiness can soften hardness and induce moist precipitation. There is also a sixth flavor, blandness, which has a water-disinhibiting action.

gallbladder: The bowel that stands in interior-exterior relationship with the liver. The gallbladder's main function is to secrete bile, which is formed from an excess of liver *qì*. The gallbladder is also a curious organ, because its bile is considered "clear fluid" rather than waste in Chinese medicine. A bitter taste in the mouth may be a sign of gallbladder disease. It is also said that the gallbladder governs decision, which means that the ability to maintain balanced judgment in the face of adversity is attributed to the gallbladder. When gallbladder *qì* is weak and timid, there are signs such as lack of courage and decision, timidity, doubt and suspicion, and frequent sighing.

gatherings: See concretions, conglomerations, accumulations, and gatherings.

glomus: A localized, subjective feeling of fullness and blockage. In the chest, glomus may be associated with a feeling of oppression in severe cases; hence the terms fullness in the chest, distention in the chest, glomus in the chest, and oppression in the chest are largely synonymous. In the abdomen, glomus is the sensation of a lump that cannot be detected by palpation.

harmonization: One of the eight methods; a method of adjusting functions within the human body that is used when an evil is at mid-stage penetration or there is disharmony between *qì* and blood or between the organs, and methods such as sweating, ejection, precipitation, warming, clearing, dispersion, and supplementation cannot be applied.

harmonize: To coordinate one element of the body with the rest of the body.

heart: The organ located in the chest and surrounded by the pericardium. The heart governs the blood and vessels, stores the spirit, and opens at the tongue. It belongs to fire in the five phases, along with its paired organ *(yáng)*, the small intestine.

heart impediment: A disease of the heart characterized by pain and suffocating oppression that is caused by stasis obstruction of the heart vessels.

heart vexation: A feeling of unrest or irritability that focuses in the heart region; a subjective feeling of heat and disquietude in the chest. Vexation is commonly observed in either vacuity or repletion heat.

heat: 1. The opposite of cold. Heat is the manifestation of the sun and fire. Hot weather (and artificially heated environments) cause sweating, and without an adequate increase in fluid intake, thirst. There may be vexation and other discomforts naturally attributed to heat by the individual. In a healthy person, these natural responses abate upon exposure to cooler temperatures. 2. The external evils known as fire and summerheat manifesting in the body in pathological signs such as high fever, fear of heat, desire for coolness, thirst, red face, red eyes, reddish urine, red tongue with yellow coating, and rapid pulse. 3. Any condition manifesting with signs similar to those of fire and summerheat that is the result of *yīn* vacuity, the transformation of external evils passing into the interior, or the transformation of *yáng qì* as a result of affect damage. 4. One of the eight parameters under which any of the above pathological conditions are classified. 5. Heat effusion or subjective sensations of heat that may or may not be classified as heat among the eight principles.

impediment: 1. Blockage, as in throat impediment. 2. Blockage of the channels arising when wind, cold, and dampness invade the fleshy exterior and the joints, manifesting in signs such as joint pain, sinew and bone pain, and heaviness or numbness of the limbs. See also wind impediment, cold impediment, damp impediment.

irascibility: Proneness to anger. Anger is the mind of the liver, and irascibility is seen in patterns such as ascendant liver *yáng*, binding depression of liver *qì*, and five minds forming fire.

kidney: Either of the two viscera located in the small of the back, on either side of the spine; the two kidneys as a single functional unit. The kidney belongs to water in the five phases, along with its paired organ *(yáng)*, the urinary bladder. The kidney governs water, stores essence, governs reproduction, is the root of early heaven, governs the bone and engenders the marrow, has its blood in the heart of the head, and opens at the ears and at the two *yīn*.

knocks and falls: 1. Blows, collisions, collapses, or falls from heights, especially when resulting in injury. 2. Any injury resulting from knocks and falls. Injuries from knocks and falls include stasis swelling (bruises), cuts and grazes, sprains, bone fractures, dislocations, and damage to the bowels and viscera.

large intestine: One of the six bowels; an organ that stands in exterior-interior relationship with the lung and whose function is to receive waste passed down from the small intestine and form it into stool before discharging it from the body. Thus, the large intestine is said to govern the transformation and conveyance of waste.

liver: The viscus located on the right side of the body, beneath the diaphragm. The liver is an interior organ and is connected by channels to the gallbladder, which is its corresponding exterior organ. In the five phases, the liver belongs to wood. The liver stores the blood and governs free coursing, the sinews, and the making of strategies. It also governs fright and is averse to wind. It opens at the eyes, and its bloom is in the nails. The liver stores the blood, meaning that the liver can retain blood and regulate the amount of blood flowing throughout the body. The liver governs free coursing, meaning that it makes *qi* course freely around the body, ensuring normal mental and emotional activity as well as the secretion and discharge of bile. Impairment of this function leads to binding depression of liver *qi*, very often associated with rashness, impatience, and irascibility, for which reason it is often said that the liver is the unyielding viscus.

liver depression: A pattern resulting from binding depression of liver *qi*.

liver-gallbladder damp-heat: A disease pattern arising when the liver's free coursing is impaired, owing either to internal damp-heat stemming from excessive consumption of fatty or sweet foods or to externally contracted damp-heat. The chief signs are alternating heat [effusion] and [aversion to] cold, bitter taste in the mouth, rib-side pain, abdominal pain, nausea and vomiting, abdominal distention, aversion to food, yellowing of the skin, and yellow or reddish urine. Stool tends to be dry if heat is more pronounced than dampness, and sloppy if dampness is more pronounced than heat. The tongue coating is yellow and slimy. The pulse is rapid and stringlike.

liver *qi* invading the spleen: A form of liver-spleen disharmony in which liver free coursing is excessive and liver *qi* moves cross counterflow and affects the spleen. Liver *qi* invading the spleen is characterized by headache, irascibility, bitter taste in the mouth, oppression in the chest and rib-side, glomus and fullness after eating, sloppy diarrhea, and a moderate stringlike pulse. This pattern differs from liver *qi* invading the stomach by a predominance of spleen signs, such as distention and diarrhea.

liver-wind stirring internally: Liver-wind arises from extreme *yīn-yáng* and *qi*-blood imbalance. In extreme cases, ascendant liver *yáng*, liver-fire flaming upward, and insufficiency of liver *yīn* and/or blood may all stir liver-wind. The chief signs of liver-wind stirring internally are severe dizziness, headache with pulling sensation (iron-band headache), tension and stiffness in the neck, tingling or numbness in the limbs, or twitching of the sinews and flesh. In severe cases, there may be pulling of the face and eyes, trembling lips, tongue, and fingers, inhibited speech, or unsteady gait. In more severe cases, there may be convulsions or tetanic reversal.

lung: Viscus located in the chest, connecting with the throat and opening into the nose. The lung is interior and is connected by its channel to the large intestine, which is the corresponding exterior organ. In the doctrine of the five phases, the lung belongs to metal. The main functions of the lung are governing *qi*, regulation of the waterways, and the governing of the exterior of the entire body. The lung governs *qi*, meaning that the lung is responsible for breathing and the production of the true *qi*. The idea that the lung governs the regulation of the waterways refers to the action of lung *qi* with regard to water metabolism. The depurative, downbearing action of lung *qi* carries water downward to the bladder and prevents accumulation of water *qi* in the body. Hence, it is also said that the lung governs movement of water and the lung is the upper source of water. Disturbance of the function can give rise to inhibited urine and water swelling.

maculopapular eruption: Eruption of macules or papules. Macules are colored (usually red) patches that vary in size and are not raised above the surface of the skin. Papules are like grains of millet in shape and size (or may be larger) and raised above the surface of the skin. The appearance of maculopapular eruptions in externally contracted heat (febrile) disease indicates heat penetrating the blood-construction. In internal damage miscellaneous diseases, they usually indicate blood-heat.

major chest bind: A disease pattern arising when inappropriate application of precipitation for an unresolved exterior pattern in greater *yáng (tài yáng)* disease causes the heat evil to fall inward and combine with phlegm and water. Major chest bind is characterized by fullness and hardness as well as pain in the chest, stomach duct, and umbilical region that is too tender to be touched.

mounting: Any of the various diseases characterized by pain or swelling of the abdomen or scrotum.

nourish: See supplementation.

opening the orifices: A method of treatment used to address clouded spirit and coma due to evil obstructing the orifices of the heart. Opening the orifices employs acrid, aromatic, penetrating medicinals to penetrate the heart and free the orifices, repel foulness, and open blocks.

outthrust: The spontaneous or induced forcing of evils to and through the exterior of the body, including those that provoke maculopapular outthrust (outbreak of rash) on so doing.

panting: Hasty, rapid, labored breathing with discontinuity between inhalation and exhalation, in severe cases with gaping mouth, raised shoulders, flaring nostrils, and inability to lie down. Panting is a manifestation of impaired diffusion and downbearing of lung *qì*. Since the lung is the governor of *qì* and the kidney is the root of *qì*, panting is associated primarily with disease of the lung and or kidney. Panting occurs in repletion and vacuity.

phlegm: A viscid substance traditionally understood to be both a product and a cause of disease. Phlegm may gather in the lung, from which it can be expelled by coughing. However, phlegm as it is understood in Chinese medicine has a broader meaning than does sputum of Western medicine. In Chinese medicine, phlegm denotes a viscous fluid that can accumulate anywhere in the body, causing a variety of diseases (including stroke, epilepsy, and scrofula), but which in the absence of expectoration are usually characterized by a slimy tongue coating and a slippery or slippery, stringlike pulse. [As you can see, the concept of phlegm in Chinese medicine is far reaching. I encourage you to not only read the *Practical Dictionary of Chinese Medicine* for more information, but also to explore other material to further your understanding of this important concept.]

phlegm-rheum: Accumulation of fluid in the body. "Phlegm" denotes thick pathological fluids, whereas "rheum" denotes thinner pathological fluids. In practice, the term phlegm-rheum has two specific meanings: 1. Any form of rheum (i.e., thin fluid) arising as a result of lung, spleen, or kidney disturbances that prevent the normal transportation and transformation of fluid, treated by warming and supplementing the spleen and kidney to secure the root and address the branches; 2. One of the four rheums. Rheum lodged in the stomach and intestines. Phlegm-rheum is characterized by sloppy stool, poor appetite, ejection of foamy drool, and emaciation occurring in obese people. In some cases, there may be heart palpitations and shortness of breath.

plum-pit *qì*: Dryness and a sensation of a foreign body present in the throat which can be neither swallowed nor ejected. The intensity of the signs fluctuates. The main cause is binding depression of liver *qì*.

precipitation: One of the eight methods. The stimulation of fecal flow to expel repletion evils and remove accumulation and stagnation.

***qì* depression:** One of the six depressions. *Qì* stagnation that arises when affect-mind binding depression causes binding depression of liver *qì*. See binding depression of liver *qì*.

***qì* stagnation:** Decrease in the normal activity of *qì* that is attributed to the obstructive effect of mental and emotional problems, external injury, evil *qì* (cold, dampness), static blood, or *qì* vacuity, and that is capable of causing static blood, water-damp, or phlegm-rheum. *Qì* stagnation is characterized by distention, fullness, and oppression in the affected area.

rectifying *qì*: Correction of any morbidity of *qì* (*qì* stagnation, *qì* counterflow, *qì* vacuity, *qì* fall), especially to treat *qì* stagnation or *qì* counterflow.

repletion: The opposite of vacuity. See vacuity and repletion.

resolve: To terminate (disease patterns), eliminate (evils), or free (parts of the body from evils).

right *qì*: True *qì*, especially in opposition to diseases. Right *qì* is the active aspect of all components, including the organs, blood, fluids, and essence and the above-mentioned forms of *qì* in maintaining health and resisting disease.

small intestine: One of the six bowels. The small intestine holds the office of reception (i.e., it receives grain and water that has been decomposed in the stomach). It further transforms food, extracting nutrients for the body, and governs the transformation of matter and the separation of the clear [from the] turbid. The small intestine stands in interior-exterior relationship with the heart, and belongs to fire of the five phases.

snivel: Snivel is the humor of the lung. Abnormalities of the nasal mucus indicate either lung vacuity or nondiffusion of the lung *qi* due to the presence of evil.

source *qi*: The basic form of *qi* in the body, made up of a combination of three other forms of *qi*: the essential *qi* of the kidney; *qi* of grain and water, derived through the transformative function of the spleen; and air (great *qi*) drawn in through the lung. It is the basis of all physiological activity.

spirit: 1. (In the narrow sense) that which is said to be stored by the heart and return to the abode of the heart during sleep, to be disquieted in conditions of heart palpitations, susceptibility to fright, heart vexation, and insomnia, and to be clouded in wind stroke or when evils enter the pericardium. The Chinese concept of spirit describes that which normally makes us conscious and alert during the day and becomes inactive during sleep; thus it corresponds to the concept expressed by the English word "mind" in the sense of the mental capacity to think, feel, and respond. 2. (In a wider sense) that which is said to present in individuals with healthy complexion, bright eyes, erect bearing, physical agility, and clear, coherent speech.

spleen: The organ that lies against the lower face of the stomach. The spleen is ascribed the function of assimilating nutrients from food in the stomach to make *qi*, blood, and fluids. It is associated with earth in the five phases. The spleen governs movement and transformation of grain and water and distribution of its essence.

stanching bleeding: Any of the various methods of treatment used to address bleeding. Different medicinals are employed, depending on whether the bleeding occurs in cold or heat patterns.

stasis: 1. Sluggishness or cessation of movement (of the blood), specifically of the blood. 2. Static blood. See blood stasis.

static blood: Blood affected by stasis (i.e., blood that does not move freely, stagnates in the vessels, or accumulates outside the vessels).

stomach: 1. The bowel standing in exterior-interior relationship with the spleen. The stomach is the place where food collects after it enters the body, before it passes to the intestines, and where it is broken down so that its "essence" (nutrients) can be absorbed into the body. Traditionally, the stomach's function of controlling appetite and receiving food is referred to as "the stomach governs intake" and its function of breaking down food is called "the stomach governs decomposition."

stomach duct: The stomach cavity and adjoining sections of the small intestine and gullet. The stomach duct is divided into the upper, center, and lower stomach ducts.

strangury: A disease pattern characterized by urinary urgency; frequent, short, painful, rough voidings; and dribbling incontinence. Strangury is attributed to damp-heat gathering and pouring into the bladder. In persistent conditions or in elderly or weak patients, the cause may be center *qi* fall and kidney vacuity and impaired *qi* transformation.

summerheat: Hot summer weather as a cause of disease, or the disease caused by such weather. Distinction is made between summerheat-heat and summerheat-damp. Summerheat-heat is caused by exposure to the heat of summer; this is known as "summerheat stroke" and is what English-speakers normally call sunstroke or heatstroke. Summerheat-damp refers to certain externally contracted diseases occurring in hot weather; in China these were once loosely called "summerheat disease" and include "summerheat warmth," which is equivalent to infectious encephalitis B.

supplementation: One of the eight methods; a method of treatment derived from the principles, "vacuity is treated by supplementation," and "detriment is treated by boosting." Supplementation is the method that supplies insufficiencies of *yīn* and *yáng*, blood and *qi*, and organ functions. When right *qi* is too weak to expel an evil, the method of supplementation can restore right *qi* to normal strength, helping it to eliminate the evil; hence the principle, "by supporting right, evils are dispelled." There are four fundamental objects of supplementation: *qi*, blood, *yīn*, and *yáng*.

toxin: 1. Any substance that is harmful to the body when eaten or entering the body through a wound or the skin, such as lacquer toxin or pitch toxin. The toxin of animals is called venom. 2. Any virulent evil *qì* (e.g., toxic *qì*), which denotes scourge epidemic *qì*; occasionally, a disease caused by such (e.g., seasonal toxin). 3. Evil *qì* that causes painful reddening and swelling, suppuration, or weeping discharge. 4. A label for certain conditions of external medicine (e.g., cinnabar toxin; innominate toxin swelling).

transformation: Change, usually of a gentle or gradual nature (relative to transmutation, which is sudden or major change). Transformation implies progressive (productive) and regressive (destructive) change, and in the former case is frequently rendered as formation. Hence, fire formation refers to the natural transformation of evils or *yáng qì* into fire (progressive change), whereas transforming phlegm refers to a method of treatment to eliminate phlegm (i.e., regressive change). Transformation often specifically refers to digestion.

triple burner: One of the six bowels, comprising upper, middle, and lower burners. The hand lesser *yáng (shào yáng)* triple burner channel passes through all three burners, linking up with many of the organs. The triple burner is an exterior organ, and its corresponding interior organ (for the purposes of acupuncture only) is the pericardium. The nature of the triple burner has always been a subject of disagreement. The following three points, however, seem to be well established: 1. The triple burner refers to specific body areas; 2. the triple burner represents the waterways; 3. the triple burner is also a concept in pattern identification.

upbear: To raise or cause to rise.

vacuity and repletion: Vacuity is emptiness or weakness; repletion is fullness or strength. Vacuity is weakness of right *qì* (the forces that maintain the health of the body and fight disease), whereas repletion is strength of evil *qì* or accumulation of physiological products within the body such as phlegm-rheum, water-damp, static blood, and stagnant *qì*. Vacuity patterns may be due to such causes as a weak constitution or damage to right *qì* through enduring illness, loss of blood, seminal loss, great sweating, or invasion of an external evil (*yáng* evils readily damage *yīn* humor, and *yīn* evils readily damage *yáng qì*).

vexation: See heart vexation.

welling-abscess: 1. Synonym: external welling-abscess. A large suppuration in the flesh characterized by a painful swelling and redness that is clearly circumscribed, and that before rupturing is soft and characterized by a thin shiny skin. 2. Synonym: internal welling-abscess. A suppuration in the chest or abdomen affecting the organs, probably so-called because it shares many of the *yáng* qualities of external welling-abscess, except for its location in the body.

wind: 1. One of the six *qì*, and natural movement of air. 2. Synonym: wind evil. One of the six excesses; wind as a cause of disease; a *yáng* evil. The nature of wind as an evil and its clinical manifestations are similar to those of the meteorological phenomenon from which it derives its name: It comes and goes quickly, moves swiftly, blows intermittently, and sways the branches of the trees. 3. Internal wind, i.e., wind arising within the body by the following pathomechanisms: liver-wind stirring internally, which occurs when liver *yáng* and liver-fire transform into wind, manifesting in dizziness, tremor, and convulsions; extreme heat engendering wind, arising in externally contracted disease such as fright wind and manifesting in convulsions, stiffness of the neck, arched-back rigidity, etc.; blood vacuity engendering wind, arising when great sweating, great vomiting, great diarrhea, major loss of blood, damage to *yīn* in enduring illness, or kidney-water failing to moisten liver-wood causes desiccation of the blood that deprives the sinews of nourishment and insufficiency of liver *yīn* that leaves *yáng* unsubdued and allows liver-wind to scurry around internally.

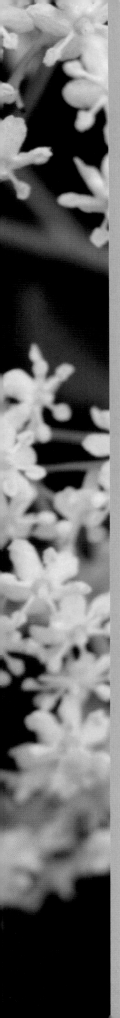

NOTES

INTRODUCTION

1. Yi-ren Liu, *The Heart Transmission of Medicine,* Trans. Yáng Shou-zhong (19th century CE; reprint, Boulder, CO: Blue Poppy Press, 1997), 11.

UNDERSTANDING WESTERN HERBS FROM THE CHINESE MEDICAL PERSPECTIVE

1. Jingfeng et al. *Advanced Textbook on Traditional Chinese Medicine and Pharmacology,* 1 (Beijing, China: New World Press, 1995), 70–71.

2. Ibid.

3. Bob Flaws, *Chinese Medicinal Wines and Elixirs* (Boulder, CO: Blue Poppy Press, 1994), 11.

4. Ibid., 3, 6.

5. Ibid., 6.

HERBAL MEDICINE MAKING

1. Michael Moore, *Medicinal Plants of the Pacific West* (Santa Fe, NM: Red Crane Books, 1993).

HERBS THAT RESOLVE THE EXTERIOR

1. Michael McGuffin et al., eds., *American Herbal Products Association's Botanical Safety Handbook* (Boca Raton, FL: CRC Press, 1997).

HERBS THAT CLEAR HEAT

1. A. W. Priest and L. R. Priest, *Herbal Medication: A Clinical and Dispensary Handbook* (1983; reprint, Essex, UK: The C.W. Daniel Company, Ltd., 2000), 99.

2. Daniel E. Moerman, *Native American Ethnobotany* (Portland, OR: Timber Press, 1998), 524.

3. Simon Mills and Kerry Bone, *Principles and Practice of Phytotherapy: Modern Herbal Medicine* (Edinburgh: Churchill Livingston, 2000), 195.

4. *Biol Pharm Bull* 22, no. 6 (1999), 602–5.

5. Shen De-Hui, Wu Xiu-Fen, and Nissi Wang, *Manual of Dermatology in Chinese Medicine* (Seattle: Eastland Press, 1995).

6. Ibid.

7. Beatrice H. Krauss, *Plants in Hawaiian Medicine* (Honolulu, HI: The Bess Press, 2001).

8. Yi-ren Liu, *The Heart Transmission of Medicine,* Trans. Yáng Shou-zhong (19th century CE; reprint, Boulder, CO: Blue Poppy Press, 1997), 80.

9. Moerman, *Native American Ethnobotany,* 234.

10. Ibid.

11. Ibid., 205.

12. Michael Moore, *Medicinal Plants of the Pacific West* (Santa Fe, NM: Red Crane Books, 1993).

13. Moerman, *Native American Ethnobotany,* 533–34.

14. Ibid., 534.

HERBS THAT PRECIPITATE

1. V. K. Chesnut, *Plants Used by the Indians of Mendocino County, California* (1902; reprint, Ukiah, CA: Mendocino County Historical Society, 1974), 368.

HERBS THAT DRAIN DAMPNESS

1. Daniel E. Moerman, *Native American Ethnobotany* (Portland, OR: Timber Press, 1998), 241–42.

2. William Salmon, *Botanologia: The English Herbal or History of Plants,* Vol. II (London: printed by I. Dawks for H. Rhodes and J. Taylor, 1710).

3. Moerman, *Native American Ethnobotany,* 579.

4. Ibid., 580.

HERBS THAT DISPEL WIND AND DAMPNESS

1. Michael McGuffin et al., eds., *American Herbal Products Association's Botanical Safety Handbook* (Boca Raton, FL: CRC Press, 1997), 152–54.

2. Ibid., 103.

3. Simon Mills and Kerry Bone, *Principles and Practice of Phytotherapy: Modern Herbal Medicine* (Edinburgh: Churchill Livingston, 2000), 106.

4. Daniel E. Moerman, *Native American Ethnobotany* (Portland, OR: Timber Press, 1998), 243.

5. Ibid., 244.

HERBS THAT TRANSFORM PHLEGM AND STOP COUGHING

1. V. K. Chesnut, *Plants Used by the Indians of Mendocino County, California* (Ukiah, CA: Mendocino County Historical Society, 1974), 382. [Orig. pub. 1902.]

2. Daniel E. Moerman, *Native American Ethnobotany* (Portland, OR: Timber Press, 1998), 109.

3. Simon Mills and Kerry Bone, *Principles and Practice of Phytotherapy: Modern Herbal Medicine* (Edinburgh: Churchill Livingston, 2000), 216.

4. Moerman, *Native American Ethnobotany,* 252.

HERBS THAT AROMATICALLY TRANSFORM DAMPNESS

1. Daniel E. Moerman, *Native American Ethnobotany* (Portland, OR: Timber Press, 1998), 371–72.

2. Ibid., 372.

3. Ibid., 371.

4. Michael Moore, *Medicinal Plants of the Pacific West* (Santa Fe, NM: Red Crane Books, 1993), 239.

5. Moerman, *Native American Ethnobotany,* 371.

HERBS THAT RECTIFY QÌ

1. Simon Mills and Kerry Bone, *Principles and Practice of Phytotherapy: Modern Herbal Medicine* (Edinburgh: Churchill Livingston, 2000), 328.

2. Aviva Romm, personal communication, 2004.

3. Mills and Bone, *Principles and Practice of Phytotherapy,* 303.

4. Nigel Wiseman and Feng Ye, *A Practical Dictionary of Chinese Medicine* (Brookline, MA: Paradigm Publications, 1998), 294, 606.

5. Ibid., 104.

6. Ibid., 73.

7. Ibid., 10.

8. Ibid., 631.

9. Daniel E. Moerman, *Native American Ethnobotany* (Portland, OR: Timber Press, 1998), 162–63.

HERBS THAT REGULATE BLOOD

1. Rudolf Fritz Weiss, *Herbal Medicine,* Trans. A. R. Meuss (Beaconsfield, UK: Beaconsfield Publishers, Ltd., 1988), 170.

2. Virgil J. Vogel, *American Medicinal Plants* (Norman: Univ. of Oklahoma Press, 1970), 275.

3. Daniel E. Moerman, *Native American Ethnobotany* (Portland, OR: Timber Press, 1998), 92.

4. Weiss, *Herbal Medicine,* 169.

5. Moerman, *Native American Ethnobotany,* 595.

6. Vogel, *American Medicinal Plants,* 296.

7. Nicholas Culpeper, *Culpeper's Complete Herbal and English Physician* (1826; reprint, Barcelona: Printer Industria Gráfica s.a., 1981), 99.

8. M. Grieve, *A Modern Herbal* (1931; reprint, New York: Dover Publications, 1971), 556.

9. William H. Cook, *The Physio-Medical Dispensatory: A Treatise on Therapeutics, Materia Medica, and Pharmacy, in Accordance with the Principles of Physiological Medication* (1869; reprint, Portland, OR: Eclectic Institute, 1985), 506.

10. Michael Moore, *Medicinal Plants of the Pacific West* (Santa Fe, NM: Red Crane Books, 1993), 216–17.

11. Moerman, *Native American Ethnobotany,* 146.

12. Ibid.

13. Ibid.,144.

14. Ibid.

15. Ibid.,145.

HERBS THAT SUPPLEMENT

1. William H. Cook, *The Physio-Medical Dispensatory: A Treatise on Therapeutics, Materia Medica, and Pharmacy, in Accordance with the Principles of Physiological Medication* (1869; reprint, Portland, OR: Eclectic Institute, 1985), 481.

2. Simon Mills and Kerry Bone, *Principles and Practice of Phytotherapy: Modern Herbal Medicine* (Edinburgh: Churchill Livingston, 2000), 439.

3. Ibid.

4. Ibid.

5. M. Grieve, *A Modern Herbal* (1931; reprint, New York: Dover Publications, 1971).

6. Ibid., 507.

7. R. A. Jack, *British Medical Journal* 4, no. 48. (1971).

8. Margarita Artschwager Kay, *Healing with Plants in the American and Mexican West* (Tucson: University of Arizona Press, 1996).

6. Ibid.

HERBS THAT STABILIZE AND BIND

1. Daniel E. Moerman, *Native American Ethnobotany* (Portland, OR: Timber Press, 1998), 352.

2. William H. Cook, *The Physio-Medical Dispensatory: A Treatise on Therapeutics, Materia Medica, and Pharmacy, in Accordance with the Principles of Physiological Medication* (1869; reprint, Portland, OR: Eclectic Institute, 1985), 571.

3. Ibid., 573.

HERBS THAT CALM THE SPIRIT

1. Daniel E. Moerman, *Native American Ethnobotany* (Portland, OR: Timber Press, 1998), 228.

2. Harvey Wickes Felter and John Uri Lloyd, *King's American Dispensatory,* 18th ed., 3rd rev., (1898; reprint, Sandy, OR: Eclectic Medical Publications, 1983), 1441.

3. Moerman, *Native American Ethnobotany,* 524.

4. Virgil J. Vogel, *American Medicinal Plants* (Norman: Univ. of Oklahoma Press, 1970), 367.

5. Thomas Brendler et al., eds. *Herb CD* (Stuttgard, Germany: Medpharm Scientific Publishers Birkenwaldstr, 2001).

6. Nicholas Culpeper, *Culpeper's Complete Herbal and*

English Physician (1826; reprint, Barcelona: Printer Industria Gráfica s.a., 1981), 80.

7. M. Grieve, *A Modern Herbal* (1931; reprint, New York: Dover Publications, 1971), 708. Rudolf Fritz Weiss, *Herbal Medicine,* Trans. A. R. Meuss (Beaconsfield, UK: Beaconsfield Publishers, Ltd., 1988), 250.

8. Michael Moore, *Medicinal Plants of the Pacific West* (Santa Fe, NM: Red Crane Books, 1993), 155–60.

9. Simon Mills and Kerry Bone, *Principles and Practice of Phytotherapy: Modern Herbal Medicine* (Edinburgh: Churchill Livingston, 2000), 542.

10. Brendler et al., *Herb CD.*

11. Ed Johnston and Helen Rogers, eds., *Hawaiian 'Awa: Views of an Ethnobotanical Treasure* (Hilo, HI: Association for Hawaiian 'Awa), 2006.

12. Ibid.

13. E. S. Craighill Handy and Elizabeth Green Handy, *Native Planters in Old Hawai'i: Their Life, Lore, and Environment,* rev. ed. (Honolulu, HI: Bishop Museum Press, 1991).

14. W. Arthur Whistler, *Polynesian Herbal Medicine* (Lawai, HI: National Tropical Botanical Garden, 1992).

15. Moerman, *Native American Ethnobotany,* 588.

16. Brendler et al., *Herb CD.*

17. Culpeper, *Complete Herbal,* 32.

18. Weiss, *Herbal Medicine,* 315.

19. Ibid., 123.

20. Ibid., 168.

HERBS THAT EXTINGUISH WIND

1. Daniel E. Moerman, *Native American Ethnobotany* (Portland, OR: Timber Press, 1998), 312.

APPENDIX 1

1. Michael Moore, *Medicinal Plants of the Pacific West* (Santa Fe, NM: Red Crane Books, 1993), 293.

2. Dan Bensky, Steven Clavey, and Erich Stöger, trans., *Chinese Herbal Medicine: Materia Medica,* 3rd ed. (Seattle: Eastland Press, 2004).

3. Ibid.

4. Dan Bensky, and Andrew Gamble, trans., *Chinese Herbal Medicine: Materia Medica* (Seattle: Eastland Press, 1993).

5. Christopher Hobbs, *Medicinal Mushrooms: An Exploration of Tradition, Healing & Culture,* 2nd Ed. (Santa Cruz, CA: Botanica Press, 1995).

6. Bensky et al., *Chinese Herbal Medicine.*

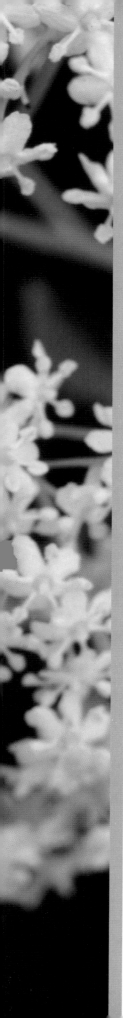

BIBLIOGRAPHY

Bean, Lowell John, and Katherine Siva Saubel. *Temalpakh: Cahuilla Indian Knowledge and Usage of Plants*. Morongo Indian Reservation, CA: Malki Museum Press, 1972.

Bensky, Dan, and Andrew Gamble, trans. *Chinese Herbal Medicine: Materia Medica*. Seattle: Eastland Press, 1993.

Bensky, Dan, Steven Clavey, and Erich Stöger, trans. *Chinese Herbal Medicine: Materia Medica*. 3rd ed. Seattle: Eastland Press, 2004.

Blakley, Tim, and Lee Sturdivant. *Medicinal Herbs in the Garden, Field and Marketplace*. Friday Harbor, WA: San Juan Naturals, 1999.

Blumenthal, Mark, et al., eds. *The Complete German Commission E Monographs: Therapeutic Guide to Herbal Medicines*. Boston, MA: Integrative Medicine Communications, 1998.

British Herbal Medicine Association. *British Herbal Pharmacopoeia*. Bournemouth, UK: British Herbal Medicine Association, 1983.

Brendler, Thomas, et al., ed. *Herb CD*. Stuttgard, Germany: Medpharm Scientific Publishers Birkenwaldstr, 2001.

Chesnut, V. K. *Plants Used by the Indians of Mendocino County, California*. 1902. Reprint, Ukiah, CA: Mendocino County Historical Society, 1974.

Cook, E., ed. *Remington's Practice of Pharmacy,* 6th ed. Easton, PA: The Mack Publishing Co., 1936.

Cook, William H. *The Physio-Medical Dispensatory: A Treatise on Therapeutics, Materia Medica, and Pharmacy, in Accordance with the Principles of Physiological Medication*. 1869. Reprint, Portland, OR: Eclectic Institute, 1985.

Culbreth, David M. R. *A Manual of Materia Medica and Pharmacology,* 7th ed. Philadelphia: Lea and Febiger, 1927.

Culpeper, Nicholas. *Culpeper's Complete Herbal and English Physician*. 1826. Reprint, Barcelona: Printer Industria Gráfica s.a., 1981.

Duke, James A., and Steven Foster. *A Field Guide to Medicinal Plants: Eastern and Central North America*. Boston: Houghton Mifflin Company, 1990.

Ellingwood, Finley, and John Uri Lloyd. *American Materia Medica, Therapeutics and Pharmacognosy*. 1919. Reprint, Sandy, OR: Eclectic Medical Publications, 1983.

Erichsen-Brown, Charlotte. *Medicinal and Other Uses of North American Plants: A Historical Survey with Special Reference to the Eastern Indian Tribes*. Mineola, NY: Dover Publications, 1989. (First published in 1979 as *Uses of Plants for the Past 500 Years* by General Publishing Company, Ltd., Toronto.)

Felter, Harvey Wickes, and John Uri Lloyd. *King's American Dispensatory*, 18th ed., 3rd rev. 1898. Reprint, Sandy, OR: Eclectic Medical Publications, 1983.

Flaws, Bob. *Chinese Medicinal Wines and Elixirs*. Boulder, CO: Blue Poppy Press, 1994.

Foster, Steven, and Christopher Hobbs. *A Field Guide To Western Medicinal Plants and Herbs*. Boston: Houghton Mifflin Company, 2002.

Green, James. *The Male Herbal: Health Care for Men and Boys*. Freedom, CA: The Crossing Press, 1991.

Grieve, M. *A Modern Herbal*. 1931. Reprint, New York: Dover Publications, 1971.

Griggs, Barbara. *Green Pharmacy: The History and Evolution of Western Herbal Medicine*. Rochester, VT: Healing Arts Press, 1991.

Gunther, Erna. *Ethnobotany of Western Washington: The Knowledge and Use of Indigenous Plants by Native Americans*, rev. ed. Seattle: Univ. of Washington Press, 1973.

Gutmanis, June. *Kāhuna Lāʻau Lapaʻau: Hawaiian Herbal Medicine*. Waipahu, HI: Island Heritage Publishing, 1976.

Hamel, Paul B., and Mary U. Chiltoskey. *Cherokee Plants and Their Uses—A 400 Year History*. Sylva, NC: Herald Publishing Co., 1975.

Handy, E. S. Craighill, and Elizabeth Green Handy. *Native Planters in Old Hawaiʻi: Their Life, Lore, and Environment*, rev. ed. Honolulu, HI: Bishop Museum Press, 1991.

Harding, A. R. *Ginseng and Other Medicinal Plants*, rev. ed. Columbus, OH: A.R. Harding, 1936.

Hickman, James C., ed. *The Jepson Manual: Higher Plants of California*. Berkeley: Univ. of California Press, 1993.

Hitchcock, C. Leo, and Arthur Cronquist. *Flora of the Pacific Northwest: An Illustrated Manual*. Seattle and London: Univ. of Washington Press, 1973.

Hobbs, Christopher. *Foundations of Health: The Liver and Digestive Herbal*. Capitola, CA: Botanica Press, 1992.

———. *Medicinal Mushrooms: An Exploration of Tradition, Healing, & Culture*, 2nd ed. Santa Cruz, CA: Botanica Press, 1995.

Hoffmann, David. *The New Holistic Herbal*. Rockport, MA: Element, Inc., 1992.

Hutchins, Robert Maynard, ed. *Great Books of the Western World: Volume 10: Hippocrates and Galen*. London: Encyclopaedia Britannica, Inc., 1952.

Jiangsu New Chinese Medicine College. *Grand Dictionary of Chinese Medicinals*, 13th ed. (*Zhōng Yào Dà Cí Diǎn*). Shanghai: Shanghai Science and Technology Publishing House, 2004.

Jingfeng et al. *Advanced Textbook on Traditional Chinese Medicine and Pharmacology*, 1 (Beijing, China: New World Press, 1995).

Johnston, Ed, and Helen Rogers, eds. *Hawaiian ʻAwa: Views of an Ethnobotanical Treasure*. Hilo, HI: The Association for Hawaiian ʻAwa, 2006.

Kay, Margarita Artschwager. *Healing with Plants in the American and Mexican West*. Tucson, AZ: University of Arizona Press, 1996.

Kenner, Dan, and Yves Requena. *Botanical Medicine: A European Professional Perspective*. Brookline, MA: Paradigm Publications, 1996.

Keville, Kathi. *Herbs for Health and Healing*. Emmaus, PA: Rodale Press, Inc., 1996.

Kindscher, Kelly. *Medicinal Wild Plants of the Prairie: An Ethnobotanical Guide*. Lawrence, KS: Univ. Press of Kansas, 1992.

Krauss, Beatrice H. *Plants in Hawaiian Medicine*. Honolulu, HI: The Bess Press, 2001.

Liu, Yi-ren. *The Heart Transmission of Medicine*, 19th century CE Trans. Yáng Shou-zhong. Boulder, CO: Blue Poppy Press, 1997.

Lyle, T. J. *Physio-Medical Therapeutics, Materia Medica and Pharmacy*. 1897. Reprint, Boulder, CO: North American Institute of Medical Herbalism and Bergner Communications, 2002.

Maisch, John M. *A Manual of Organic Materia Medica,* 2nd ed. Philadelphia: Lea Brothers & Co., 1885.

McGuffin, Michael, et al., eds. *American Herbal Products Association's Botanical Safety Handbook*. Boca Raton, FL: CRC Press, 1997.

Mills, Simon, and Kerry Bone. *Principles and Practice of Phytotherapy: Modern Herbal Medicine*. Edinburgh: Churchill Livingston, 2000.

Millspaugh, Charles F. *American Medicinal Plants*. 1892. Reprint, New York: Dover Publications, 1974.

Moerman, Daniel E. *Native American Ethnobotany*. Portland, OR: Timber Press, 1998.

Moore, Michael. *Medicinal Plants of the Desert and Canyon West*. Santa Fe, NM: Museum of New Mexico Press, 1989.

———. *Medicinal Plants of the Pacific West*. Santa Fe, NM: Red Crane Books, 1993.

———. *Medicinal Plants of the Mountain West,* rev. ed. Santa Fe: NM: Museum of New Mexico Press, 2003.

———. *Principles and Practice of Constitutional Physiology for Herbalists*. Albuquerque, NM: Southwest School of Botanical Medicine, n.d.

Murphey, Edith Van Allen. *Indian Uses of Native Plants,* 1959. Reprint, Ukiah, CA: Mendocino County Historical Society, 1987.

National Association of Medical Herbalists. *The Medical Herbalist,* Vol. 11. Great Britain. National Association of Medical Herbalists, 1937.

The National Formulary of Unofficial Preparations. Baltimore: American Pharmaceutical Associations Press, 1888.

Priest, A. W., and L. R. Priest. *Herbal Medication: A Clinical and Dispensary Handbook*. 1983. Reprint, Essex, UK: The C.W. Daniel Company Ltd., 2000.

Radford, Albert E., Harry E. Ahles, and C. Ritchie Bell. *Manual of the Vascular Flora of the Carolinas*. Chapel Hill: The University of North Carolina Press, 1968.

Reynolds, James E. F., ed. *Martindale: The Extra Pharmacopoeia,* 29th ed. London: The Pharmaceutical Press, 1989.

———. *Martindale: The Extra Pharmacpoeia,* 31st ed. London: The Pharmaceutical Press, 1996.

Salmon, William. *Botanologia: The English Herbal or History of Plants,* 2. London: printed by I. Dawks for H. Rhodes and J. Taylor, 1710.

Scudder, John M. *Specific Medication and Specific Medicines*. Cincinnati: Wilstach, Baldwin & Co., Printers, 1870.

Seymour, Frank Conkling. *The Flora of New England*. Rutland, VT: The Charles E. Tuttle Company, 1969.

Sionneau, Philippe. *Pao Zhi: An Introduction to the Use of Processed Chinese Medicinals*. Trans. Bob Flaws. Boulder, CO: Blue Poppy Press, 1995.

Shen De-Hui, Wu Xiu-Fen, and Nissi Wang. *Manual of Dermatology in Chinese Medicine*. Seattle: Eastland Press, 1995.

Svenson, Henry K., and Robert W. Pyle. *The Flora of Cape Cod: An Annotated List of the Ferns and Flowering Plants of Barnstable County, Massachusetts*. Brewster, MA: The Cape Cod Museum of Natural History, 1979.

Sweetman, Sean C., ed. *Martindale: The Extra Pharmacopoeia,* 33rd ed. London: The Pharmaceutical Press, 2002.

The Revolutionary Health Committee of Hunan Province. *A Barefoot Doctor's Manual,* rev. ed. Trans. Yu, Titus, Lam Wah Bong, and Kwok Chui. Seattle, WA: Madrona Publishers, 1977.

Tierra, Michael. *The Way of Herbs*. Santa Cruz, CA: Unity Press, 1980.

———. *Planetary Herbology: An Integration of Western Herbs into the Traditional Chinese and Ayurvedic Systems*. Twin Lakes, WI: Lotus Press, 1988.

Unschuld, Paul U. *Medicine in China: A History of Ideas*. Berkeley: University of California Press (Ltd.), 1985.

Uphof, J. C. *Dictionary of Economic Plants*. New York: Hafner Publishing Co., 1959.

Vogel, Virgil J. *American Medicinal Plants*. Norman: Univ. of Oklahoma Press, 1970.

Wagner, Warren L., Derral R. Werbst, and S. H. Sohmer. *Manual of the Flowering Plants of Hawai'i,* rev. ed. Honolulu, HI: Univ. of Hawai'i Press and Bishop Museum Press, 1999.

Weed, Susun S. *Wise Woman Herbal for the Childbearing Year.* Woodstock, NY: Ash Tree Publishing, 1986.

Weiss, Rudolf Fritz. *Herbal Medicine.* Trans. A. R. Meuss. Beaconsfield, UK: Beaconsfield Publishers Ltd., 1988.

Whistler, W. Arthur. *Polynesian Herbal Medicine.* Lawai, HI: National Tropical Botanical Garden, 1992.

WHO Monographs on Selected Medicinal Plants. Geneva: World Health Organization, 2002.

Wiseman, Nigel, and Feng Ye. *A Practical Dictionary of Chinese Medicine.* Brookline, MA: Paradigm Publications, 1998.

Wood, George B., and Franklin Bache. *The Dispensatory of the United States of America,* 12th ed. Philadelphia: J. B. Lippincott and Company, 1866.

———. *The Dispensatory of the United States of America,* 13th ed. Philadelphia: J. B. Lippincott and Company, 1872.

Wood, Horatio C., and Joseph P. Remington. *The Dispensatory of the United States of America,* 20th ed. Philadelphia: J. B. Lippincott and Company, 1918.

Wood, Horatio C., Joseph P. Remington, and Samuel P. Sadtler. *The Dispensatory of the United States of America,* 17th ed. Philadelphia: J. B. Lippincott and Company, 1894.

Wren, R. C. *Potter's New Cyclopaedia of Botanical Drugs and Preparations.* Saffron Walden, UK: The C. W. Daniel Company Limited, 1988.

Yeung, Him-che. *Handbook of Chinese Herbs and Formulas.* Rosemead, CA: Institute of Chinese Medicine, 1985.

Zhang Ji. *Shang Han Lun.* 2nd century CE Trans. Mitchell, Craig, Feng Ye, and Wiseman. Brookline, MA: Paradigm Publications, 1999.

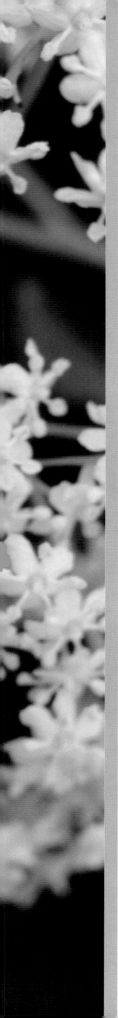

INDEX

intestines
  binding, 187
  clearing heat in, 209–10
  damp-heat in, 74, 75
  large, 238
  small, 240
irascibility, 192, 237
irritability, 111

Jade Windscreen Powder, 44, 51, 98
jaundice, 69, 73, 83
joint pain, 52, 121, 123, 124, 129,
  148, 155
joints, swollen, 41, 46, 60, 83, 109,
  123
joint stiffness, 116, 121

kava *(Piper methysticum)*, 21–22, 191,
  203–5
kidney inflammation, 128, 138
kidneys
  described, 237–38
  stabilizing, 187
  supplementing, 181, 183, 189
kidney stones, 127
knocks and falls, 155, 238
Kudzu *(pueraria lobata, P. montana)*,
  219

large intestine, 238
Latin names for herbs, 5, 227–32
laxatives, 83, 86, 107, 109
leaky gut syndrome, 103
lesions, healing, 114
ligustrum lucidum (privit), 218
liniments, 121, 155
lin syndrome, 113, 128, 129
lip balm, 26
liquid extracts, 21, 23, 24
liver
  coursing, 37, 91, 146, 200, 206, 209,
    235
  damp-heat in, 83–84
  depression, 89, 90–91, 194, 200,
    201, 206

detoxifying, 177–78
heat, 33, 69, 198
hyperactivity, 234
liver qi invading the spleen, 238
regeneration, 91
stimulants, 75, 86
strengthening, 189
vacuity, 177
wind, 212–15, 238
liver-fire
  clearing, 60, 61, 106
  invading the lungs, 86, 87, 107–8
liver-gallbladder damp-heat, 73, 74,
  78, 80, 86, 89, 238
liver-gallbladder depression, 192
Lobelia *(Lobelia inflata)*, 11, 212–15
local herbs, viii, ix–x, 17
lonicera japonica (honeysuckle), 33,
  218
loquat *(eriogotrya japonica)*, 217
lower-burner damp-heat, 93, 98, 119,
  128–29, 138
lumbar pain, 148
lung
  described, 238
  heat, 134, 136
  supplementing, 179
  yin, 138
lung qi
  circulating, 52
  diffusing, 131–32, 137, 213
  restraining, 187
  supplementing, 50
lycopodium clavatum (clubmoss), 218
lyme disease, 103
lymphatics, 93, 95
lymphatic swelling, 97
lymph congestion, 67
lymph nodes, swollen, 69, 111, 117
lymph tonics, 104

maceration tinctures, 21–22
maculopapular eruption, 61, 238–39
má huáng, 57
Major Qi-Coordinating Decoction, 64

mammary welling-abscess, 67
marsh mallow *(Althaea officinalis)*,
  169, 179–80
mastitis, 147, 148, 151
materia medica
  Chinese materia medica, 8–9
  construction and use of, 10–12
  cultivated versus wildcrafted herbs,
    17–18
  herbal preparations, 13–15
  herb quality, 16–17
  overview, 4–6
  Western materia medica, 8–10
MDMA (ecstasy), 127
meadowsweet *(Filipendula ulmaria)*,
  59, 63–64
medicine-making techniques
  benefits of, 19
  decoctions, 21
  fluidextracts, 23
  infused oils, 25–26
  infusions, 20
  liquid extracts, 23–24
  mix-fried medicinals, 27
  poultices, 24
  powdered extracts, 26–27
  salves, 26
  suppositories, 24–25
  tinctures, 21–23
menopausal symptoms, 148
Menses-Stabilizing Decoction, 147
menstrual bleeding, excessive, 37, 116,
  158, 163
menstrual cramps, 125
menstrual cycle, 146, 147, 151, 158,
  161, 162, 193
middle burner, 75, 77, 141
migraine headaches, 61
milk thistle *(Silybum marianum)*, 169,
  177–78
Minor Bupleurum Decoction, 97
mint *(mentha arvensis)*, 218
mix-fried medicinals, 27, 48, 171
Modify Minor Bupleurm Decoction,
  90

Books of Related Interest

HEALING WITH CHINESE HERBS
by Richard Hyatt

THE HEALING CUISINE OF CHINA
300 Recipes for Vibrant Health and Longevity
by Zhuo Zhao and George Ellis

HERBAL EMISSARIES
Bringing Chinese Herbs to the West: A Guide to Gardening,
Herbal Wisdom, and Well-Being
by Steven Foster and Yue Chongxi

THE BOOK OF GINSENG
And Other Chinese Herbs for Vitality
by Stephen Fulder, Ph.D.

MEDICAL HERBALISM
The Science and Practice of Herbal Medicine
by David Hoffmann, FNIMH, AHG

THE HERBAL HANDBOOK
A User's Guide to Medical Herbalism
by David Hoffmann

THE FAMILY HERBAL
A Guide to Natural Health Care for Yourself and Your Children
from Europe's Leading Herbalists
by Barbara & Peter Theiss

HEALTH FROM GOD'S GARDEN
Herbal Remedies for Glowing Health and Well-Being
by Maria Treben

ADAPTOGENS
Herbs for Strength, Stamina, and Stress Relief
by David Winston and *Steven Maimes*

PRICKLY PEAR CACTUS MEDICINE
Treatments for Diabetes, Cholesterol, and the Immune System
by Ran Knishinsky

Inner Traditions • Bear & Company
P.O. Box 388 • Rochester, VT 05767
1-800-246-8648 • www.InnerTraditions.com

Or contact your local bookseller